Plague, Print, and the Reformation

This book surveys a neglected set of sources, German plague prints and treatises published between 1473 and 1573, in order to explore the intertwined histories of plague, print, medicine, and religion during the Reformation era. It argues that a particularly German reform of healing flourished in printed texts during the Renaissance and Reformation as physicians and clerics devised innovative responses to the era's persistent epidemics. These reforms are "German" since they reflect the innovative trends that originated in or were particularly strong within German-speaking lands, including the rapid growth of vernacular print, Protestantism, and new interest in alchemy and the native plants of northern Europe that were unknown to the ancients. Their reforms are also "German" in the sense that they unfolded mainly in vernacular print, which encouraged physicians to produce local knowledge, grounded in personal experience and local observations as much as universal theories. This book contributes to the history of medicine and science by tracing the growth of more empirical forms of medical knowledge. It also contributes to the history of the Renaissance and Reformation by uncovering the innovative contributions of various forgotten physicians. This book presents the broadest study of German plague treatises in any language.

Erik A. Heinrichs is an associate professor of history at Winona State University, Minnesota.

The History of Medicine in Context
Series Editors: Andrew Cunningham and Ole Peter Grell
Department of History and Philosophy of Science
University of Cambridge
Department of History
Open University

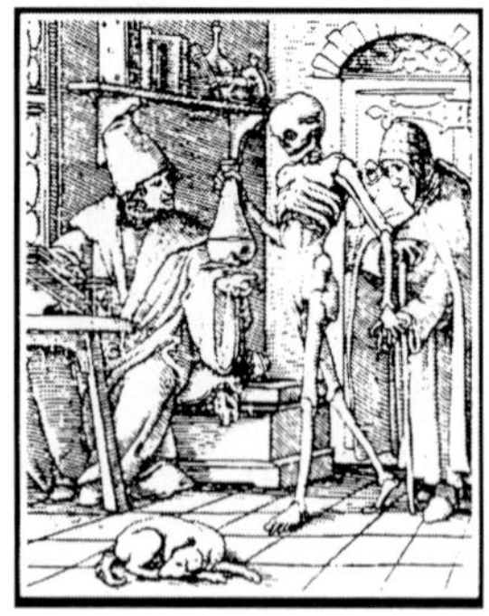

A full list of titles in this series is available at www.routledge.com/history/series/HMC

Titles in the series include:

From Clinic to Concentration Camp
Reassessing Nazi Medical and Racial Research, 1933–1945
Edited by Paul Weindling

Medicine, Natural Philosophy and Religion in Post-Reformation Scandinavia
Edited by Ole Peter Grell and Andrew Cunningham

Medicine, Trade and Empire
Garcia de Orta's Colloquies on the Simples and Drugs of India (1563) in Context
Palmira Fontes da Costa

The Political and Social Dynamics of Poverty, Poor Relief and Health Care in Early-Modern Portugal
Laurinda Abreu

The World of Plants in Renaissance Tuscany
Medicine and Botany
Cristina Bellorini

Plague, Print, and the Reformation
The German Reform of Healing, 1473–1573
Erik A. Heinrichs

Plague, Print, and the Reformation

The German Reform of Healing, 1473–1573

Erik A. Heinrichs

Routledge
Taylor & Francis Group
LONDON AND NEW YORK

First published 2018
by Routledge
2 Park Square, Milton Park, Abingdon, Oxon OX14 4RN

and by Routledge
711 Third Avenue, New York, NY 10017

Routledge is an imprint of the Taylor & Francis Group, an informa business

British Library Cataloguing-in-Publication Data
A catalogue record for this book is available from the British Library

Library of Congress Cataloging-in-Publication Data
A catalog record for this title has been requested

ISBN: 978-1-472-47314-1 (hbk)
ISBN: 978-1-315-60069-7 (ebk)

Typeset in Sabon
by Out of House Publishing

MIX
Paper from responsible sources
FSC® C013604
www.fsc.org

Printed and bound by CPI Group (UK) Ltd, Croydon, CR0 4YY

To Julie, Elsa, Clara, Sofie, and Willa

Contents

Figures

Acknowledgments

This book's earliest beginnings date to 1999, when I first encountered German plague treatises as an undergraduate student at Marquette University. Ronald Zupko recommended that I explore the library's microfilm collection of plague texts when I sought a paper topic in his medieval history class. I am forever grateful to Prof. Zupko for this tip, as well as for inspiring an engineering student to become an historian in the first place. Only later, in graduate school at Harvard University, did I return to these sources and realize their untapped potential. I would also like to express deep gratitude to my graduate advisers, who gave generous support for my doctoral project of surveying German plague literature. They include Steven Ozment and Katharine Park of Harvard University, as well as Robert Jütte of the Institute for the History of Medicine at the Robert Bosch Foundation.

My work has been supported by doctoral fellowships from Harvard University, as well as postdoctoral fellowships from the Herzog August Bibliothek in Wolfenbüttel (Lower Saxony) and the Leibniz Institute of European History in Mainz (Rhineland-Palatinate). The German-American Fulbright Commission supported one wonderful year of research in rare book rooms across southern Germany at a time before all of the texts even appeared in online catalogs, much less in full-text online format. The Harvard Graduate Society provided a summer research grant that allowed me to camp in the forests outside Leipzig while I campaigned in the archives by day. Support from the German Historical Institute Doctoral Seminar in Berlin also allowed brief forays into the libraries of northern Germany. My early research and *Bildung* benefitted greatly from a year at the University of Innsbruck after my undergraduate studies, supported by the Austrian-American Fulbright Commission. More indirect, but essential, support came from the universities where I taught as an adjunct or visiting professor after earning my Ph.D.: the University of Massachusetts-Lowell, Bridgewater State University, and Benedictine College. This book never would have come to completion without the enduring institutional support of Winona State University. Finally, special thanks belong to the *Sixteenth Century Journal*, which first published Chapter 4 on Caspar Kegler as an article in 2012.

I bear great debts to other historians who have encouraged my work through friendship, consultation, or criticism over the years: Patrick Baker, Adam Beaver, Ann Blair, Alix Cooper, John Noël Dillon, William Eamon, John Gagné, Chad Gunnoe, Philip Haberkern, Amy Houston, Daniel Jütte, Elaine Leong, Mary Lindemann, Laura Lisy-Wagner, Matthew Lundin, Elizabeth Mellyn, Erik Midelfort, Bruce Moran, Heinz Noflatscher, Alisha Rankin, John Romano, Ulinka Rublack, Jole Shackelford, Eugene Tesdahl, Heléna Tóth, Demmy Verbeke, and others. Personal thanks for hosting me on trips to Germany belong to Bruno and Hilde Gödde and family, Alexia D'Arco, Pam Bromley, and Kris Neville. Unending thanks for their support belong as well to Ronald and Kathleen Heinrichs, Gretchen Heinrichs and Matt Schaefer, and David and Beth Swanberg, as well as my colleagues and students at Winona State in the great state of Minnesota. And, finally, I owe the greatest debt to my wife Julie and our daughters Elsa, Clara, Sofie, and Willa, who shared the burdens and excitement of producing this book. This book is dedicated to them.

Introduction

Reading German plague treatises from the first century of print is like stepping into a room full of secret treasures. While the disruptive brilliance of Paracelsus (1493–1541) has long dominated the history of early modern German medicine, one finds little trace of him among the hundreds of such sources published up to 1573. Instead one finds a number of largely forgotten physicians, such as Johann Vochs (1440s? – ?) and Caspar Kegler (ca. 1461–1537), who appear as the innovative reformers of this important era of change. While Reformation historians often assume that physicians generally did not contribute to the religious reform, one finds various physicians attempting to shape piety during the late Middle Ages and Reformation. While historians of medicine emphasize the universal dimensions of late medieval thought on plague, one finds physicians grappling with the plague's origins and solutions on a regional or local level, even promoting a "German" understanding of bodies and cures.[1] And, while some historians emphasize the derivative or static nature of early modern plague literature, German sources reveal a dynamic story of physicians pursuing novel ideas and medicines. This book attempts to uncover the treasures long hidden in this enormous body of sources to promote a fuller understanding of early modern German medicine, the Renaissance, and the Reformation.

This book presents the broadest study of German plague treatises and related printed plague texts thus far in any language. It focuses mainly on the vernacular plague treatises of German-speaking lands, but broadens the investigation at times to include some Latin treatises written by German authors as well as contemporary religious texts. German plague treatises reveal new perspectives on a number of great changes under way between 1473 and 1573. Certainly, their natural medical content gives valuable insight into how contemporaries sought to prevent and cure the plagues of the time. Yet historians can appreciate the full value of plague treatises only by taking a broad cultural perspective, which allows one to grasp the era's wide field of innovations. Looking beyond a narrow sort of medical history reveals how medicine, religion, cultural identity, and the new print technology affected each other amid the concerns of the Renaissance and Reformation. In the century after the birth of the printed plague monograph, in 1473, these various changes became interconnected and together had a dramatic impact on plague advice. Such cultural changes challenged, if not overturned, long-held assumptions in medicine and religion and deserve to be included in the broader narratives of the Renaissance, Reformation, and early modern revolutions in medicine and science. Plague treatises, therefore, are not a "boring" or static body of sources, as some have described this genre.[2] They are, rather, more dynamic and innovative than historians have allowed.[3]

Pestilential epidemics were a perennial problem in late medieval and early modern Europe. Recurring "pestilence" (*Pestilentz*) was among the cruelest realities of life in the late Middle Ages, and yet the coming century held no relief. As a new global age dawned in the decades around 1500, epidemics flourished in forms new and old. Central Europe in particular experienced a series of epidemics in the early sixteenth century that some viewed not only as highly unusual, but even as novel and a possible sign of the End Times. Among the more unsettling epidemics was the mysterious French Disease, which appeared in central Europe by 1496, joining the other plagues of 1494–96, 1504–07, 1519–21, 1534–36, and 1562–65.[4] Amid these epidemics came another equally mysterious sickness, the English Sweating Sickness, which struck continental Europe in 1529 after earlier outbreaks in England. Due to their prevalence, destructiveness, and mysterious origin, such epidemics presented some of the greatest spiritual, medical, and social challenges of the era.

This book focuses on the written advice that university-trained physicians gave for preventing and curing these epidemics, and particularly the epidemics described as *Pestilentz* or something similar.[5] Physicians' plague treatises formed a loose medical genre that existed in a range of academic and popularized forms. If taken in a broad sense, "plague" is the best translation for *Pestilentz*, since it is more evocative today than "pestilence" and conforms to historians' traditional use of the term to describe these historical epidemics. The term "plague" here denotes a broad and vague category of epidemics that contemporary physicians used and should not imply a specific retro-diagnosis of plague in modern medical terms.[6] To contextualize physicians' advice, this book considers all other forms of printed media that offered solutions to these plagues, including the work of clerics, surgeons, artists, and printers. Such sources include religious literature, single-leaf broadsides, and civic health regulations, as well as printed literature on other more specific pestilential sicknesses, such as the French Disease and English Sweating Sickness.[7] This approach allows a broad consideration of ideas about prevention and healing in general, including their natural and spiritual components.

Historians could write numerous books on the medical and cultural changes evident in German printed plague media since this body of sources is so vast.[8] Yet one of the most striking, if also overlooked, themes that run through these sources is the growth of a particularly German movement that set out to reform the spiritual and natural components of plague advice during the first half of the sixteenth century. The specifically "German" identity of this reform is rooted in an emerging German cultural patriotism on the eve of the Reformation, first evident in the 1507 plague text by Cologne physician Johann Vochs.[9] In this influential Latin treatise, Vochs began to promote indigenous medicines and Church reform as a liberation of "Germania" from insidious foreign interests, cultural and commercial. Amid the Reformation, such ideas inspired other physicians to adopt Vochs's regional perspective and join his quest for finding specifically "German" medicines. The use of the term "German" here is not anachronistic, but draws on the terms that contemporary physicians used to describe German-speaking lands, including "*Germania*," "*deudschen Landen*," and "*Deudscher Nation*," as well as "*Deutsche*" for Germans themselves.

Vochs's 1507 plague treatise was merely the start of a broad German reform of healing that encompassed other changes and innovations under way in the first half of the sixteenth century. All of these trends are "German" to the extent that they originated in German-speaking lands and were particularly important there: the rapid growth of print and especially vernacular print, the Protestant Reformation, and new interest in the native plants of northern Europe, some of which were unknown to ancient scholars. Alchemy was one other important source of change within plague medicine, and, although it did not have a specifically German origin, it was particularly important for medical thought and printed literature in German-speaking lands.[10] All of these sources of innovation combined in German plague treatises and reinforced each other to some extent as physicians sought new approaches to the puzzling epidemics. For example, reforming physicians in this period did some or all of the following in their plague treatises: promoted so-called "German" medicines, embraced the potential of vernacular print to popularize their ideas, invented or marketed alchemical novelties, and encouraged Protestant rhetoric on medical and spiritual issues, even repeating Martin Luther's statements. Overall, Luther played a much larger role in this reform than Paracelsus, whom historians have too often portrayed as the sole hero of German medical reform.[11] From the perspective of plague treatises, Luther is the "Luther of physicians," rather than Paracelsus (also known as Philippus Aureolus Theophrastus Bombastus von Hohenheim).

Vernacular print provided an essential medium for nurturing this German reform of healing, much as vernacular print played an important role in the growth and spread of the Reformation. Vernacular print was particularly prevalent in German-speaking lands as the homeland of print and Protestantism. Moreover, vernacular print had profound and sometimes surprising effects on plague advice. By writing in the German regional vernaculars for an audience imagined to be broader than before, university-trained physicians began to produce a more local sort of medical knowledge, grounded in the local marketplace and personal experience as much as the universal theories of ancient scholars. Physicians also adopted content from contemporary religious advice, and sometimes even became preachers in their own right. By presenting their profession as attuned to popular expectations and the environmental realities of northern Europe, German physicians sought to strengthen their social authority among this broader audience. This process of making universal knowledge local also had the effect of boosting the epistemic value of personal experience in the production of medical knowledge. The medical and cultural innovations of the early sixteenth century thereby encouraged the empirical values that played such an important role later during the Scientific Revolution, when scholars more broadly sought to invert the traditional relationship between theory and experience.[12] In certain cases explored here, German physicians and botanists began to champion reliance on personal experience as more important than the guidance of universal theory. In this way, the German physicians explored here were at the leading edge of change in the early modern sciences as they questioned the traditional path to medical knowledge.

Physicians are important subjects for historians of early modern science since their duties often included practice in addition to philosophical reasoning. Although their discipline was rooted in ancient theories, university-trained physicians attended to private patients and took on more civic responsibilities over time. Rulers of church and state especially sought out physicians' medical advice for themselves and the larger community during the late medieval and early modern eras. In German-speaking lands it became increasingly common for cities and towns during the fifteenth and sixteenth centuries to hire a physician at public expense. The powers of these appointed physicians also grew over time. During the sixteenth century such appointed physicians claimed to oversee the community's broader health system, including the regulation of the lower medical professions.[13] The rise of physicians to greater social power between the fifteenth and sixteenth centuries is one factor behind the great upswing in German plague literature, since writing a plague treatise became a common way for city physicians to advise the broad population upon the approach of an epidemic. One historian has even argued that the resulting flood of medical information resulted in a "new order of knowledge" within German civic life, as physicians and medical information became more prevalent and influential by the early sixteenth century.[14]

Much like the practical side of the physicians' profession, place matters in the history of medicine and science. Lands north of the Alps were (and are) very different from the lands to the south, where Europe's academic medical traditions originated. As one travels away from the Mediterranean, cultural and environmental differences mount. German lands in particular had special features that shaped the growth of the medical sciences there in the late medieval and early modern periods. These include a cultural identity that sought some measure of independence from southern cultures during this period, a burgeoning religious reform movement directed against Roman authority and traditions, and a very different environmental context that included plants and other medical resources that were unknown to the ancients. This special transalpine context encouraged German physicians to pursue new knowledge by departing from ancient medical traditions, rooted as they were in the lands and peoples of the Mediterranean and Near East. Since the special characteristics of German plants and environments could be known only through personal experience, it became fundamental in constructing this new knowledge.

In various ways explored here, German physicians began to experiment with their received medical traditions as they became more sensitive to the differences between northern and southern Europe, and as they sought to increase their social or economic standing within the local community. While doing so, German physicians sought to make medical teachings more relatable to local realities and began to note their own observations and trials. Such practices fit into a broader European trend in the sixteenth century that encouraged observational practices based on direct personal experience. In her history of observational practices in the sixteenth century, historian Gianna Pomata finds that the idea of *observatio* became an important epistemic category that began to bridge disciplines between the 1530s and 1570s. Some plague treatises bear traces of similar observational practices, and even anticipate the development of the *observationes*, a new genre of medical writing that grew during the 1560s. Both plague treatises and the *observationes* were often written by the same kinds of authors, town and court physicians, who emphasized their healing successes rather than medical doctrine as the source of their legitimacy. Print played an important role in the development of both forms of literature, as it enabled the broad distribution of novel information gained from hard-won experience, and therefore played an important role in fostering medical change.[15] Certainly, observation and experience played a role in earlier plague treatises of the fourteenth and fifteenth centuries, yet one can detect a new emphasis on experience in some of the plague treatises of the early sixteenth century, and especially in the texts that physicians wrote with a strong ego perspective.[16] Such innovative plague authors who had a stronger appreciation for personal experience and novelty include Johann Vochs, Caspar Kegler, Johann Reusch (1490s? –1543), and Tarquinius Schnellenberg (? –1561), among others explored here.

An introduction to plague treatises and plague medicine

This book's core set of sources consists of 392 vernacular German plague monographs printed between 1473 and 1573.[17] Most of these sources are plague treatises of varying degrees of popularization. This figure, also includes texts that focus on religious advice for plague, however, many of which claim to offer "spiritual medicine," as well as texts that announce civic rules for epidemics, although they did not become common in print until after the 1560s. Plague treatises were typically written by university-trained physicians according to a scholastic literary form established in the fourteenth century.[18] After a brief introduction or dedication to patrons, the author discusses the causes and signs (portents) of a plague, then turns to preventative and curative medicine. For most late medieval and early modern plague treatises, recipes and instructions comprise the single largest element of the texts. Plague treatises appeared in a wide variety of lengths, corresponding to how broad the desired audience was intended to be. Some of the shortest treatises comprise four pages or fewer, whereas the longer works can extend to hundreds of pages. Shorter works fit the description of pamphlets or leaflets that aimed to reach a broad audience, similar to uses of popular print for propaganda purposes during the German Reformation.[19] The translation and popularization of plague manuscripts in the fifteenth and sixteenth centuries had little overall effect on the traditional literary structure, although content and authorship changed over time. The content of these treatises often appears repetitive since the authors typically derive much of their medical content from the same authoritative texts. Yet a careful reading of a broad set of treatises reveals novel elements that are valuable for understanding historical change within early modern medicine and culture.

Physicians' plague treatises became a widespread medical genre in 1348 in the wake of the Black Death. Historians know this genre by various names, including plague tracts, plague pamphlets, and *Pestschriften*, as well as the late medieval literary forms *consilia* and *practica*. One of the first historians to attempt an extensive survey of physicians' plague treatises was the German historian Karl Sudhoff.[20] Since his survey ended at the year 1500, however, and did not address the religious content of the texts, it left many texts and issues unexplored, especially in the age of print. Besides filling this gap in history, this book also aims to encourage comparative studies of plague treatises from across Europe and Ottoman lands.[21] Comparisons of plague literature across cultural and linguistic boundaries will provide new avenues of inquiry into early modern medicine and society, especially given the importance of a specifically "German" identity within some German plague treatises.

To understand plague medicine and how it changed over time, one must first understand ancient medical theory and the impact of the Black Death of 1348. Traditional Galenic medicine viewed sickness as an individual problem, resulting from an imbalance of a person's four bodily humors, caused most often by immoderate bodily regimen. Plague outbreaks in the later Middle Ages challenged this theoretical basis, however, since plague seemed to be a novel phenomenon unknown to Greek and Roman physicians, including Hippocrates and Galen. With little ancient precedent to follow, physicians of the fourteenth and fifteenth centuries categorized the Black Death within Avicenna's discourse on pestilential fever, adding their own discussions of poison, contagion, and swellings to the thought of this eleventh-century Persian physician. These physicians turned to poison rather than humoral imbalance to explain the sickness, since it affected all regardless of age, wealth, and health and seemed to spread from person to person through occult means. More specifically, late medieval physicians believed that pestilential poisons were spread in harmful vapors unleashed during planetary conjunctions and earthquakes, and more generally from foul smells created by putrefaction and waste.[22] Such poisons seemed to corrupt the entire atmosphere, explaining why entire communities suffered together. Despite this transformation of ancient medical theory, Galenic understandings did not disappear, since the four humors helped to explain how sicknesses unfold after pestilential poisons enter the body. For many physicians, the basic problem existed in superfluous humors inside the body that were corrupted by the horrible poison from outside the body.

It is important to recognize the wide range of aids and treatments for body and soul that physicians offered in their plague treatises. First and foremost were often repentance and reconciliation with God, since physicians often listed God's wrath for human sins as a primary cause of plague. Spiritual advice also sometimes included other aids, such as prayers to saints, aimed at placating God's anger. Late medieval physicians saw no conflict between using spiritual and natural measures alongside each other, but, rather, seemed to view the two as complementary responses. After the spiritual advice, physicians focused on understanding the natural and earthly causes of plague and their solutions. Physicians sought to prevent the harm of poisons by purifying the air with fragrant smoke or herbs, and recommended bloodletting and specific preventative medicines. Important to both prevention and cure was maintaining a moderate bodily regimen by regulating the body's use of the six *res non naturales*: air, sleep and waking, food and drink, rest and exercise, excretion and retention, and the emotions.[23] These six things were considered "non-natural" since they affected the human body but were not a constituent part of the body itself. For those who fell ill, curative treatments sought to draw out the poisons or correct the corrupted humors through purging, sweating, bloodletting, and taking special medicaments, such as the ancient antidotes theriac and mithridate, which were compounded from many exotic ingredients.[24] Treatments for buboes and swellings included topical treatments or even surgical incision in the attempt to neutralize or extract the foul substances.[25] A closer examination of the content and structure of one plague treatise from 1517 follows in Chapter 1.

Plague epidemics, like any crisis, brought out the best and worst in people, encouraging both charity and self-promotion. Physicians especially took advantage of the plague for self-promotion and community service, using plague treatises to advertise services and medicines while also attempting to protect the community. Apothecaries too likely benefitted from this literature since most of the recipes contained therein required too many special ingredients or were too complex for home preparation. Most recipes therefore necessitated a trip to the local apothecary shop. Physicians' efforts to promote their own professional expertise reflected the difficult audience that they faced, since the majority of the public did not necessarily need or desire the help of learned, university-trained healers.[26] Early Europeans may have desired the quick and effective remedies of more popular healers, especially in times of crisis, rather than the regimens of physicians, which required considerable discipline of diet and behavior. Early modern cities and towns had a variety of healers who were more numerous and approachable for the broad population than university-trained physicians. Besides physicians, other professional healers who enjoyed recognition from local authorities included apothecaries, surgeons, barbers, bath attendants, and midwives, all of whom learned their trade through apprenticeships. The lowest ranks of the hierarchy of healers were filled by those with no official recognition. These folk healers and empirics were often self-taught and included resident healers, male and female, including clerics, noblewomen, and peasants, as well as traveling peddlers and wayfarers. Traveling healers of any category attracted charges of being quacks and charlatans when their activities attracted negative attention from local healers.[27] Since competition among healers was intense in the early modern city, physicians took every chance they could to promote their profession. As plague treatises reveal, physicians even developed new religious arguments in favor of using natural medicine and consulting doctors. In their efforts to promote themselves in new ways, natural healers of the sixteenth century even went so far as to place their "mandate and power to heal on a plane with religion."[28]

In 1473 the first monograph devoted to plague appeared in print in the southern German city of Ulm, the first such work to appear in all of Europe.[29] This text was a plague treatise, composed by the Ulm city physician Heinrich Steinhöwel drawing on a vernacular manuscript he had written earlier in 1446.[30] Although plague advice appeared in print earlier in various forms, the use of metal movable type to produce a plague monograph ushered in a new era of medical communication.[31] Suddenly it became much easier and cheaper to provide detailed information to the broad public on preventing and curing the epidemics. Vernacular print especially brought about a new phase in the popularization of medicine in Europe by greatly expanding the aims, content, and print volume of medical literature of all sorts.[32]

The authors of vernacular plague literature typically addressed a broad audience, imagined as including medical professionals, high and low, and the literate authorities of church and state, as well as the middling classes of early modern German towns, sometimes described as the "common man." Post-mortem inventories of personal libraries show that plague literature was in the hands of physicians, surgeons, and students, and presumably was also owned by merchants and artisans.[33] Readers sought plague literature to expand their knowledge of treatments, recipes, and preventative practices, especially physicians, surgeons, and apothecaries, who desired a range of treatments to meet the needs of their customers.

This literature was also embedded in local institutional and commercial contexts. Among other things, authors informed readers of medicines available at the local pharmacy and helped authorities reinforce the community's standards of spiritual and material order, especially as the authorities developed and promoted plans to separate the sick from the healthy during epidemics. As consumer items, printed plague literature was closely connected to economic trends as well, as printers and booksellers sought to market material that responded to the anxieties of the growing literate population. Shrewd printers stayed ahead of an epidemic, publishing their works well before its arrival, allowing printers and booksellers to sell the products to a population unattenuated by flight. The fear and uncertainty that gripped a city when rumors of a nearby plague circulated provided a prime atmosphere in which to sell the product.

The underlying ethos of plague treatises was active, since physicians, magistrates, and clerics hoped that the broad population would respond to their advice in order to avert catastrophe for the body, soul, and community. For this reason passivity itself was the target of many authors, as were the beliefs that supported it, such as the notion that natural medicine offends God or the fatalistic beliefs that a person's hour of death is preordained and unchangeable. Authors affirmed an active response to plague since they viewed passivity as utterly dangerous. This ethos is apparent in the 1519 plague treatise by the Swiss physician and reformer Joachim von Watt (Vadianus), as he included the common saying "God helps those who help and care for themselves."[34] Furthermore, the literary form of the recipe itself assumes an active reader response, thereby reinforcing the active ethos that underlies the genre.[35]

Printed plague literature also extended to oral culture, thereby reaching to various levels of society. Clerics' plague texts recorded sermons that were preached from pulpits and sometimes contained common prayers and songs for home use to dispel fear and strengthen faith. The advice that physicians gave in print was also what one may have heard in a visit to the doctor, surgeon, or apothecary. Some early plague texts were even composed in verse, making it easier for the surgeon or lay reader to commit the information to memory, and possibly repeat to others. Furthermore, authorities sometimes ordered the oral spread of physicians' advice in the attempt to reach the entire community. For example, the Bavarian Dukes Ludwig and Wilhelm ordered that Johann Rhomming's 1530 pamphlet on the English Sweating Sickness be read aloud to the public.[36] Thus even the non-literate population may have been familiar with the plague advice from physicians and clerics.

The number of German plague publications is vast – so vast, in fact, that German lands may even lead all other parts of Europe in the publication of plague texts. This survey has uncovered 943 vernacular German plague monographs printed between 1473 and 1682, after which publication and epidemics abruptly slowed to a halt. This figure does not include single-leaf broadsides or texts written in Latin. Although there are no complete publication histories of plague literature in any particular area, German-speaking lands seem to be rivaled only by Italian-speaking lands in total output.[37] Historian Samuel Cohn Jr. counted 609 plague texts published in Italian-speaking lands during the sixteenth century, although this figure includes Latin-language works.[38] By comparison, German lands produced at least 588 vernacular plague monographs in the sixteenth century, not including texts in Latin. One reason for the large publication numbers in German- and Italian-speaking lands is likely the political fragmentation, since each town published texts to protect and organize its own people, rather than relying on books and instructions imported from elsewhere.

Geographical publication trends show printed plague literature starting in southern German-speaking lands and expanding northward during the sixteenth century. Between 1473 and 1550 publication was centered in Augsburg, Nuremberg, and Leipzig, and included to a lesser extent the other print centers of Strasbourg, Ulm, Mainz, Regensburg, Ingolstadt, Basel, and Vienna. Between 1520 and 1550 expansion to the north and east unfolded as more printers established themselves in Wittenberg, Hanover, Magdeburg, Dresden, Frankfurt an der Oder, and Lübeck. During the second half of the sixteenth century plague literature appeared in most German-speaking regions, as print blossomed in cities such as Frankfurt am Main, Heidelberg, Hamburg, Bremen, Danzig, Tübingen, Innsbruck, Jena, and Breslau and somewhat later in Rostock, Halberstadt, and Brunswick.[39]

Publication trends by decade reveal vernacular plague literature rising sharply during the Protestant Reformation in the 1520s, peaking in the 1560s, and remaining prolific through the 1620s (Figure 0.1). Over half of all plague publications appeared in years marked by widespread epidemics: 1521, 1529–30, 1562–66, 1575–77, 1581–85, 1597–98, 1606–07, 1625–26, and 1679–81. The greatest blossoming of plague literature appeared between 1562 and 1566, when ninety-three editions appeared. This peak suggests a connection to the worsening climate and overall health in German lands in the 1560s.[40] Although the numbers of publications dropped after the 1560s, vernacular plague literature remained a mainstay of printers into the 1640s, after which publication rates dropped substantially. The exception is one last flourish that coincided with the widespread epidemics in central Germany, Austria, and Bohemia between 1679 and 1683.[41]

Briefly, the format and content of plague treatises underwent significant changes in their first century of printed publication. The fifty years between 1473 and circa 1520 saw the birth of the printed vernacular plague pamphlet and initial attempts to popularize medieval medical lore in print. Noteworthy additions and adaptations of these decades included title page illustrations and greater spiritual rhetoric among some physicians. These pamphlets aimed to provide entire communities, and sometimes specifically the "common man," with helpful advice to withstand the epidemic. While this attempt to reach the "common man" was new, much of the medical

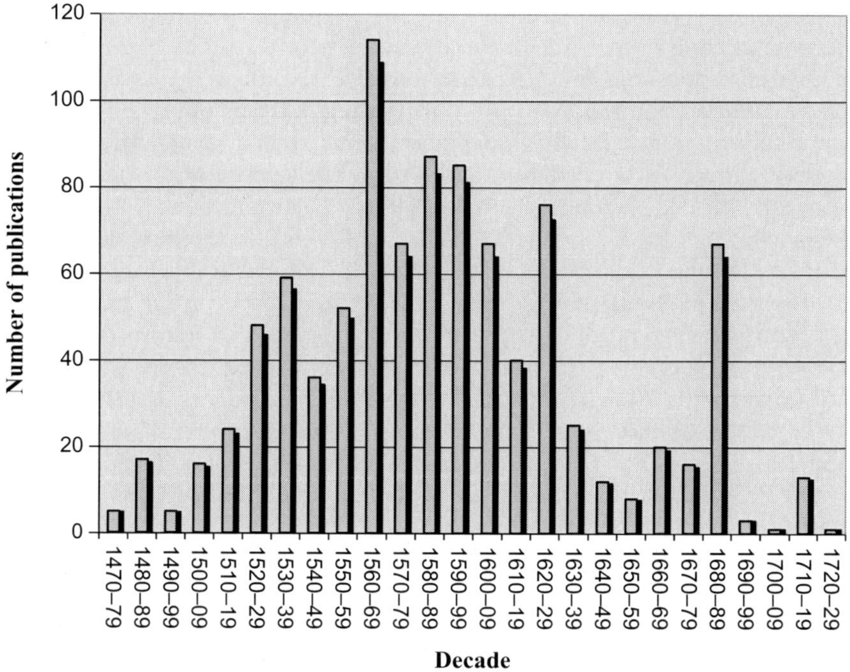

Figure 0.1 Publication of German vernacular plague literature by decade, 1473–1729

content resembles that of fifteenth-century plague manuscripts. Plague literature by clerics was rare in this period, since prints devoted to spiritual plague prevention were typically very short and focused on consoling images or words. Magistrates appear in plague treatises in this period not because they sought to regulate behavior during epidemics but because they urged their appointed physicians to compose advice literature for the broad community.

The first decade of the Protestant Reformation marks an important turning point in printed plague literature as new elements appear in authorship, civic context, and content. Authors more commonly wrote from a personal perspective, discussing specific experiences using medicines and personal views pertaining to religion and current affairs. Physicians began to preach more often, drawing moral lessons from the plagues, condemning sin, and urging moral improvement. This period parallels the heyday of the vernacular propaganda of the Protestant Reformation. Some plague authors even joined the religious debates of the 1520s and adopted new methods to popularize their views.[42] Specifically Protestant perspectives appeared in vernacular medical literature by the end of the 1520s. This new wave of popularization also encouraged a new commercialization of natural medicines for plague. Authors made new attempts to sell novel medicines to the common man and even to medicate the lowest orders of society through the male head of household, the *Hausvater*. Attention to the plague's contagious nature proliferated in the literature during the 1520s, as physicians became more aware of public health issues, paralleling their rise to greater social authority within cities. The first attempt to publicize civic or territorial rules for conduct during plague was Johann Salius's 1521 pamphlet, intended for Austrian lands.[43] In this way, the 1520s appear as a watershed decade for reforms to the medical, spiritual, and political response to plague.

By the mid-sixteenth century physicians' plague literature in many cases was becoming longer, full of detailed content devoted to natural medicine, sometimes with greater scholarly flair. During this expansion of medical detail between 1520 and circa 1560, physicians and magistrates began to treat plague as more of a local phenomenon, traceable to specific local origins, although this remained compatible with the attribution of the plague to divine wrath. Pictures and rhyming verse disappeared from the literature, as authors and printers seemed to turn away from attempts to appeal to the most popular audience. Some physicians noted the expanding length of plague pamphlets and resisted the trend for the sake of common readers. In 1550 the physician of Brunswick, Anthoni Nigri, complained that bookshops were stuffed with plague literature and yet attracted few buyers. Attributing their unpopularity to expanding length, Nigri condensed his advice to fifteen pages.[44] Nigri's actions countered the dominant trend, however, and by the 1560s most plague treatises were over fifty pages long, while some reached gigantic proportions. Some of the longest plague pamphlets appeared in 1564, including Jakob Theodorus's 816-page tome and Sebastian Mayr's 293-page work.[45] Plague pamphlets with fewer than twenty pages became less common by the 1580s.

A fitting end for this book's timeframe comes in the 1560s and 1570s as a specifically "German" identity became less of a cultural concern in the plague treatises of German physicians. The end of this trend coincided with the start of other new trends. A new era of public health was beginning at this time, as printed civic plague mandates became increasingly common, following early publications by Vienna in 1541 and Nuremberg in 1562. These sources are different from plague treatises since they command rather than recommend a certain response, although enforcement was notoriously lax.[46] Change in medical content also came after 1560 as physicians began to refer to Paracelsus specifically when discussing the merits of new chemical medicines. The first plague pamphlets to discuss new sorts of chemical medicines include the work of Georg Phaedro (1562) and Johann Vogt (1564), following the first publication of Paracelsus's corpus of writings in the 1560s.[47] After the 1560s references to medicines containing arsenic, antimony, and sulfur become more common, although these new sorts of medicines never supplanted traditional Galenic medicine. Spiritual content also changed in this decade as the continuing divergence of the religious confessions in German lands brought more references to religious ideas that were specific to a particular confession.

Chapter outline

This book surveys plague texts from the first century of print and interprets their changes in terms of a specifically "German" reform of healing, both spiritual and natural. Chronologically, it covers the period between 1473 and circa 1573, although at times it follows trends and texts into the early seventeenth century. The narrative arc of this book pursues the birth, growth, and demise of a German cultural identity within printed plague advice, while also assessing the impact of the Renaissance and Reformation, the expansion of vernacular print, and the increasing reliance on personal experience among German physicians. These particularly German reform movements combined together in many cases to have lasting effects on the spiritual and natural medical content of plague advice, as well as on medical thought and practice more broadly.

Chapter 1 explores plague texts from the late Middle Ages in order to understand the effects of vernacularization, under way since 1348, as well as the effects that print had on the popularization process, under way since 1473. This chapter reveals how dynamic German plague texts were in the decades before the Reformation as authors sought to reach a broader audience and thereby shape ideas about natural and spiritual health within society. Some German physicians even resembled preachers as they sought to shape piety on the eve of the Reformation. This chapter also provides a detailed exploration of both the natural and spiritual medicine of the late Middle Ages in order to lay the groundwork for understanding the changes brought by the Renaissance and Reformation.

Chapter 2 investigates the innovative thought of Johann Vochs, who introduced a new sort of German medical localism in 1507 in order to protect Germans from harmful foreign ideas, medicines, and commercial interests. His Latin plague treatise of 1507 promotes German medicines for German bodies, known through experience more so than scholarly texts, and thus marks the beginning of a specifically German reform of healing. Underlying Vochs's thought is a new German cultural patriotism that had been developing among German humanists, interpreted in this chapter as part of a broader Renaissance discovery of northern Europe. His patriotism is also expressed in his criticism of the Roman Church, as was increasingly common among German humanists on the eve of the Reformation.

Chapter 3 explores the intersection of plague, medicine, and the Protestant Reformation by examining the plague treatises of the 1520s, as well as the printed religious literature of this revolutionary decade. This chapter argues that plague and medicine belong at the center of Reformation history, since their story provides important insights to the Reformation's agents, appeal, and cultural impact. It uncovers a movement made of physicians and reforming clerics, including Martin Luther, who worked during the 1520s to reimagine the era's spiritual and natural response to plague in the hopes of finding more powerful sources of healing or protection. This disparate group of reformers found common cause in omitting saints from healing traditions and in strengthening religious arguments for the use of natural medicine. Thus, during the 1520s the German reform of healing broadened to include the new Protestant agenda of the time, even if not all physicians acted out of Protestant conviction. Overall, this reform of healing represents an important branch of the Reformation, providing new perspectives on its cultural breadth and impact.

Chapter 4 uncovers the life and work of the Leipzig physician Caspar Kegler, who wrote the most reprinted plague treatises of sixteenth-century German lands. Although he is not well known to history, this chapter argues that Kegler and his descendants were among the first to develop and market a more "modern" sort of brand-name medicine in the marketplaces of central Europe, if not in all of western Europe. Kegler's innovations were both commercial and medical, as he pursued alchemical experimentation in his quest for new and more powerful medicines. Kegler's work fits into the broader German reform of healing as he introduced commercial innovations to vernacular print and deemphasized traditional learned authority as he cultivated personal experience in the field and laboratory.

Chapter 5 pursues the full flourishing of the German reform of healing within plague texts by exploring some of the more popular works produced after 1530. Plague texts written by the physicians Johann Reusch, Tarquinius Schnellenberg, Jodocus Willich, and Ernst Reuchlin show the varied and lasting impact of Johann Vochs and the Protestant reformers. These later plague texts reveal how innovative trends from Renaissance humanism, Protestantism, and vernacular print blended after 1530 to give German plague treatises their own character, and sometimes even encouraged non-traditional views of plague. These later plague texts also reveal that a considerable shift in the foundations of medical knowledge continued, as physicians cultivated environmental observation and particular knowledge known through experience.

Notes

1 Ann Carmichael first traced issues related to the "emerging particular within the 'Universal' Pestilence" in mainly French and Italian plague literature up to 1500: Ann G. Carmichael, "Universal and Particular: The Language of Plague, 1350–1500," in *Pestilential Complexities: Understanding Medieval Plague*, Ed. Vivian Nutton (London: Wellcome Trust Centre, 2008): 17–52, esp. 33 and 52.

2 Colin Jones describes early modern French plague literature as "extremely boring, indeed quite stupendously tedious," although he also argues for the historical value of these texts: Colin Jones, "Languages of Plague in Early Modern

France," in *Body and City: Histories of Urban Public Health*, Eds. Sally Sheard and Helen J. Power (Aldershot, UK: Ashgate, 2000): 41–49, at 43. On their "endless repetitiveness" and "rebarbativeness," see: Colin Jones, "Plague and Its Metaphors in Early Modern France," *Representations* 53 (1996): 97–127, at 101. Paul Slack similarly describes the medical content in English plague literature as "conventional and derivative": Paul Slack, *The Impact of Plague in Tudor and Stuart England* (Oxford: Clarendon Press, 1985), 24.

3 On the innovations of sixteenth-century Italian plague literature: Samuel K. Cohn, Jr., *Cultures of Plague: Medical Thinking at the End of the Renaissance* (Oxford: Oxford University Press, 2010). For a similar emphasis on historical change and innovation in plague treatises over a broader period: Erik A. Heinrichs, "The Live Chicken Treatment for Buboes: Trying a Plague Cure in Medieval and Early Modern Europe," *Bulletin of the History of Medicine* 91 (2017): 210–232.

4 Jean-Noël Biraben, *Les hommes et la peste en France et dans les pays européenes et méditerranéens*, Vol. I (Paris: Mouton, 1975), 407–415. More specific to German lands, evidence of widespread epidemics appears in various local histories and chronicles. To name just a few: *Die Chroniken der deutschen Städte vom 14. Bis ins 16. Jahrhundert*, Vols. 4, 5, 22, 23 (Leipzig: S. Hirzel, 1865–1917); Carly Seyfarth, *Das Hospital St. Georg in Leipzig durch acht Jahrhunderte 1212–1940*, Vol. I (Leipzig: Georg Thieme Verlag, 1939), 65; Richard Bauer, Ed., *Geschichte der Stadt München* (Munich: C. H. Beck, 1992), 123.

5 "Pestilentz" appears as the most common term in vernacular literature to describe these epidemics. Other variations of the term considered here include: Pestilencz, Pestilenz, Pestilentzie, Pestilentzseuch, Pestilentzseuche, Pestilentzzeite, Pestilentie, Pest, Pestis, Peste, Pestseuche. This study also tracks and considers literature that uses other related terms: Gifftigen Seuche, Gift, Infection, Im lauff des sterbens, Jetzigen Leufften, sterblichen leüff, and their variant spellings.

6 Cultural historians are correct in highlighting this uncertainty and the panoply of terms early modern Europeans used to describe these various plagues and pestilences. Mary Lindemann, *Medicine and Society in Early Modern Europe* (Cambridge: Cambridge University Press, 2010), 42–43. See also: A. Lynn Martin, *Plague? Jesuit Accounts of Epidemic Disease in the 16th Century* (Kirksville, MO: Sixteenth Century Journal Publishers, 1996).

7 On the French Disease in northern Europe: Jon Arrizabalaga, John Henderson, and Roger French, *The Great Pox: The French Disease in Renaissance Europe* (New Haven, CT: Yale University Press, 1997), 88–112.

8 There are few books devoted to these sources. Among the studies that examine a broad source base or that take a broad chronological of geographical perspective are: Thilo Esser, *Pest, Heilangst und Frömmigkeit: Studien zur religiösen Bewältigung der Pest am Ausgang des Mittelalters* (Altenberge: Oros, 1999); Petra Feuerstein-Herz, Ed., *Gotts verhengnis und seine straffe: Zur Geschichte der Seuchen in der Frühen Neuzeit* (Wolfenbüttel: Herzog August Bibliothek, 2005); Joachim Telle, Ed., *Pharmazie und der gemeine Mann: Hausarznei und Apotheke in deutschen Schriften der frühen Neuzeit* (Wolfenbüttel: Waisenhaus-Buchdruckerei und Verlag, 1982).

9 Johann Vochs, *De pestilentia Anni p[raese]ntis et ei[us] cura* (Magdeburg, 1507).

10 Rudolf Hirsch, "The Invention of Printing and the Diffusion of Alchemical and Chemical Knowledge," *Chymia* 3 (1950): 115–141, esp. 118–119.

11 Charles Webster has pointed out the problems of viewing Paracelsus as a "lone prophet" of reform: Charles Webster, "Paracelsus: Medicine as Popular Protest," in *Medicine and the Reformation*, Eds. Ole Peter Grell and Andrew Cunningham (London: Routledge, 1993): 57–77.

12 Just one recent example of this vast historiography on the Scientific Revolution: Pamela H. Smith, *The Body of the Artisan: Art and Experience in the Scientific Revolution* (Chicago: University of Chicago Press, 2004), 11–20.

13 Manfred Stürzbecher, "The Physici in German-Speaking Countries from the Middle-Age to the Enlightenment," in *The Town and State Physician in Europe from the Middle Ages to the Present*, Ed. Andrew W. Russell (Wolfenbüttel: Herzog August Bibliothek, 1979): 123–129.

14 Mariusz Horanin, "Die Pest in Augsburg um 1500: Die soziale Konstruktion einer Krankheit," Ph.D. thesis, Georg-August-Universität Göttingen, 2011, esp. 171–172.

15 Gianna Pomata, "Observation Rising: Birth of an Epistemic Genre, 1500–1650," in *Histories of Scientific Observation*, Eds. Lorraine Daston and Elizabeth Lunbeck (Chicago: University of Chicago Press, 2011): 45–80, esp. 59.

16 On observation and experience in plague treatises from before 1500: Melissa P. Chase, "Fevers, Poisons, and Apostemes: Authority and Experience in Montpellier Plague Treatises," in *Science and Technology in Medieval Society*, Ed. Pamela O. Long (New York: New York Academy of Sciences, 1985): 153–171; Cohn, *Cultures of Plague*, 10–15.

17 This figure does not include the single-leaf broadsides, Latin plague treatises, and general medical compendia, although these sources are also considered here. This figure includes later editions of plague monographs.

18 Cohn finds evidence of this literary form from earlier in the fourteenth century, predating the Black Death: Cohn, *Cultures of Plague*, 1.

19 Hans-Joachim Köhler, Ed., *Flugschriften als Massenmedium der Reformationszeit* (Stuttgart: Klett-Cotta, 1981).

20 Sudhoff's studies of individual plague texts appeared in twenty installments over a fourteen-year period. Karl Sudhoff, "Pestschriften aus den ersten 150 Jahren nach der Epidemie des 'schwarzen Todes' 1348" I–XX, *Archiv für Geschichte der Medizin* 4, 5, 6, 7, 8, 9, 11, 14, 16, 17 (1911–1925). See also: Arnold C. Klebs and Karl Sudhoff, *Die Ersten Gedruckten Pestschriften* (Munich: Verlag der Münchener Drucke, 1926).

21 On Italy: Cohn, *Cultures of Plague*. On England: Slack, *The Impact of Plague*. On France: Jones, "Languages of Plague"; Joël Coste, *Représentations et comportements en temps d'épidémie dans la littérature imprimée de peste (1490–1725)* (Paris: Editions Champion, 2007).

22 Chase, "Fevers, Poisons, and Apostemes."

23 Lindemann, *Medicine and Society*, 14.

24 Christiane Nockels Fabbri, "Treating Medieval Plague: The Wonderful Virtues of Theriac," *Early Science and Medicine* 12 (2007): 247–283.

25 Heinrichs, "The Live Chicken Treatment."

26 Martin Gnann, "Populäres Heilen im kulturellen Umfeld der Vormoderne," Ph.D. thesis, Eberhard-Karls-Universität Tübingen, 1994, esp. ch. 2.

27 Robert Jütte, *Ärzte, Heiler und Patienten: Medizinischer Alltag in der frühen Neuzeit* (Munich: Artemis & Winkler Verlag, 2013), 17–32; Lindemann, *Medicine and Society*.

28 Steven Ozment, *Magdalena and Balthasar* (New Haven, CT: Yale University Press, 1989), 125.
29 Klebs and Sudhoff, *Die Ersten Gedruckten Pestschriften*, 59–66.
30 Gerd Dicke, "Heinrich Steinhöwel," in *Die deutsche Literatur des Mittelalters: Verfasserlexikon*, Vol. IX, Ed. Wolfgang Stammler (Berlin: Walter de Gruyter, 1995): 258–278; Ortrun Riha, "Vom mittelalterlichen 'Hausbuch' zur frühneuzeitlichen 'Hausväterliteratur': Medizinische Texte in Handschrift und Buchdruck," in *Die Gleichzeitigkeit von Handschrift und Buchdruck*, Eds. Gerd Dicke and Klaus Grubmüller (Wiesbaden: Harrassowitz Verlag, 2003): 203–227.
31 Esser, *Pest, Heilangst und Frömmigkeit.*
32 Telle, *Pharmazie und der gemeine Mann.*
33 Michael R. Hackenberg, "Private Book Ownership in Sixteenth-Century German-Language Areas," Ph.D. thesis, University of California, Berkeley, 1983.
34 "Wā ein gemeiner spurch ist / das der mensch im selb helffen vnd fürsehen sol / so helffe im gott ouch": Joachim von Watt, *Ein kurtz und trüwlich underricht / wider die sorgklich kranckeyt der Pestilētz / nach aller notturfft vnd ordnung so in söllichem fal / betracht uñ gehaltē werden mag: neulich ußgan gen / uñ zů nutz gemeyner Lantschafft der eydgenoschafft zůsamen bracht im xv. hundert vnd xix. Jar* (Basel: Adam Petri, 1519), sig. B2r.
35 Joachim Telle, "Das Rezept als literarische Form: Bausteine zu seiner Kulturgeschichte," *Medizinische Monatsschrift* 28 (1974): 389–395.
36 Rhomming was the city physician of Landshut. John L. Flood, "'Safer on the battlefield than in the city': England, the 'sweating sickness', and the continent," *Renaissance Studies* 17 (2003): 147–176.
37 Paul Slack identified 153 English vernacular medical works published between 1486 and 1604. Only twenty-three of these works are plague monographs, while most are general medical books that have a section on plague. Slack, *The Impact of Plague*, 23. Similar numbers of French vernacular plague pamphlets are explored by Joël Coste. See: Coste, *Représentations et comportements.*
38 Cohn, *Cultures of Plague*, 27.
39 Naturally, one cannot name all the cities where plague pamphlets were produced. This information is meant to illustrate broad trends, rather than a specific geographical periodization.
40 Wolfgang Behringer gives 1570 as the culmination of this general social crisis, based largely on a study of weather. Wolfgang Behringer, "Die Krise von 1570: Ein Beitrag zur Krisengeschichte der Neuzeit," in *Um Himmels Willen: Religion in Katastrophenzeiten*, Eds. Manfred Jakubowski-Tiessen and Hartmut Lehmann (Göttingen: Vandenhoeck & Ruprecht, 2003): 51–156.
41 Edward A. Eckert, "The Retreat of Plague from Central Europe, 1640–1720: A Geomedical Approach," *Bulletin of the History of Medicine* 74 (2000): 1–28, esp. 15–17.
42 Steven Ozment, "The Social History of the Reformation: What Can We Learn from Pamphlets?" in *Flugschriften als Massenmedium der Reformationszeit*, Ed. Hans-Joachim Köhler (Stuttgart: Klett-Cotta, 1981): 171–203, esp. 177. Köhler argues that the Reformation pamphlet reached its full potential for propaganda after 1520: Hans-Joachim Köhler, "The Flugschriften and Their Importance in Religious Debate: A Quantitative Approach," in *Stars and the End of the World in Luther's Time*, Ed. Paola Zambelli (New York: Walter de Gruyter, 1986): 153–175, 156.

43 Johannes Salius (Hans Saltzman), *Ein nutzliche ordnu-g vnd regime-t wider die Pestilentz durch Doctor Hansen Saltzman vo- Steir / des Durchleichtigisten Fuersten vnnd herren herrn Ferdinanden Ertzhertzogen von Osterreych. c. Leybartzt. dem gemainenn man zw nutz furchtperlich gemacht* (Vienna: Johannes Singriener, 1521).

44 Anthoni Nigri, *Regiment Antonij Nigri / der Artzneien Doctoris vnd Leibartzt / der Erbaren Stadt Braunschweig / Inhaltendt / wie sich wider die Pestiletz zubewaren / auch den jenen die damit begriffen / hülff zu reichen* (Hanover: Henningk Rüdem, 1550), sig. A1v.

45 These pamphlets were published in a smaller size, roughly 105mm by 160mm, while many earlier works measure around 150mm by 190mm. Although the size of the pages was generally shrinking in this period, the great growth of page numbers indicates that an actual growth in content was under way. Jacob Theodorus Tabermontanus, *Gewisse vnnd erfahren Practick / Wie man sich mit Göttlicher hülff / vor der Pestilentz hüten vnd bewaren / vnnd so einer damit behafft / wie demselben zuhelffen. Es seyen alte oder junge / arme oder reiche leuth. Gepracticiert vnd beschrieben in Anno 1551. 52. vnd nachfolgende Jar...* (Heidelberg: Johann Mayer, 1564). Sebastian Mayr, *Ein newer nutzlicher / vnd grundtlicher Tractat / von der Pestilentz / Item wesen / vrsachen / fürsehung und Cur. Darinn auch vil schädlicher jrthumb / wölche in der gemeinen Cur im schwanck gehn / entdeckt vnd widerlegt werden / der massen bißher nie geschehen ist* (Tübingen: Ulrich Morharts, 1564).

46 In some cities, plague mandates began to emerge through collaboration between physicians and magistrates in the 1520s and existed in manuscript form. For the Austrian context, see: Heinz Flamm, *Die ersten Infektions- oder Pest-Ordnungen in den österreichischen Erblanden, im Fürstlichen Erzstift Salzburg und im Innviertel im 16. Jahrhundert* (Vienna: Verlag der Österreichischen Akademie der Wissenschaften, 2008). Among the first Nuremberg prints to command behavior is: *Ains Erbern Raths der Stadt Nürmberg / vernewete Gesetz und Ordnung / in gegenwertigen sterbsleufften diß M.D.LXII. Jars auffgericht* (1562). For a comparative perspective on enforcement, see: Martin Dinges, "Süd-Nord-Gefälle in der Pestbekämpfung: Italien, Deutschland und England im Vergleich," in *Das europäische Gesundheitssystem: Gemeinsamkeiten und Unterschiede in historischer Perspektive*, Eds. Wolfgang U. Eckart and Robert Jütte (Stuttgart: Steiner, 1994): 19–51.

47 Georg Phaedro, *GE. PHAEDRONIS RHODOCHAEI MEDICI HAlopyrgice siue Iatrochemica pestis epidemicae curatio. Oder Warhaffte Cur der erschröcklichen sucht der Pestilentz / an den Hochwürdigsten in Gott Fürsten vnd Herrn Johann Jacob Ertzbischoff zů Saltzburg rc* (Ingolstat, 1562). Johannes Vogt, *Ein nutzliche anzeigung gebrauchter Artzneyen / von gelerten Doctoribus in der hohen Not der Pestilentz / wie die Exempla außweisen / auch yetzunder zů Straßburg in der hohen Not in Brauch geordnet: Bey jnen Diastimios vnd precipitatis cum Auro genannt / die beide fast einer Würckung / Ich aber habs mein Aurum vitae / auch Confectionem vitae ettlich vnd dreissig Jar in meinen Schrifften genannt vnd gebraucht: Die Ertzney würt gebraucht wider allerley verborgne vnbekannte / wie sie genannt mügen werden / Kranckheitten...* (Ulm: Oßwald Gruppenbacher, 1564).

1 Printed plague literature in the late Middle Ages, 1473–1519

Between 1473 and 1519 plagues threatened German-speaking lands roughly once a decade, striking various cities around 1473, 1483–85, 1494–96, and 1504–07.[1] German physicians, clerics, and printers responded to contemporary fears by embracing the new print technology to popularize their medical and spiritual guidance. For physicians, this first flourish of printed plague treatises began with Heinrich Steinhöwel's vernacular work of 1473, the first printed plague monograph in all of Europe. This chapter explores a variety of plague texts produced before and after this introduction of print in order to understand how plague advice changed, considering especially the trends of popularization and vernacularization. Another purpose of this chapter is to provide a detailed portrait of the wide array of natural and spiritual medicine that late medieval authors recommended for plague, especially before the changes of the Reformation era. While physicians' plague treatises written in the German vernacular form the core set of sources, this chapter also considers printed religious devotional literature and single-leaf broadsides, as well as a small number of manuscript sources written in German or Latin since 1348.

Surprising trends appear from this survey of late medieval plague texts. While plague treatises have a reputation for being formulaic and repetitive, some reveal innovation and authentic social engagement. In cases explored here, some German physicians even sought to shape medicine and piety on the eve of the Reformation, beginning their participation in such debates well before the social and cultural turbulence of the 1520s. On natural medicine, popularization in vernacular print brought physicians to change the tone and content of traditional scholastic advice by speaking more often about personal experience and incorporating some non-traditional remedies. On spiritual topics, physicians engaged and even sought to shape the surging piety of the fifteenth century.[2] The importance of spiritual content to the plague treatise genre is immediately apparent in the rich illustrations that grace the title pages of plague treatises in the decades before the Reformation. Multiple title pages of this era depict the plague's spiritual causes or cures, such as the title page of Philippus Culmacher's treatise of circa 1495 (Figure 1.1), as explored further below.

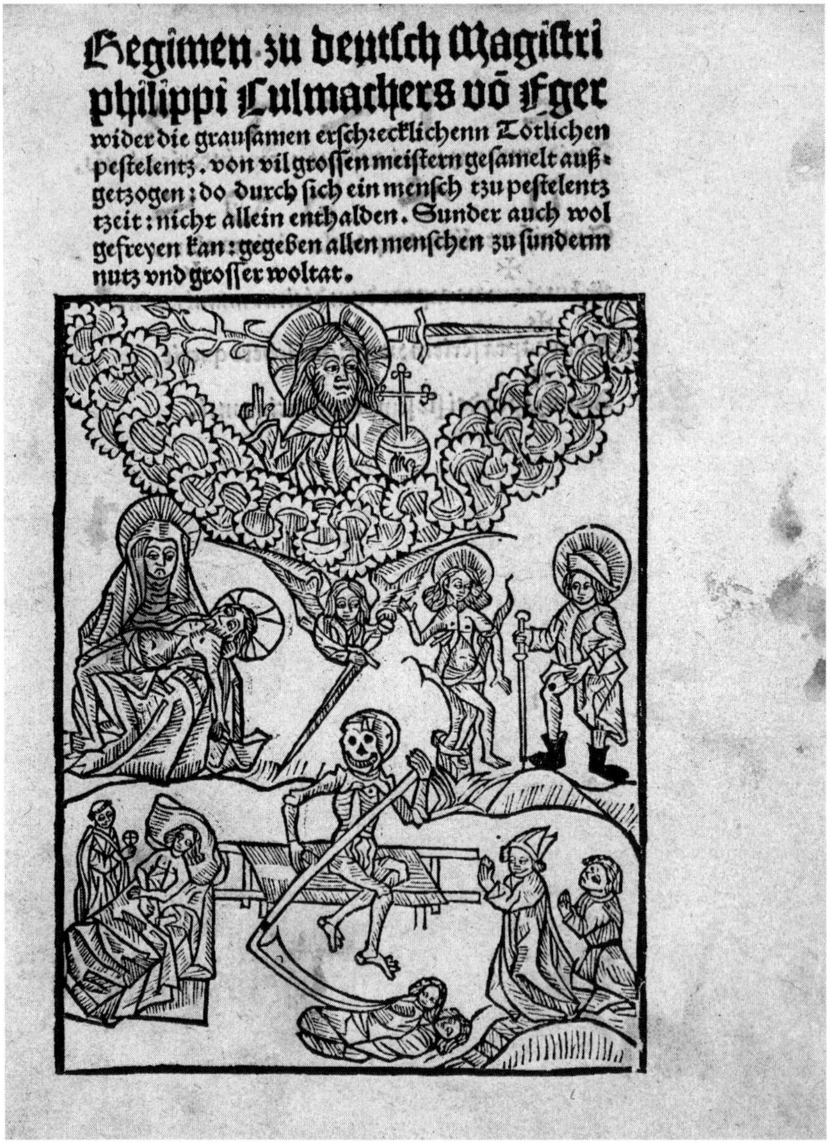
Regimen zu deutſch Magiſtri
philippi Culmachers võ Eger
wider die grauſamen erſchrecklichenn Totlichen
peſtelentz. von vil groſſen meiſtern geſamelt auß-
getzogen: do durch ſich ein menſch tzu peſtelentz
tzeit: nicht allein enthalden. Sunder auch wol
gefreyen kan: gegeben allen menſchen zu ſunderm
nutz vnd groſſer woltat.

Figure 1.1 The panoply of late medieval spiritual medicine for plague

Title page illustration: Philippus Culmacher, *Regimen zu deutsch Magistri philippi Culmachers*... (Leipzig: Martin Landsperg, ca. 1495)

commons.wikimedia.org/wiki/File:P._Culmacher,_Regimen_wider_die_pestilenz;_Wellcome_L0021401.jpg

Spiritual advice was arguably the most dynamic element of German plague treatises in the decades before the Reformation, even as physicians retained the genre's traditional focus on natural medicine. This spiritual advice was neither superficial nor formulaic, but played an important role in popularizing physicians' advice in print. The health of the soul was of great concern within society at large, and therefore a strategic choice for physicians aiming to speak to a broad audience. Plague especially carried powerful spiritual and cultural meaning within early modern societies, due to the traditional biblical association between plague and divine punishment. For these reasons, the spiritual content of physicians' plague treatises grew in both words and images as physicians addressed a broader audience. Some physicians, such as the Augsburg physician Ambrosius Jung, were so enthusiastic about their spiritual messages that they began to resemble contemporary preachers. Furthermore, physicians' spiritual advice changed with broader trends in preaching on the eve of the Reformation in German-speaking lands. After 1500 a new phase of popularization began, in which physicians stopped emphasizing divine anger and moral reform but focused their spiritual messages on what was presumably more popular: fast and easy "spiritual medicines." This represents a shrewd attempt to popularize plague advice further and demonstrates how the boundary between plague texts and contemporary religious devotional literature was porous even before the Reformation.

Notable changes to natural medicine began to appear in the first decades of print as well, continuing the trends of vernacularization that had been developing since 1348. In general, vernacular authors refer to personal experience and observations more often and thereby deemphasize learned authorities as they promote their medical solutions. Some of the popularized plague treatises also mention the newer alchemical medicines of the time more often than their peers. Furthermore, their writing descends more often from the level of universal theory to include more observations about the local environment, especially when discussing the origins of plague. All of these changes in tone and content are reflected in the more personal voice that vernacular authors adopt as they speak more specifically to a local audience that would not necessarily appreciate scholarly discourse. Admittedly, a clear ego perspective was never common in plague treatises at any point, as one might expect of a genre with roots in late medieval scholastic thought. Distinct personal statements do appear more frequently, however, as vernacular print established itself after 1473, and as the texts became even more popularized with the full flourishing of vernacular print during the 1520s, as explored in Chapters 3 and 4. By adding personal perspectives, the more original authors of the time achieved greater success on the book market, while also promoting a greater appreciation for personal experience within the production of medical knowledge.

It is important to note that nearly all German authors of plague literature writing before the 1520s did not emphasize their medicine or advice as having a particularly "German" character. Even though they were writing in German, or, rather, a late medieval regional dialect, authors did not yet employ a German cultural identity to frame their ideas about the causes and solutions to the plague. The obvious exception is Johann Vochs, who in 1507 developed this approach as part of a German cultural movement, as explored in Chapter 2. For the most part, however, German physicians before the Reformation did not present their ideas and remedies as somehow distinct from the plague advice found in other parts of Europe. This trend is rooted in the universal character of medical learning at the time, and, more specifically, reflects the universal scope of contemporary theories about the causes and cures of plague.

Popularizing advice: Vernacular and Latin treatises between manuscript and print

The trend of popularizing plague advice was not an invention of print, however, but began at the onset of the Black Death in 1348. The popularizing trends of the late fifteenth century were therefore just amplifications of trends established earlier. Between the Black Death and 1473, physicians and surgeons throughout western Europe wrote many manuscripts to advise learned and lay audiences. While many early treatises appeared in Latin, some early authors wrote in the regional vernacular, thus pioneering the process of reaching out to a broader audience within society. Vernacular texts were sometimes very different from their academic cousins in both their medical and spiritual content, since their imagined audiences were different. As physicians and other medical authors sought to appeal to the broader community, they incorporated more aid and guidance for the soul. In this way, they tapped into the surging piety of the late Middle Ages to calm troubled souls as well as to protect the bodies. The plague-specific piety that they incorporated into their texts was also somewhat new, having grown since 1348.

Differences in the content of Latin and vernacular plague treatises are apparent among the very first treatises written in 1348. One of the most influential Latin plague treatises of 1348, the report of the Paris medical faculty, is fairly reticent on the spiritual cause and solutions to the plague.[3] Writing for the French King Philippe VI and an educated audience in general, the Paris medical scholars mention the plague's supernatural origins almost as an afterthought. Only at the end of the first section do the Paris masters state that plague can occur in accordance with divine will, but do not mention divine punishment or sin, much less offer detailed spiritual advice.[4] As was typical of text-based scholastic medicine at the time, appeals to experience and local observations are also minimal in the Paris text compared to later treatises, and especially later vernacular texts. The Paris physicians do describe some local signs that portend a coming pestilence, such as recent unseasonable weather, but are careful to cite authorities or "wise men" to demonstrate the relevance of their observations. As one might expect of the late Middle Ages, the Paris masters do not assume that their observations carry epistemic weight on their own.[5]

The first vernacular plague treatise, however, contrasts strongly with the Paris masters on such points. Writing for the town of Lerida in 1348, the Catalan physician Jacme d'Agramont included substantial personal comments on his local environment, not to mention more spiritual content. For example, d'Agramont mentions that Lerida has been healthier since the poplar trees by the city fountain were cut down, supporting his idea that tall trees prevent a cleansing ventilation from wind. He also reflects on why particular streets and parts of town seem to experience plague more often, such as the bridgehead, the monastery of friars, the tripe butchery, and the marketplace, often finding the answer in the level of filth within the locality.[6] Furthermore, d'Agramont's spiritual content includes long Bible verses to support the plague's origin as a divine punishment for sins, as well as its remedy: "The supreme remedy in such a case is to acknowledge our sins and our failings by hearty repentance and oral confession by works and acts and thus is given satisfaction to God by a true repentance."[7] D'Agramont's emphasis on works and acts is a characteristically Catholic expression of repentance, which was standard for the time. As explored in Chapter 3, this emphasis on human actions came under sharp attack later during the Reformation, and even within plague treatises.

Academic and vernacular plague treatises were never so sharply separated, however, that they form two distinct genres. Furthermore, these differences between the first Latin and vernacular plague treatises became less sharp over time as more physicians gained direct experience with the sickness. The relative lack of experience in some of the earliest Latin plague texts does not necessarily mean that physicians were deemphasizing their own experience in favor of ancient, textual knowledge on the issues. One problem during the first epidemic of 1348 was that not many authors had direct experience with the sickness. Historian Samuel Cohn, Jr., has shown that the authors of fifteenth-century Latin plague texts began to mention experience more often as they became more experienced in dealing with the sickness, and even recorded some healing successes. Hence some authors of late medieval Latin manuscripts became eager to share their experiences, and sometimes even claimed superiority over the ancients in treating a general epidemic. Such confidence in experience seems to have waned for some physicians by the mid-fifteenth century, however, as the pestilences continued and confounded prior solutions.[8]

The shift from manuscript to print in the later fifteenth century encouraged the divergence between Latin and vernacular plague advice on such issues. Authors' efforts to address a broad, often local audience brought vernacular plague pamphlets to resemble more d'Agramont's writing rather than the stiff academic discourse of the Paris medical faculty. Given the prevalence of printing presses in German-speaking towns during the later fifteenth century, German authors were at the forefront of attempts to appeal to the expectations of the "common man." Vernacular authors found themselves walking a fine line between establishing their learned authority through scholarly discussion, on the one hand, and appealing to the practical interests of the audience, on the other, by relating tried-and-true remedies and stories of healing successes. Authors writing in the vernacular also sought to instruct or even discipline their readers on the spiritual issues of plague's causes and responses. By tapping into the plague-specific piety that grew in the decades after the Black Death, authors were able to provide a wide variety of channels for divine mercy.

Print itself did not create the impulse to broaden the audience of plague treatises. The importance of the vernacular manuscript tradition is even apparent in the case of the first printed plague monograph, written by the Ulm city physician Heinrich Steinhöwel (1412–1478). Steinhöwel's plague treatise was the first of any text to be printed in Ulm, appearing on Johann Zainer's press in 1473.[9] While historian Karl Sudhoff claimed that this text was composed specifically for printed publication, the discovery of a predecessor text, a 1446 vernacular manuscript, has diminished this claim.[10] More importantly, this 1446 manuscript reveals that Steinhöwel was reaching out to a broad audience well before print, as he included both a "lower medicine and teaching" (*ringen erczny vñ ler*) for people unpracticed in medical arts as well as information for people with more training and resources.[11] The manuscript format limited the text's potential to spread knowledge, however, as compared to the later printed format. The fact that only one copy of Steinhöwel's 1446 manuscript is known today indicates that its reach was likely not extensive.

Sudhoff was right to some extent, however, since Steinhöwel did make significant changes to the 1446 manuscript to prepare it for print. Steinhöwel's 1473 monograph was more than a medieval manuscript set in moveable metal type, but continued the process of reaching out to an imagined broad audience.[12] The text's preface, for example, offers new spiritual content and addresses the "common man" for the first time. The 1473 monograph states that Steinhöwel's intended audience is both the "common man" (*gemein man*) and young surgeons still learning their trade.[13] These additions strengthen his prior commitment to providing a less scholarly medicine and show that the literary trope of addressing the "common man" entered German plague literature at the birth of printed works. Steinhöwel's 1473 text was the first of what became a long tradition of vernacular plague pamphlets that spoke to the "common man," whom authors believe needed help as plague threatened.[14] The appeal to the "common man" grew along with the vernacular book market, lasting within medical literature into the eighteenth century.[15]

The shift from manuscript to print also brought more spiritual content to Steinhöwel's text. Steinhöwel's 1473 work is fairly long at eighty pages, which gives space to dwell on the moral lessons of plague as well as to provide copious spiritual remedies and appeals to saints. In his opening pages Steinhöwel mentions that if a plague comes as the scourge of God there is no better medicine than "proper confession, true regret, and holy penance."[16] While Steinhöwel did not specify that confession should be made to a priest, such things were understood within the late medieval context.[17] Although similar lines of anger and repentance appear in the 1446 manuscript, what was new to print was a long prayer to St. Sebastian as well as a small image of the saint in an illumination of the text's first letter. Steinhöwel seeks a certain and lasting solution for plague through St. Sebastian's intercession with God and Jesus, as seen in his prayer:

> Oh Saint Sebastian, how great is your faith. Pray for us to the lord Jesus Christ, that he save us from the evil outbreak of pestilence. Pray for us Sebastian, holy martyr for Christ, that we should be counted worthy of Jesus's promise. Almighty, eternal God, on account of the merit of your most holy and precious martyr Sebastian you have called back and taken away humanity's pestilence. Look upon your eager supplicants, that all who say this prayer reverently in the face of the evil *Pestilentz*, and all harm to body and soul, be saved through his prayer, through the lord Jesus Christ, your son who lives and reigns with you in eternity, of God's Holy Spirit, through all worlds, amen.[18]

In addition to this prayer, Steinhöwel recommends fasting and alms giving as ways to gain the saint's favor, as was typical for late medieval piety. Within the context of an expanding audience and an emerging plague piety after the Black Death, Steinhöwel was incorporating conventional spiritual advice into his pamphlet. Thanks to print, however, this information became easier to reproduce. Steinhöwel's 1473 work set the standard for printed plague treatises and was the most reprinted such work within the first decade. Between 1473 and circa 1482 his text appeared in print at least five times in three different cities: Ulm, Esslingen, and Nuremberg.[19]

One other important contemporary print confirms that adding spiritual content was a broader trend during the shift from manuscript to print.[20] Around 1482 two editions of a classic medieval plague manuscript by the fourteenth-century French physician Johannes Jacobi appeared in print in Nuremberg, one in Latin and one in German. Much like Steinhöwel's text, Jacobi's work gained notable spiritual additions as a printed vernacular text. For example, when the Latin Jacobi text recommends repentance as the highest remedy for pestilence, the vernacular Jacobi adds more sentences that describe how exactly a person should confess to clear the conscience. Furthermore, a different part of Jacobi's text acquired spiritual significance that was not present in the Latin edition. According to ancient medical wisdom, the Latin Jacobi gives the following on how to regulate emotions for optimal plague protection:

> Levity of the heart is a great remedy for the health of the body. A way to guard one's life in times of plague is to not fear death, but to hope to live for a long time without anxiety and fear of the pestilence, death or danger.[21]

The vernacular edition, by contrast, sacralizes this secular advice through some notable biblical additions:

> The joy of the heart without sin is a good remedy for the health of the body. For this reason a person must lighten his conscience of sin. Prepare as given above and live as safely and happily as one can without a need to fear. As the wise Solomon said, a constant spirit is similar to a continual banquet. One may add, a sad man has an evil, burdened conscience and lives in constant fear of terrible things. In contrast, only an unburdened conscience can be happy and courageous in God and that is the best remedy against the pestilence.[22]

The translator of this passage adds sin, repentance, and a biblical reference to what had been secular, ancient wisdom about the health benefits of a good mood. Jacobi's Latin plague text was one of the most widely distributed plague treatises of late medieval western Europe and appeared in print in many European cities before 1500.[23]

Print also unleashed the power of the image, and especially spiritual images, to raise interest in physicians' texts. Many plague treatises printed before the Reformation feature saints on their title pages, especially the saints who had acquired a specific connection to plague, such as Sts. Sebastian and Roch. In fact, title pages themselves were new to these printed plague monographs starting around 1494. The title page of *A True Medicine and Treasure of Life* of 1494 is among the earliest and features a large illustration of St. Sebastian, the late Roman Christian martyr (Figure 1.2). While this text is mainly devoted to natural medicine, it is clear that the publisher was borrowing an image similar to those that had been appearing for two decades in printed spiritual broadsides on plague. One such example counts among the earliest printed single-leaf broadsides on plague, which appeared in Augsburg at roughly the same time as Steinhöwel's 1473 pamphlet (Figure 1.3). Intended to provide only spiritual solutions to plague, this broadside features a powerful God who sheaths a sword, likely in response to Sts. Sebastian and Roch praying for the sick people who lie before them. German-language prayers to both saints make up the lower third of the page and recall the saint's stories of holiness, suffering, and personal sacrifice.[24] The juxtaposition of suffering saints with suffering humans in this image also highlights the soteriological function of suffering within late medieval piety.[25] Not only did saints provide avenues for divine intercession, but they also provided the laity with models of what could be gained through suffering, namely a purification of the soul. Many believed that one could atone for sins and gain divine favor by suffering through a divine trial such as plague, much like Sts. Sebastian and Roch.

Most striking is the broad variety of late medieval "spiritual medicine" help available in late medieval plague prints, as illustrated in the title page image of Philippus Culmacher's plague treatise of circa 1495 (Figure 1.1).[26]

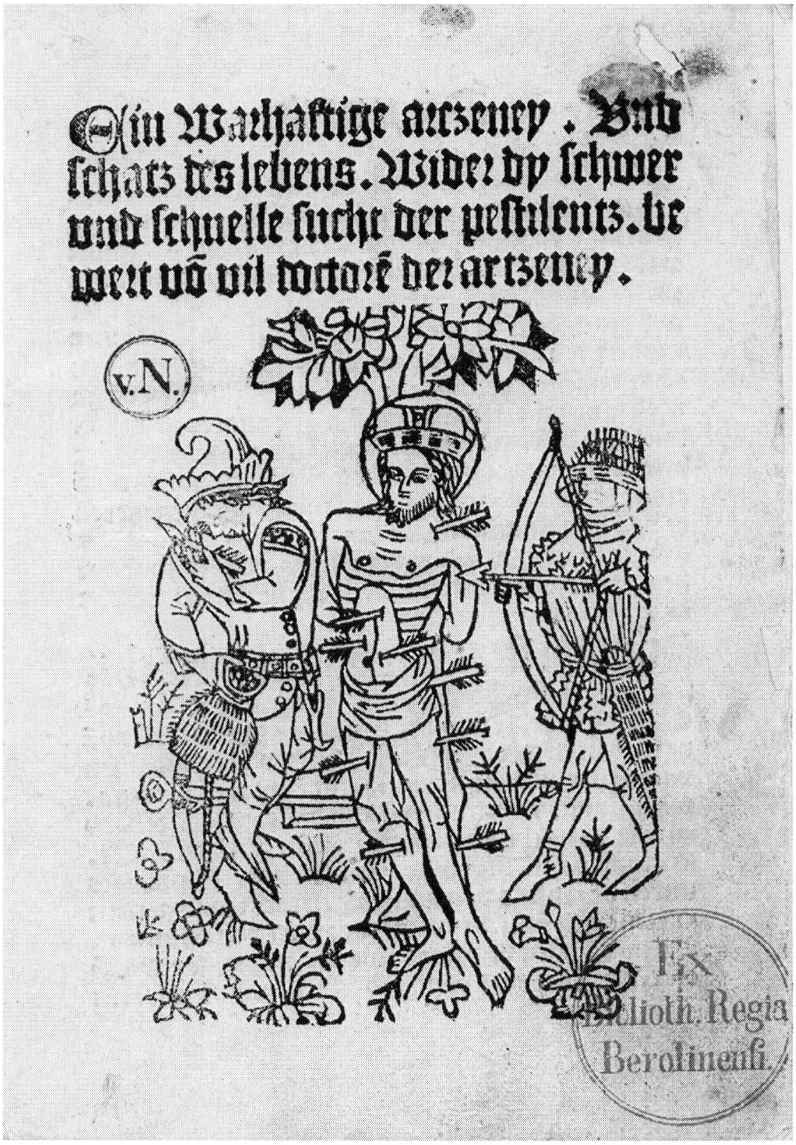
Ein Warhaftige arczeney. Und
schatz des lebens. Wider dy schwer
und schnelle sucht der pestilentz. be
wert vō vil doctorē der artzeney.
v.N.
Ex
Biblioth. Regia
Berolinensi.

Figure 1.2 St. Sebastian

Title page illustration: *Ein Warhaftige arczeney. Und schatz des lebens…* (Erfurt: Hannßen Sporer, 1494)

Staatsbibliothek zu Berlin – Preußischer Kulturbesitz

Call number: Inc. 1120 (reproduced with permission)

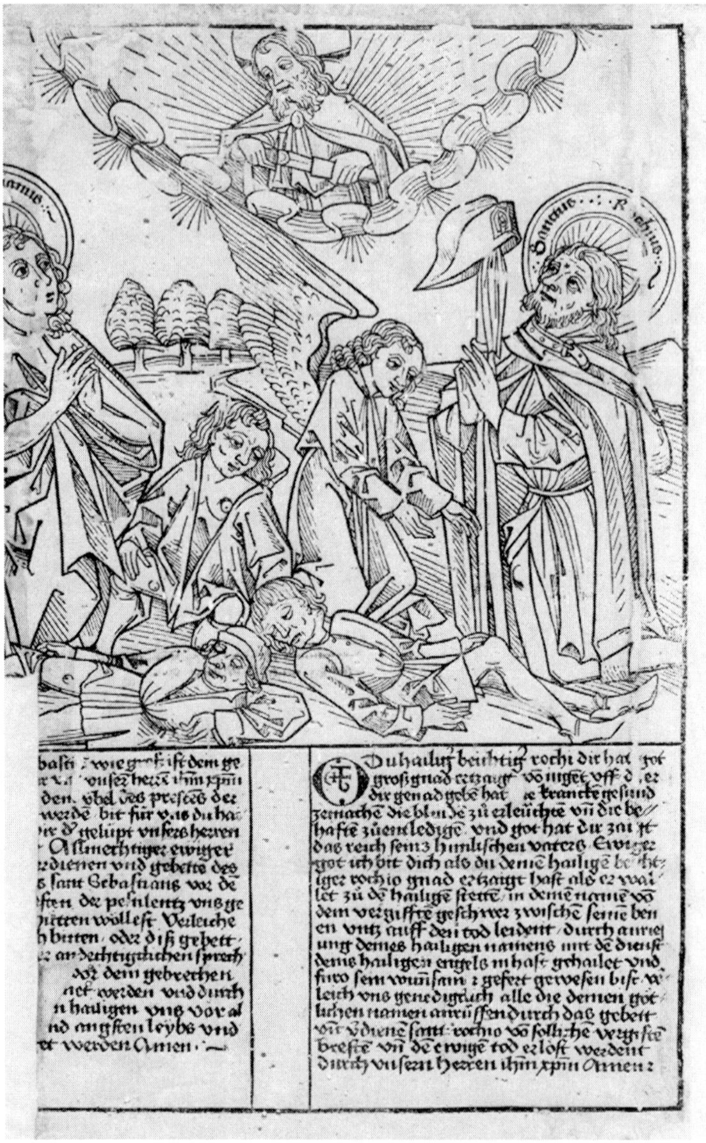

Figure 1.3 Angry God, Sts. Sebastian and Roch with suffering humans [single-leaf broadside: Pestblatt] (Augsburg: s.n., ca. 1473)

Boston Medical Library in the Francis A. Countway Library of Medicine

Call number: Rare Books Ballard 526 (reproduced with permission)

The key theme of this image is the balance between divine punishment and spiritual remedies, as it depicts a balance of divine anger and mercy.[27] Frightening scenes of a judging God, an angel of death, and a threatening skeleton are flanked by the spiritual remedies of this world, including the Eucharist, repentance, and prayer to Jesus, Mary, and Sts. Sebastian and Roch. How a person negotiates this balance of good and evil, judgment and mercy, depends upon an individual's choice from this array of spiritual options.

The printer Martin Landsperg likely added this dramatic title page in order to enliven Culmacher's content, which focuses on natural medical advice, delivered in a "somewhat stiff manner of popularizing," as Karl Sudhoff put it.[28] Culmacher does not include personal stories or references to experience to help gain the trust or sympathy of the audience, but mainly repeats the sayings of scholars, such as Hippocrates, Aristotle, and Avicenna. Two unusual elements, however, make the text remarkable: a spiritual incantation on the verso of the title page, and a later reference to an "elixir of life," one of the first references to an alchemical remedy. Such additions indicate that vernacular texts composed for print were more likely to contain a wider variety of ways to combat plague, since they were better able to straddle academic and more popular approaches to protection and healing. Culmacher discusses his "elixir of life" in the final chapter of his text, as an addendum to the genre's normal literary structure. Here Culmacher mentions a wondrous remedy that draws on a fifth element of nature, attained through distillation, and recorded by the great philosophers among their secrets.[29] Culmacher does not discuss how to make this elixir, however, and does not advertise where one can find it. At the time it was unusual for physicians trained at universities to discuss alchemical procedures and remedies, since this topic fell outside their own learned tradition.

More surprising is the incantation "Ananizapta" that appears on the verso of Culmacher's title page. This apotropaic saying describes its own use and function, as apparent below. The name "Ananizapta" originates from the first letters of the Latin words in the first two verses:

> Antidotum nazareni auferat necem intoxicacionis. /
> Sancrificet alimenta pocula trinitas alma. /
> Est mala mors capta: dum dicitur ananizapta. /
> Ananizapta ferit mortem: que ledere querit. /
> Ananizapta dei sit semper medicina mei.[30]

Translated as:

> The antidote of the Nazarene takes away death by poisoning. /
> May the Trinity sanctify the cup of nourishment. /
> Evil death is captured: therefore Ananizapta is spoken. /
> Ananizapta strikes dead that which tries to harm. /
> May the Ananizapta of God always be my medicine.

This saying appeals to the power of Jesus ("the Nazarene") and the Trinity in order to ward off poisons. There is evidence that this incantation was not uncommon during the late Middle Ages, since it was inscribed above Ingolstadt's medieval city gates as well as over the sacristy door of the court chapel at Meran.[31] Such incantations did attract criticism, however. In his prose plague tract of 1482 the Nuremberg surgeon Hans Folz warns against healing methods that are tainted by magic, characters, and blessings on account of their irreligion (*vnglauben*).[32] It is unclear, however, if Folz would have found this incantation objectionable, since it is essentially a Christian blessing. In any case, the inclusion of this incantation reveals Culmacher, or perhaps his printer, incorporating protective elements from a more popular tradition, and from outside the learned medical tradition.

By elaborating on the spiritual causes and solutions to the plague, physicians and printers were keeping pace with trends in preaching and devotional literature in the later fifteenth century. It is well known that this was a time of heightened piety and devotion within Western Christendom. The fifteenth century also saw a great increase in vernacular religious literature that aimed to shape the piety of the lower clergy and laypeople who lacked theological training. Such literature included handbooks for pastoral care, thematic sermons, and devotional literature of all sorts, including catechisms and prayer books.[33] Thus, as German plague literature underwent the transformations of vernacularization and the shift from manuscript to print, it began to share some elements of popular religious literature, which was going through a similar process of popularization in the fifteenth century.

Of all late medieval German plague authors, the Augsburg physician Ambrosius Jung (1471–1548) was the most interested in preaching moral reform and was one of the most successful early authors. Most importantly, since Jung published Latin and vernacular plague pamphlets nearly simultaneously in 1494, his work allows direct comparison and offers insight into the processes of vernacularization and popularization in print. Jung's translation of knowledge from his elite Latin learning into the vernacular was clearly an attempt to reform the common man's soul in addition to answering the physical needs of a broad audience.

Jung wrote both his Latin and vernacular plague pamphlets in 1494 at the age of twenty-three, after he had become the personal physician to the bishop of Augsburg and the cathedral chapter. Although Jung stepped tentatively into the new media, his 1494 vernacular pamphlet initiated a lifelong interest in vernacular plague literature. Jung revised his original vernacular pamphlet twice during the Protestant Reformation to produce pamphlets that were influential into the 1560s. The Augsburg printer Hans Schönsperger aided the success of Jung's text, as he added an illustrated title page and formatted it into clear sections. The title page image of both Latin and vernacular pamphlets depicts the young doctor presenting his work to his patrons, the lords of the cathedral chapter (Figure 1.4). As Jung bends

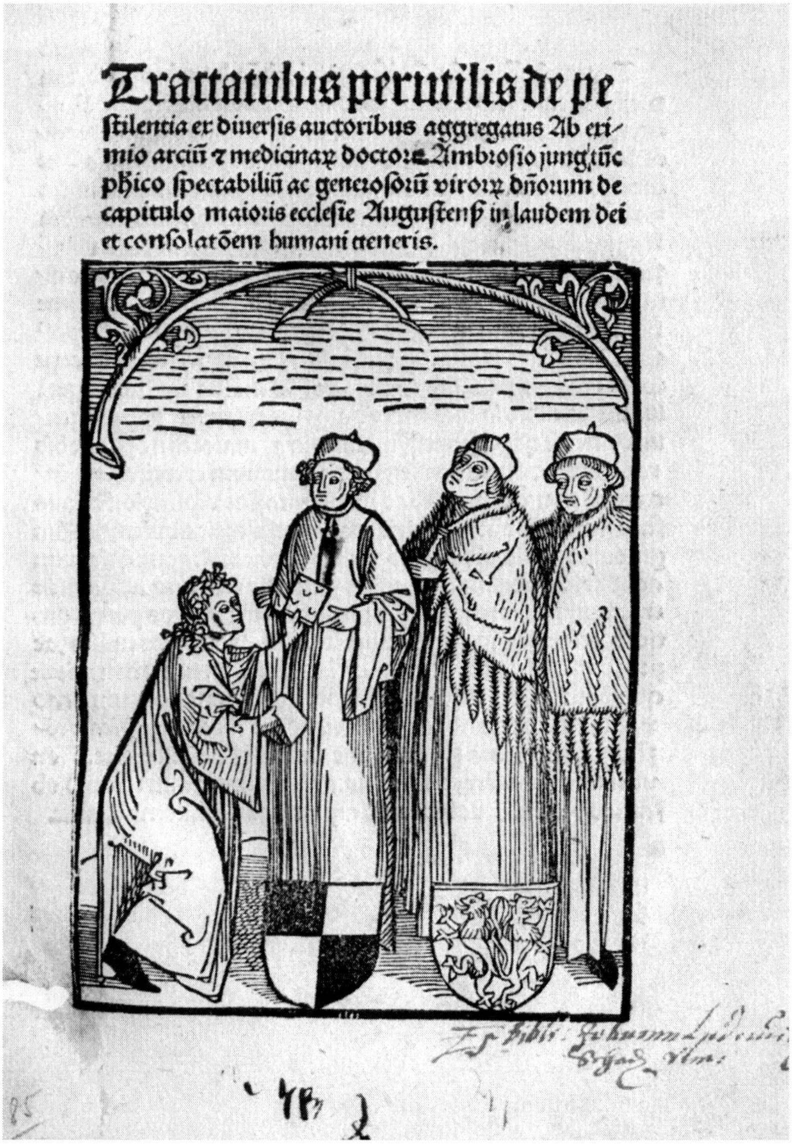
Tractatulus perutilis de pe
stilentia ex diuersis auctoribus aggregatus Ab exi-
mio arciũ ꝛ medicinarꝫ doctore Ambrosio jung tũc
phẏsico spectabiliũ ac generosorũ virorꝫ dñorum de
capitulo maioris ecclesie Augustenß in laudem dei
et consolatõem humani generis.

Figure 1.4 Ambrosius Jung and the Augsburg Cathedral chapter

Title page illustration: Ambrosius Jung, *Tractatulus perutilis de pestilentia ex diuersis auctoribus aggregatus...* (Augsburg: Hans Schönsperger, 1494)

Boston Medical Library in the Francis A. Countway Library of Medicine

Call number: Rare Books Ballard 419 (reproduced with permission)

his knee before his splendid patrons, the image emphasizes the status and power of the church officials. This obsequious pose likely embarrassed Jung later in his life, given his behavior during the Reformation, as discussed in Chapter 3.

The differences between Jung's Latin and vernacular pamphlets of 1494 lie more in their content than in their length or format. Jung opens his Latin pamphlet with a fawning dedication to his patrons, while the preface of his vernacular pamphlet describes his work as intended for the comfort and aid of all common humanity (*gemeynten menscheyt*).[34] Jung's first venture into the production of vernacular medical literature was tentative. The vernacular dedication reveals his doubts about the ability of German to express the ideas and recipes of ancient medicine:

> If you, the reader of this little book, find it lacking, you can refer to the Latin work, which is longer and more thorough. Also, do not let Latin information and recipes lead you astray because it is not possible to put many things into German. I included this information in the book since I did not want to hide anything.[35]

This passage indicates that Jung did not have great faith in the precision of the German language for communicating technical information, but also reveals his assumption that some of his readers could read Latin as well. The former view stands in stark contrast to later champions of the German vernacular for technical writing, such as Paracelsus and Walther Hermann Ryff. The fine line that Jung walked between the integrity of his technical information and popularization is reflected in his recipes. Jung's vernacular pamphlet keeps many recipes in Latin, avoiding the problems of translation.[36] But, while he guards the integrity of his recipes, Jung also accommodates people of modest means and those who read only German by offering alternative recipes in the vernacular that use simpler ingredients.

A close analysis of the spiritual content of Jung's vernacular pamphlet reveals that his preaching, absent from his Latin pamphlet, fits the model of late medieval sermons on divine anger and mercy. In fact, Jung's vernacular writing offers an extraordinary glimpse into the piety of a late medieval physician.[37] Jung's vernacular rhetoric even lapses into the unusual form of an imagined dialogue with a sinner. Jung's preaching attempts to balance divine anger and judgment with the promise of divine mercy, much like other late medieval German preachers, including Johannes Geiler von Kaysersberg of Strasbourg (1445–1510).[38] Divine punishment for sins was real and frightening in such sermons, but it was offset with equivalent emphasis on Christian promises of mercy and redemption.

Jung opens his discussion of the plague's origins by focusing on divine punishment and the causes of divine wrath: a lack of good works and love for God alongside much infidelity, falsehood, and deception.[39] To remedy the spiritual situation, Jung encourages his readers to seek a "spiritual medicine" (*geystliche artzney*) from the spiritual fathers of the Holy Scriptures and confessor priests. The spiritual medicine here is confession for all who have "wounded themselves deeply" with sin. At this point Jung launches his dialogue with a sinner – a rhetorical approach that was highly unusual in plague treatises:

> What is worse than being accustomed to sin? You say, "I do not know what I have done." Then say what good you have done. This issue is not my own creation, but rather comes from the worthy and spiritual fathers of the Holy Scriptures. With them, I say, have you defied and sinned against God and your fellow humans? Then repent by first turning yourself to God with a repentant heart, with a remorseful expression of confession and complete acts of atonement and penance with the intention thereafter of keeping the commandments of God. Perhaps the Almighty God sees the thought and good will of your heart and forgives you, but do not deceive Him. You err. But as far as you are righteous, you will find mercy.[40]

Jung's statements on sin and confession are traditional in form and theology as they emphasize good works, the acts of contrition and penance, and the role of the confessor priest. Furthermore, the fact that he addresses people who may give a half-hearted confession ("but do not deceive Him") suggests that he is targeting those of lukewarm piety, who desire the mercy of God but resist submitting themselves to full repentance.

While confession is the only spiritual solution to plague that Jung describes specifically as "medicine," he also recommends additional help from heavenly intercessors. Jung states that the audience can turn to the clergy for prayers to the Virgin Mary, St. Sebastian, and St. "Eurochus" (St. Roch), from whom a person can acquire great results. Jung even advises that parents teach their children songs that are prayers to saints. Although Jung promotes the cult of the saints, he does not recommend some practices, such as ascribing apotropaic powers to physical copies of prayers. Jung condemns parents' practice of hanging written prayers around the necks of children to protect them from harm.[41] Rather, he advises people to first unite themselves with God, then to use the protection of natural medicine.[42]

The differences between Jung's 1494 Latin and vernacular works highlight the differences in the texts' assumptions about the interests and needs of laypeople as opposed to scholars. Dialogues with sinners do not appear in his 1494 Latin work, which, overall, has shorter sections on the spiritual responses to plague. Moreover, there are no references to saints as mediators in the Latin work, with the exception of Mary, who appears once.[43] Another difference is that the condescending tone of the vernacular pamphlet carried into Jung's discussion of medical issues as well, since he sometimes speaks directly to the "ignorant." Jung introduces his section on preventative medicine with an attack on fatalism: "You ignorant man, this much you can say – it is possible to protect the human body from the plague."[44] Elsewhere Jung attacks the beastly life of those who do nothing about the bad smells in their homes and bodies: "[T]hus in your unreasonable life you are like a beast."[45] Most offensive to Jung were the people who blame the plague on God's cruelty, rather than examining their own filthy ways. Clearly, Jung's 1494 vernacular pamphlet reflects the physician's mission to encourage moral reform and counter medical passivity in the broader population.

Jung's 1494 vernacular work also introduces a religious justification for natural medicine itself. This reflects the increasing complexity of the rhetorical aims of the plague pamphlets, as physicians began to press their case on the importance of natural medicine. To fight medical passivity and promote his profession, Jung cites the Book of Sirach (Ecclesiasticus):

> Thus says Ecclesiasticus. The work of medicine (*artzney*) is His mercy, not a test of God. You say, yes, [previously] I went just the same in the name of God. But you are a rational person, not a beast. Use your reason. God created medicine out of the Earth for all living people, and a prudent person does not neglect it.[46]

The Bible thus reveals God's command to humans to use natural medicine. Not only does this construct an irreproachable foundation for the physician's profession, it also strengthens the social position of physicians as the mediators of this divine healing power. Although Jung was the first author to use this justification in a printed vernacular plague pamphlet, the appeal to Ecclesiasticus was common in manuscripts and appears in other printed genres.[47]

Jung's strong moral tone reveals that vernacular preaching in plague literature was not a product of the Reformation but, rather, had been present since the late fifteenth century. His rhetorical tone was new to plague writing, however. Rather than simply recommending recipes and practices for the prevention and cure of plague, Jung commands change at the personal level. He seeks to reform his audience of its bad habits, encouraging greater spiritual discipline and a steadfast acceptance of the value of natural medicine. One wonders, however, whether a broad audience was receptive to Jung's preaching or if there were more effective ways to reach the "common man." Further developments in vernacular plague texts after 1500 show authors pioneering other ways to popularize natural and spiritual advice.

A late medieval plague pamphlet and its natural medical content

A close look at one popular plague pamphlet of circa 1517 reveals the natural medical content in greater depth, as well as illustrating the complexity and goals of such late medieval texts. At a length of fifteen pages, *A True Medicine and Treasure of Life against the Heavy and Quick Scourge of the Plague* was a short plague pamphlet that targeted a broad audience

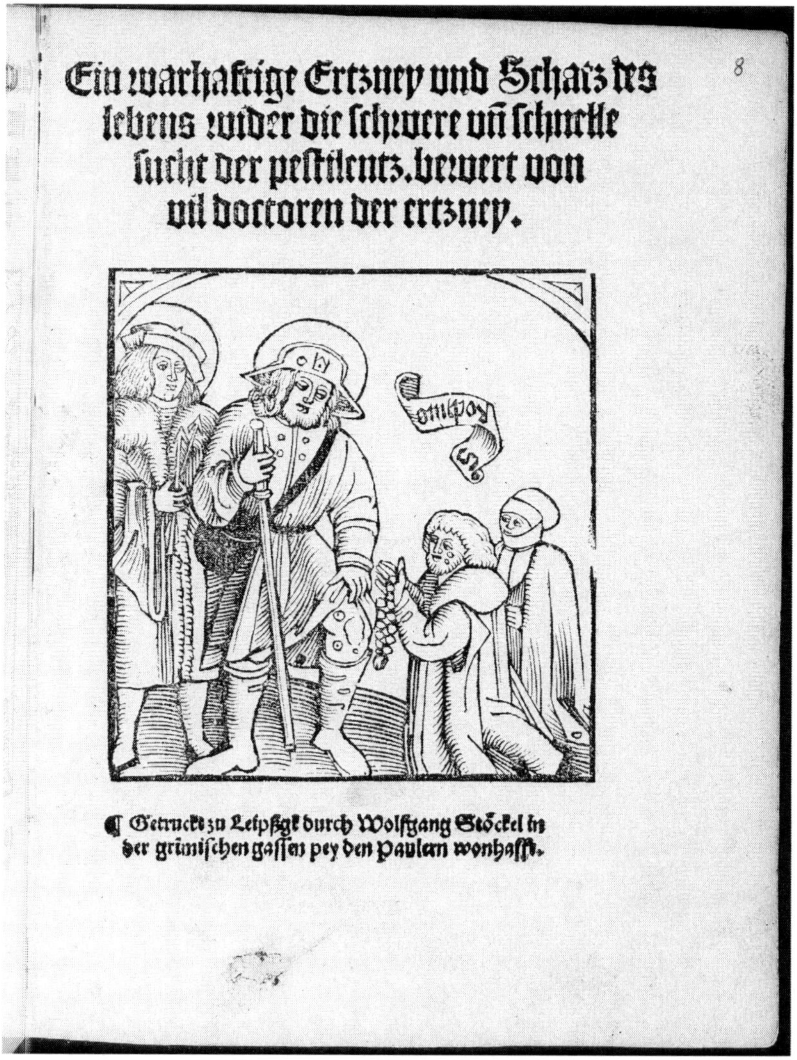

Figure 1.5 Sts. Roch and Sebastian

Title page illustration: *Ein warhaftige Ertzney und Schatz des lebens...* (Leipzig: Wolfgang Stöckel, after 1500)

Herzog August Bibliothek, Wolfenbüttel

Call number: N. 96.4 Helmst. (8) (reproduced with permission)

and succeeded on the book market. The text joined two older texts and appeared three times around 1517, twice on Wolfgang Stöckel's press in Leipzig and once on Matthes Maler's press in Erfurt.[48] These 1517 editions appeared with title page illustrations that depict the healing power of saints,

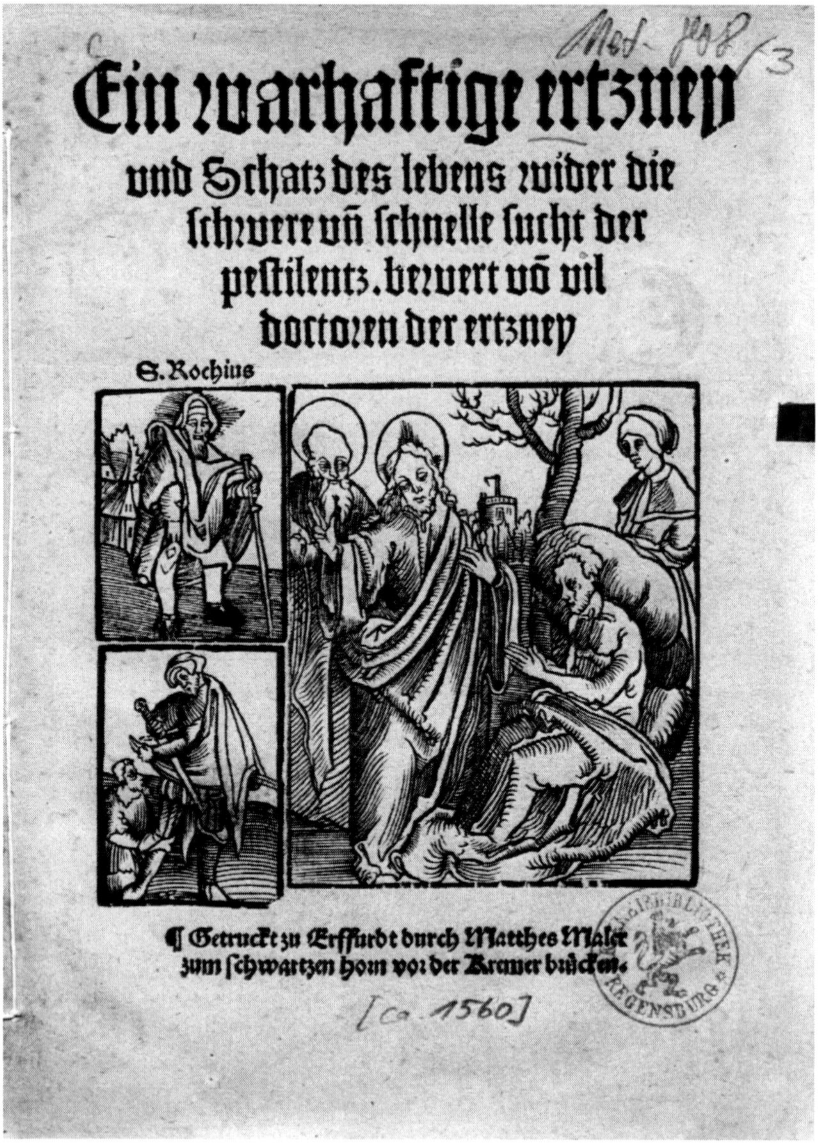
Ein warhaftige ertzney vnd Schatz des lebens wider die schwere vñ schnelle sucht der pestilentz. bewert võ vil doctoren der ertzney

S. Rochius

Getruckt zu Erffurdt durch Matthes Maler zum schwartzen horn vor der Kremer brücken.

Figure 1.6 Jesus healing the sick

Title page illustration: *Warhaftige Ertzney vñ Schatz des lebens* (Erfurt: Matthes Maler, ca. 1517)

Staatliche Bibliothek Regensburg

Call number: 999/Med.808 /3 (reproduced with permission)

common to many plague texts published before the Protestant Reformation (Figures 1.5 and 1.6). The history of this text demonstrates the many hands involved in the production of a plague pamphlet. The motives of the surgeons, physicians, and printers who created it ranged from spiritual to commercial, although an overriding concern was often to establish professional medical authority among the broader population.

The 1517 *True Medicine and Treasure of Life* is actually a compound pamphlet, the product of an unidentified editor who united two plague texts from earlier decades, both of which deserve close examination: the anonymous *Treasury of Life* (Erfurt, 1493) and a prose plague text by the surgeon and *Meistersinger* of Nuremberg, Hans Folz (Nuremberg, 1482).[49] Both texts were composed in German and are unusual among the pamphlets written between before 1520 since they contain much first-person advice and references to personal observation and experience. Such "ego" documents provide some of the most revealing information about contemporary views of plague and healing, contrasting sharply with texts by physicians, who were content to repeat ancient authorities for their more academic audience. The *Treasure of Life* was written by an anonymous author "N," who claims that everything in the text has proved useful against the sickness based on his own long experience.[50] While this approach promises a potentially innovative approach to plague, N's contribution was actually more derivative than novel. He also states that he produced his text by extracting things from the proven writings of many doctors and teachers of medicine. In 1493 the time had not come when an author could build authority primarily on his own ideas and observations, even within vernacular plague texts.

N constructs his authority in a short preface that dedicates the work to his sponsor, Herr von Linigen, the treasure-keeper of the holy church at Cologne. Since this part of the text is dedicated to a high-ranking cleric, there is no mention of the common man or a general audience, which may indicate that the text was not originally composed for printed publication. Also unusual is that N does not attribute the plague to God, nor does he mention sin or divine punishment. N places his emphasis on divine protection, which he tells his sponsor comes from God the Almighty, "your own physician."[51] Although this description of God as doctor has a long medieval tradition, its appearance here is among the first in printed vernacular plague literature.

N's medical explanation of plague illustrates how Galenic medicine incorporated a new emphasis on poisons, as N states that a person becomes sick when his or her internal complexion is similar to the complexion of the poisoned air. That is, a person's body becomes more susceptible to the poison when it has "superfluous unclean humidities," as "the great doctor Galen" states.[52] Plague etiology was more complex in the fifteenth century, however, since physicians noticed that plague affected people of the same nature and complexion in different ways. N explains this problem by appealing to the seemingly random "influence" (*anblick*) of heavenly bodies. For N, the effects of stars and planets (*gestirn*) can be localized, apparent even in how individual trees are afflicted. The reason a foggy and harmful air poisons some trees but not others of the same type is due to how the heavenly bodies glance on them.[53] N does not explain in greater detail how this mechanism works. Although the potential for receiving such a shot from the heavens could be a cause for alarm, a person could prepare the body to resist the poison by keeping it clean and free of harmful humidities.

Preventative medicine was a matter of keeping the body and home clean and keeping the body's four humors in balance: blood, phlegm, and yellow and black bile. The advice emphasizes moderation in all things pertaining to the body and mind, especially being neither too full nor too thirsty or hungry. Such advice follows the traditional six *res non naturales*, which were the foundation of medieval dietetic medicine. N gives specific instructions on what foods to avoid because they are too humid (fish) or too hot (spices such as pepper and "paradise corns"). He recommends against baths and heat, since they open the sweat pores and open the body to the poisons in the air. He also warns against sexual intercourse and bodily pleasure. Other preventative measures include bloodletting and taking medicines aimed at cooling the heart in order to protect the humoral balance. And, like many authors before the Reformation, N gives unqualified support for fleeing the plague as effective prevention. Among the unusual suggestions is one plague recipe N claims has been kept secret by physicians despite being very effective: oxisacram powder mixed with barley water, taken at daybreak once or twice a week. N's personal voice comes through in his endorsement of oxisacram powder, although he does not recommend the pills that some physicians make with it. Although authors usually do not make claims to reveal secrets, one of the most popular authors of the genre, Caspar Kegler, used this approach effectively, as Chapter 4 explores.

Curative medicine is typically directed at removing plague poisons that have entered the body and assault its vital spirits. Immediate action is essential when one detects the poisons, or, as N states, when one feels "something severe." Purgative medicines were usually the first recourse. N gives a hearty endorsement to a powder of fraxinella (*diptam*), primrose (*bibenel*), bolus armenus, and terra sigillata mixed with wine and a water of distilled tormentil root, saying that he has used it a hundred times. N also recommends immediate bloodletting and warns that drawing too little blood is more harmful than taking none at all, saying it "kills more than it heals." Although bloodletting was common in plague pamphlets into the eighteenth century, N's recommendation to draw large quantities of blood is somewhat unusual. He explains that, when one bleeds a great quantity of blood, it removes the poison from the body, whereas drawing too little blood not only fails to catch the poison but also hastens death by forcing the blood and poison to run within the body. This perilous movement carries the poison to the heart and other vital organs. N seems to assuage fears by saying that, if not all of the poison is removed with the blood, the action of bloodletting strengthens the body's resistance to the poison. N's personal, results-oriented approach is apparent at the end of his pamphlet, as he states: "I have not seen any who have died in the *Pestilentz* after taking the above medicine and bloodletting."[54]

The second text in the 1517 *True Medicine and Treasure of Life* illustrates how greatly early texts can vary, since it differs in many ways. Hans Folz, the surgeon and *Meistersinger* of Nuremberg, wrote this text in 1482 upon the request of the city patrician Anton Haller.[55] When the text was printed later that year, it was among the first plague pamphlets printed in Nuremberg. The particular strengths of Folz's text complement gaps left in the first text, producing a union text that is comprehensive in scope. Folz's text adds strong promotion of professional medical authority as well as discussion of spiritual medicine.

In the late fifteenth century it was not unusual for a surgeon to write a plague pamphlet, although after 1500 surgeons largely disappeared among the ranks of authors. This trend likely reflects the growing power of physicians, as more and more German towns appointed a city physician as the head medical authority, many smaller towns for the first time in the sixteenth century.[56] City physicians had a practical and professional interest in dominating medical advice and sought to reinforce the traditional division between surgeons and physicians – that surgeons treated the outside of the body, while physicians' sole realm was the inside of the body. Surgeons themselves were typically not trained in the more theoretical aspects of internal medicine, which required university study. This limitation did not keep some surgeons from teaching themselves the subject from scholarly medical texts, however. Folz and Hieronymus Brunschwig of Strasbourg are prime examples of learned fifteenth-century surgeons whose plague texts offered both internal and external medical advice.

Some of Folz's major concerns include justifying professional healers and attacking untrained practitioners, thus suggesting that he intended his text to have an impact on popular medical beliefs and the broader medical marketplace. Folz opens his campaign by attacking the view that a person cannot resist or flee the pestilence since it is a special punishment from God. Folz reasons that, if the pestilence cannot be stopped, then God created natural medicine in vain. Supporting his own professional authority, Folz offers a common biblical justification from the words of Solomon: "Honor the medical healer (*artzt*) for the sake of your own relief."[57]

Folz argues for the skills and products of professional healers throughout his text, including those of the apothecary, while also condemning lay healers. When prescribing the pills of Rhazes (854–925) to clean the body of its superfluous humors – a standby remedy from the medieval Persian/Arabic tradition – Folz gives the recipe in Latin specifically for apothecaries and not in German for fear of the errors that would result from home production of the medicine. This indicates that Folz was aware that his book might fall into the hands of non-Latinate lay healers. Concerns about harmful errors also come through in his complaints about vernacular medical books containing false translations of recipe ingredients, specifically the "printed German book called Ortolffus" – almost certainly a reference to the *Regimen sanitatis deutsch* by Ortolf von Baierland, first printed in Augsburg in 1472.[58] Elsewhere Folz sharpens his attack on popular healers, especially those who give out medicines to all ("both Heinz and Kunz") regardless of whether the pain is in their head or foot, and irrespective of a person's individual complexion, strength, and age. Folz condemns both buyers and sellers of such medicines and seems especially offended that these merchants prevail upon learned and unlearned alike by using lines such as these: "It helps everyone, and some for more than a year" and "There is nothing better on earth." Folz describes this as "the blind leading the blind" and relates that he has seen purgatives for sale that would sooner result in death.[59] Folz appeals to the leaders of Nuremberg to take action against such so-called healers, such as bakers, metalsmiths, coppersmiths, goldsmiths, old women, Jews, and vile country salesmen (*landt bescheyssern*) who confirm their medicines with foolish letters of testimony. As Folz's writing demonstrates, authors sought to use their vernacular plague texts to establish clear lines between legitimate and illegitimate healers.

Folz's effort to define and enforce a right and wrong plague response carries over into his treatment of the spiritual topics. Showing an interest in religious discipline, Folz states that prayers can be an effective "true medicine" against plague as long as they are free of "magic, characters, spells and other elements of irreligion (*unglauben*)."[60] The spiritual response itself is very important for preventing the plague, since Folz describes repentance, loving God, and following God's laws as the highest medicine and most sure prevention.

The anonymous editor of the 1517 *True Medicine and Treasure of Life* also contributed to the overall text by adding recipes aimed at boosting the pamphlet's popular appeal. One is a recipe directed specifically at the poor, common people that uses one of the newer and increasingly popular medicines of the era: distilled alcohol, also known as brandy or *aqua vitae*. Distilled alcohol was fairly new and controversial among physicians in the fifteenth and early sixteenth centuries, but seemed to be popular with the public. This remedy's quick and powerful effect made it highly valued among common people, yet physicians often hesitated to recommend it since it was not a traditional part of scholarly medicine and its overall benefit was far from clear. The editor's recipe calls for mixing various roots and herbs in a vessel with "the best, strongest brandy" and letting it age in the sun for a month or two. The recipe calls for drinking a tablespoon of this "good and precious medicine" before leaving the house in the morning during plague times, when the air is poisoned and foggy.[61] Chapter 4 explores further how distilled alcohol and alchemical ideas became more common in plague texts in the early sixteenth century through the work of the Leipzig physician Caspar Kegler.

Mercy, consolation, and Christo-centric piety in popular print after 1500

The moralizing tone that Jung and others brought to their pamphlets in the first decades of print was not typical of pamphlets produced after the year 1500. At this time it became more common for physicians, as well as at least one clerical author, to focus on divine mercy and grace, rather than dwelling on divine anger and moral reform. This represents a dramatic change in the equilibrium between these two sides that had existed previously in preaching and iconography. This change reflects two trends affecting print and culture around 1500: a greater emphasis on divine mercy within contemporary preaching and devotional literature, and a reduction in the average length of vernacular plague literature, which gave authors less space to discuss issues of all sorts. In creating these shorter, presumably more popular pamphlets, physicians chose to offer simple spiritual solutions rather than discuss divine anger and sin. It is possible that physicians were imitating trends within the most simple plague prints, which promoted fast and easy mercy. Printers and authors may have realized by 1500 that spiritual solutions sold more readily than lengthy moralizing, not to mention Jung's condescending tone in dealing with beastly, irrational sinners.

Historian Berndt Hamm describes the fifteenth century as a time when the quest for God's mercy ran high as war, famine, and plague brought periodic catastrophe to much of western Europe. Hamm sees a growing emphasis on divine mercy around the year 1500 in the sermons of German preachers such as Johannes von Staupitz, even though discussion of divine judgment never quite disappeared. This shift to mercy seems to have been related to the expansion of vernacular devotional literature in the fifteenth century. Messages of mercy and consolation were popularized in devotional literature that aimed to shape the piety of the lower clergy and laymen who were not trained in theology. The goal of this effort was to standardize belief and focus devotions on certain essential elements: the mercy of God, the suffering of Jesus, the intercession of Mary as a co-redeemer, and repentance.[62]

The shift of emphasis to mercy is present in some of the most popular plague prints of the late fifteenth century. Even before 1500 printed single-leaf broadsides and plague pamphlets composed in rhyming verse were less likely to mention divine anger and sin than to present spiritual help regardless of conscience.[63] An early broadside and its later printings before 1500 demonstrate this point. In a decidedly popular format, this broadside set medical and spiritual advice into rhyming verse and included images of saints. Printed first in Augsburg circa 1472 with images of St. Sebastian and St. Achatius, the text appeared again in Augsburg circa 1476 with an image of St. Sebastian only, and again in Nuremberg circa 1500 with images of both St. Sebastian and St. Roch. All of these broadsides emphasize calling out to God and St. Sebastian for mercy, but fail to mention divine punishment and sin. The Nuremberg broadside adds specific prayers to Sts. Sebastian and Roch below their images and emphasizes the help they provide.[64] The plague advice that the Nuremberg surgeon Hans Folz published in verse in 1482 reflects a similar approach. Folz does not mention divine punishment, but focuses on divine helpers, such as Mary and St. Sebastian. Folz describes St. Sebastian's help as certain: "[H]e who honors and celebrates him will be protected from the plague."[65] The producers of such popular texts probably sensed that a broad audience was less interested in discussion of the plague's origins than in immediate solutions, spiritual and natural. The common man seems to have wanted quick and easy solutions that had little impact on everyday behavior, just as he expected natural medicines to have an immediate effect.[66] To put it simply, fast mercy sold.

A survey of single-leaf broadsides reveals that printers were building a popular industry of mercy, especially after 1500, as they churned out prints that focused on merciful and healing images. Many encouraged the audience to protect body and soul through the contemplation of holy pictures and words. Reflecting the late medieval trend of the panoply of spiritual aid, some broadsides are crowded with various images for contemplation. Among the more prevalent symbols for plague protection was the Tau cross, described in these instructions from Nuremberg circa 1505:

> A Christian symbol given to the people of Israel by God through Moses for the plague of Pestilentz. In distress a person must contemplate it and say, 'Oh holy God, Oh mighty God, Oh holy merciful Jesus Christ, do not give us a bitter death.'

The Tau cross itself was one of many holy images and words that one could use for plague protection or to atone for sins. Here it appears alongside images of Jesus's *sudarium* and the holy heart of Jesus, which offer similar merit. These three images are only marginal additions to the broadside's main focus, however, which reproduces the words on Jesus's cross in Hebrew, Greek, and Latin. Reflecting the new emphasis on a Christo-centric system of mercy, this broadside states that one can gain great spiritual merit by saying and contemplating these words.[67]

It was common in the late Middle Ages to seek spiritual healing of body and soul from images as well as sacraments and relics. Robert Scribner investigated this process by examining the use of images of St. Veronica, who is a legendary saint usually depicted holding the *sudarium* with the imprint of Jesus's face. Through contemplation a believer would establish a spiritual and well as physical connection with a sacred image or object, which was seen to hold the presence of the holy being.[68] This holy spiritual presence was perceived with body and soul, bringing benefits to both. In practice, people would appeal to many different holy objects and images in the search for effective healing. A recent study of Matthias Grünewald's Isenheim altarpiece (ca. 1515) interprets his art in the context of healing, since the Antonine monastery that commissioned it was dedicated to healing the sick. The monks typically led their sick charges to the monastery church and planted them in view of holy wine, relics, and Grünewald's painted altarpiece, one panel of which depicts Jesus on the cross, suffering from an intense illness as well as crucifixion. Most interestingly, the Antonine monks may have specialized in treating Saint Anthony's Fire, a sickness viewed as a type of fiery pestilence (*pestilentia ignis*).[69]

Such depictions of the suffering Jesus in the *sudarium* and elsewhere reveal a growing Christo-centric movement within piety on the eve of the Reformation in German-speaking lands. This trend is also an expression of the era's quest for divine mercy. The title page illustration on the 1517 Erfurt edition of *The True Medicine and Treasure of Life* is one example, as Jesus appears most prominently healing the sick (Figure 1.6 above).[70] Another expression of the Christo-centric trend appears in the growing use of the metaphor of Jesus as physician in physicians' plague literature after 1500. The metaphor reached vernacular plague treatises when Johannes Jacobi's text was translated in Nuremberg circa 1482, as discussed above. Its use spread among physicians writing vernacular plague texts. The Heidelberg physician Conrad Schelling opened his 1501 work with a statement that Jesus, the "almighty, highest doctor," is the source of medicine for body and soul. Schelling's emphasis on mercy is notable:

> [H]e who will be helped will praise, honor, and give thanksgiving to the almighty, highest physician in a beneficial and humble way and will ask for the necessary medicine of soul and body as well as eternal mercy.[71]

Schelling's text lacked a moralizing tone and appeared first in Heidelberg in 1501 featuring an image of the baby Jesus with heraldry on its title page. Schelling's pamphlet was reprinted later in Speyer in 1502.[72]

The portrayal of Jesus as a heavenly doctor draws on ancient, scholarly traditions, dating to the biblical Book of Sirach (Ecclesiasticus), and was common within the writing of the early Church fathers. References appeared in Latin plague literature of the fourteenth and fifteenth centuries, such as in Nicolo de Burgo's 1382 plague tract and later versions of the Johannes Jacobi text.[73] Although Martin Luther and Protestant reformers certainly played a role in popularizing this metaphor later in the sixteenth century, it is clear that physicians played an important role in the revival of this theme in the late Middle Ages. Its growing popularity in the early sixteenth century is reflected in its frequent appearance within iconography. Jesus appears in artwork as a physician for the first time in a Dutch book of circa 1510, and later appears in two of the most important altarpieces commissioned during the papacy of Leo X (1513–1521): Raphael's *Transfiguration* and Sebastiano del Piombo's *Resurrection of Lazarus*.[74]

Jesus appears in late medieval plague literature as the merciful divine physician or as the highest example of suffering and sacrifice. These two important roles unite in one remarkable anonymous plague pamphlet printed in Oppenheim in 1511.[75] Most likely the work of a cleric, this text is significant for its Christo-centric piety and for applying a "how-to" approach of practical medical literature to spiritual medicine. Advertised as a spiritual regimen for protecting oneself from plague, the pamphlet mimics the format and content of physicians' advice by presenting spiritual recipes that encourage a sinner to imitate Christ's actions on the cross. The anonymous author was obviously aware of contemporary medical advice and used this practical approach in order to relate to a broad audience. At sixteen pages long and richly illustrated, this pamphlet is filled with prime examples of how the cultural forms of spiritual and natural healing overlapped in popular plague literature.

Divine punishment is implicit in the 1511 Oppenheim pamphlet, since it bears a title page illustration of God holding arrows and striking down humans. The text does not mention divine punishment or anger, however, but focuses on the merciful Jesus, who is described as an apothecary and founder of its spiritual recipes.[76] The author presents a series of exercises in the imitation of Christ, prescribed as "pills" for use each morning on an empty stomach. These pills "from the apothecary of Jesus" aim to build the Christian virtues of faith, hope, patience, humility, and the service of God. The author extends the medical metaphors to describe how these virtues, or "pills," work in physical terms. For example, the pill of humility "drives from you the bad blood of worldly and spiritual pride and was made by your apothecary Christ (*apotecker Christus*)..."[77] Curative spiritual exercises appear at the end of the pamphlet in the form of a "golden electuary," which follow the things Jesus did on the cross: he prayed, shouted out in a loud voice, cried, recommended his soul to God, and gave up his ghost.[78] Christians who use the recipes daily will be able to drive away the baneful, poisonous plague from body and soul, as well as attain a holy death that avoids eternal pain and gains eternal joy.[79] In other words, the author promises all the gain with little pain.

The 1511 Oppenheim pamphlet is unusual in that it depicts both God and Jesus in terms of health professionals – God as both a doctor and apothecary combined, and Jesus as an apothecary. Such an early description of Christ as apothecary counters historian Fritz Krafft's claim that the term "Christus Apotecker" emerged only in the seventeenth century and after the cultural impact of the Protestant Reformation. The profession of the apothecary was certainly deemed worthy enough in 1511 that it could be related to Christ, although the use of this metaphor certainly remained rare. To counter another tenet of Krafft's explanation of the seventeenth-century theme, it is clear that the metaphor certainly functioned within a Catholic context and did not depend upon Protestant theology for its existence.[80]

The examples from Schelling and various anonymous plague texts reveal a trend in the decades before the Reformation that singled out Jesus as the main source of spiritual healing. This Christo-centric trend would grow stronger during the Reformation, as scholars and printers began to favor more literal interpretations of the Bible and worked against traditional elements of Christianity that seemed to be unbiblical. It is important to realize that this Christo-centric trend was in place before Luther and other religious reformers rose to prominence, and was perhaps conditioned by the continual plague epidemics of the period. The search for merciful divine powers amidst what were dark and destructive times seems to have inspired a number of thinkers in this period, including some physicians.[81]

Although God's judgment attracted less interest from authors of plague literature after 1500, the iconography of a judging God remained in some later title page illustrations. Many, however, were reused images created in earlier decades. The Leipzig printer Martin Landsberg reused Culmacher's title page of circa 1495 (Figure 1.1), placing the image of the judging God on the cover of the 1506 plague pamphlet by the Leipzig physician Simon Pistoris, and again in 1517.[82] The illustration on the 1511 Oppenheim pamphlet was also reused in a different plague pamphlet from Oppenheim in 1519.[83]

Despite lingering older images of an angry God, the emphasis on mercy prevailed in both the texts and images after 1500. Most images that were new to plague treatises after 1500 did not feature a judging God in the heavens or other representations of divine anger. Furthermore, nearly all of the vernacular pamphlets published in German lands between 1501 and 1519 either emphasize divine powers as merciful helpers at the expense of divine anger or do not mention spiritual issues at all.[84] This includes vernacular pamphlets by physicians Conrad Schelling (1501, 1502), Simon Pistoris (1506, 1517), Ulrich Rülein von Calw (1507), Andres Reichlin (1512), Martin Steinpeiß (1515), Balthasar Lothwiger (1516), Heinrich Stromer (1516, 1517), Johann Engel (1518), Johann Lotzer (1519), and Sixtus Kolbenschlag (1519), as well as plague pamphlets by other anonymous authors. In nearly every case, divine punishment and sin are not explicit. Evidence from Leipzig also demonstrates that this change in the presentation of the spiritual problem of the plague texts did not result from a lack of epidemics between 1500 and 1519. The Leipzig treatises by Pistoris (1506) and von Calw (1507) each coincided with an epidemic in the city. Furthermore, the wave of plague pamphlets that appeared in Leipzig between 1516 and 1517 were written amidst fears of approaching plague, which arrived in the city in 1518.[85] None of these texts have the moralizing tone of texts written before 1500.

The declining length of the pamphlets printed after 1500 meant that there was less space for spiritual content. Most pamphlets that physicians composed after 1500 fell under twenty pages in length, whereas Steinhöwel's totaled eighty pages, Jung's thirty-five, and Culmacher's fifty-one. But, despite the shorter lengths, some authors did find ample room to discuss spiritual health. For example, the pamphlet that the physician Balthasar Lothwiger wrote for the city of Halle in 1516 is among the shortest of the decade, at eight pages. It has an unusual reference to the healing power of saints' relics, however. Lothwiger was clearly drawing upon local piety when he recommended reconciliation with God as well as calling out to Mary and all saints, especially to the saints whose "bodies and particles" reside in the church of St. Moritz, located in the center of Halle. Lothwiger's advice seems to have come in response to a recent gift of relics to the city by its princely overlord, Albrecht of Brandenburg, the Archbishop of Mainz.[86] Lothwiger's thoughts on relics dominate his spiritual advice. As he puts it, through the "help and holy medicine" that the relics offer, the audience "may be freed, protected, and cured" of the plague.[87] To foreshadow the changes that the 1520s brought, this reference to the healing power of relics is the last in plague treatises, since relics disappeared along with saints during the Protestant Reformation.

Conclusion

Through a close examination of the spiritual and natural advice found in late medieval plague texts, this chapter provides a detailed portrait of contemporary strategies for preventing and curing plague during the decades before the Reformation. This era before the social and cultural turbulence of the Reformation was not static for plague texts, however. It was an era of change, as authors explored the potential for popularizing their advice in the vernacular. This process of popularization and vernacularization, under way to some extent since 1348, changed the tone and content of contemporary plague advice. The plague advice in these texts became more diverse and less moored to traditions, as authors and printers explored new ways to appeal to a broader audience. The shift from manuscript to print around 1473 further intensified earlier efforts to engage with a broader audience, and thereby began a new era of popularization and innovation.

The most surprising element of the plague treatises composed before the 1520s is the spiritual advice. It was neither superficial nor formulaic, but played an important role in popularizing physicians' plague advice in print. Physicians in this period used vernacular plague treatises to participate in the cultural trends affecting piety towards the end of the Middle Ages, just as they tailored their natural medicine for a broader audience. As plague texts became more closely intertwined with contemporary piety and devotional literature, plague authors – including some physicians – sought to shape piety, starting a trend that would continue during the Protestant Reformation. As plague authors explored more popular formats after 1500, their spiritual advice emphasized mercy and in some cases began to focus piety on Jesus, presaging a cultural trend that would continue during the Reformation. Furthermore, as physicians began to discuss specific observations of the local environment or record their own experiences with effective recipes, the foundation of medical knowledge itself began to shift, moving towards a greater appreciation for new personal experience. It is important to recognize that these trends were established in the late Middle Ages, creating a model for ambitious physicians to follow in later decades.

Notes

1 Jean-Noël Biraben, *Les hommes et la peste en France et dans les pays européenes et méditerranéens*, Vol. I (Paris: Mouton, 1975), 407–415. Widespread epidemics are also apparent in local histories and chronicles. For Augsburg: *Die Chroniken der deutschen Städte vom 14. bis ins 16. Jahrhundert*, Vols. 4, 5, 22, 23 (Leipzig: S. Hirzel, 1865–1917). For Leipzig: Carly Seyfarth, *Das Hospital zu St. Georg in Leipzig durch acht Jahrhunderte 1212–1940*, Vol. I (Leipzig: Georg Thieme Verlag, 1939), 65. For Munich: Richard Bauer, Ed., *Geschichte der Stadt München* (Munich: C. H. Beck, 1992), 123.

2 On the strong piety in German lands in the fifteenth century: Bernd Moeller, "Religious Life in Germany on the Eve of the Reformation," in *Pre-Reformation Germany*, Ed. Gerald Strauss (New York: Harper & Row, 1972): 13–31.

3 The *Compendium de epidemia* of the medical faculty of Paris appears here: H. Emile Rebouis, *Etude historique et critique sur la peste* (Paris: Alphonse Picard, 1888), 70–145. On this text's role in standardizing late medieval plague theories, see: Gundolf Keil, "Seuchenzüge des Mittelalters," in *Mensch und Umwelt im Mittelalter*, Ed. Bernd Herrmann (Stuttgart: Deutsche Verlags Anstalt, 1986): 109–128.

4 Rebouis, *Etude historique et critique*, 92.

5 Ibid., 88.

6 This text is also the very first plague treatise overall. C.-E. A. Winslow and M. L. Duran-Reynals, "Jacme d'Agramont and the First of the Plague Tractates," *Bulletin of the History of Medicine* 22 (1948): 747–765. For an English translation of the text, see: C.-E. A. Winslow and M. L. Duran-Reynals, Trans., "Texts and Documents: Regiment de Preservacio a Epidemia o Pestilencia e Mortaldats," *Bulletin of the History of Medicine* 23 (1949): 57–89; see 68–70 for discussion of local causes of pestilence around Lerida.

7 Winslow and Duran-Reynals, "Texts and Documents," 65, 78–79.

8 Samuel K. Cohn, Jr., *Cultures of Plague: Medical Thinking at the End of the Renaissance* (Oxford: Oxford University Press, 2010), 10–15.

9 Heinrich Steinhöwel, *Undanckberkeit (alsz die altern wÿsen schriben) ist für andere laster zeschelten. So aber ich Hainricus Stainhöwel von wÿl doctor in den ercznÿen / so vil gütheit er gunst vnd nucz / ÿecy zweÿ vn zweinczig iar / von den fürsichtigen ersamen vnd wÿsen burgermiestern / rät vnd ganczer gemaind der stat Vlm / mÿnen lieben herren / enpfangen habe!* (Ulm: Johann Zainer, 1473).

10 Arnold C. Klebs and Karl Sudhoff, *Die Ersten Gedruckten Pestschriften* (Munich: Verlag der Münchener Drucke, 1926), 194. On the 1446 manuscript: Gerd Dicke, "Heinrich Steinhöwel," in *Die deutsche Literatur des Mittelalters: Verfasserlexikon*, Vol. IX, Ed. Wolfgang Stammler (Berlin: Walter de Gruyter, 1995): 258–278; Ortrun Riha, "Vom mittelalterlichen 'Hausbuch' zur frühneuzeitlichen 'Hausväterliteratur': Medizinische Texte in Handschrift und Buchdruck," in *Die Gleichzeitigkeit von Handschrift und Buchdruck*, Eds. Gerd Dicke and Klaus Grubmüller (Wiesbaden: Harrassowitz Verlag, 2003): 203–227.

11 Kantonsbibliothek St. Gallen VadSlg. Ms. 455, 44r (and 2b in 1473).

12 Klebs and Sudhoff, *Die Ersten Gedruckten Pestschriften*, 172–211. Here Sudhoff describes Steinhöwel's text and its relationship to German plague prints of 1472 that do not meet the definition of a monograph.

13 Steinhöwel, *Undanckberkeit (alsz die altern wÿsen schriben)*, 1473, 1v. Steinhöwel's 1446 manuscript: Kantonsbibliothek St. Gallen VadSlg. Ms. 455, fol. 44r.

14 This reference to the "common man" appears early in the history of this term, since most accounts have traced its rise to later decades. Rudolf Schenda's earliest example of the "common man" trope is Johann Tallat's 1497 general medical manual. Rudolf Schenda, "Der 'gemeine Mann' und sein medikales Verhalten im 16. und 17. Jahrhundert," in *Pharmazie und der gemeine Mann: Hausarzneі und Apotheke in deutschen Schriften der frühen Neuzeit*, Ed. Joachim Telle (Wolfenbüttel: Waisenhaus-Buchdruckerei und Verlag, 1982): 9–20, 10.

15 Telle, Pharmazie und der gemeine Mann, 109.

16 Steinhöwel, *Undanckberkeit,* fol. 2r.

17 Anne T. Thayer, *Penitence, Preaching and the Coming of the Reformation* (Aldershot, UK: Ashgate, 2002), 55–64.

18 Steinhöwel, *Undanckberkeit*, fol. 4r.

19 See the publication list in Klebs and Sudhoff, *Die Ersten Gedruckten Pestschriften*, 59–61.

20 The trend of increasing spiritual content was not limited to German texts. For a limited account of this phenomenon in England, see: Georg R. Keiser, "Two Medieval Plague Treatises and Their Afterlife in Early Modern England," *Journal of the History of Medicine and Allied Sciences* 58 (2003): 292–324.

21 Johannes Jacobi, *Ad honore[m] sancte & i[n]diuidue trinitatis, gloriosq[ue] virginis marie & ad utlititatem rei publice, pro [con]seruatione sano[rum] ac reformatione lapsorum…* (Nuremberg: Conrad Zeninger, ca. 1482), sig. A6r.

22 Johannes Jacobi, [Z]V lob vnd zu ere der heiligen vñ vegeteiltē trinitet. vñ der seligen erentreichen iückfrawen marien Zu gut vnd zu nucz einer ganczē gemein zu auffenthaltung der gesunden. vnd erkoberūg od widerpringūg der siechē. wil ich auß den geschriftē der namhaftigē vñ furnēstē maysterñ in d erczney etwas schreyben von dem gebrestē od pestelencz dy zu zeyten vberhand nympt… (ca. 1482), fol. 9r. An identical formulation appeared later in an anonymous Strasbourg pamphlet: Hie in disem büchlin vindest du Ein gut regimēt Für dye Pestilentz / Wer sich nach diser weyß als hie nach geschriben stad regiert / Dem getrew ich ym sol geraten werdē vñ büß wider die pestilētz Durch die gnad vnsers Herren Jhesū christi / on den nichts gůts beschehē mag (Strasburg: Mathis Hüßfuff, 1502), sig. A6r.

23 Frieder Schanze, "'Pestregiment Herrn Kamits' eine unbekannte deutsche Inkunabel," in *Gutenberg-Jahrbuch 1993* (Mainz: Gutenberg Gesellschaft, 1993): 88–90. Karl Sudhoff, "Der Pesttraktat des Magisters Johannes Jacobi zu Montpelier (1373) und seine spätere Überarbeitung," *Archiv für Geschichte der Medizin* 17 (1925): 16–32.

24 [Pestblatt], (Augsburg: s.n., ca. 1473). See also: Henry R. Viets and James F. Ballard, "Notes on the Plague Tracts in the Boston Medical Library," *Bulletin of the History of Medicine* 8 (1940): 370–380.

25 On the role of the saints in plague iconography in general, see: Christine M. Boeckl, *Images of Plague and Pestilence: Iconography and Iconology* (Kirksville, MO: Truman State University Press, 2000).

26 Philippus Culmacher, *Regimen zu deutsch Magistri philippi Culmachers von Eger wider die grausamen erschrecklichenn Totlichen pestelentz. von vil grossen meistern gesamelt außgezogen…* (Leipzig: Martin Landsperg, ca. 1495). This was probably the first printed plague monograph in Leipzig.

27 See Esser's commentary on this text and image: Thilo Esser, *Pest, Heilangst und Frömmigkeit: Studien zur religiösen Bewältigung der Pest am Ausgang des Mittelalters* (Altenberge: Oros, 1999), 40–42. Esser dates Culmacher's text to ca. 1490.

28 Karl Sudhoff, *Deutsche medizinische Inkunabeln* (Leipzig: Barth, 1908), 177–178.

29 Culmacher, *Regimen zu deutsch*, sigs. D2v–3v.

30 Ibid., sig. A1v.

31 Thilo Esser, "Die Pest – Strafe Gottes oder Naturphänomen? Eine frömmigkeitsgeschichtliche Untersuchung zu Pesttraktaten des 15. Jahrhunderts," *Zeitschrift für Kirchengeschichte* 108 (1997): 32–57, 50. On Ingolstadt and the medieval history of this incantation, see: Karl Werner, "Ananizapta – eine geheimnisvolle Inschrift des Mittelalters," *Sammelblatt des Historischen Vereins Ingolstadt* 105 (1996): 59–90.

32 *Ein Warhaftige Ertzney vñ Schatz des lebens wider die schwere vñ schnelle sucht der pestilentz. bweret von vil doctoren der ertzney* (Leipzig: Wolfgang Stöckel, 1517), sig. A4v. This text is a reprinting of Folz's 1482 work, reprinted along with another late medieval work multiple times before 1520.

33 Berndt Hamm, *The Reformation of Faith in the Context of Late Medieval Theology and Piety*, Ed. Robert J. Bast (Leiden: Brill, 2004), 19. Hamm traces this movement to the spread of a practical, consoling piety emphasized by late medieval preachers and theologians such as Jean Gerson (1363–1429), Thomas of Kempten (ca. 1380–1471), and Johannes von Staupitz (ca. 1460–1524).

34 Ambrosius Jung, *Ein außerrvelt loblich tractat vñ regiment in dem schwären zeit der pestilentz…* (Augsburg: Hans Schönsperger, 1494), sig. A1v; Ambrosius Jung, *Tractatulus perutilis de pestilentia ex diuersis auctoribus aggregatus…* (Augsburg: Hans Schönsperger, 1494).

35 Jung, *Ein außerrvelt loblich tractat…*, sig. A1v. This quotation also illustrates the lack of punctuation in early vernacular printing, following the tradition of the Latin language.

36 Ibid., sig. A6v.

37 Karl Sudhoff addressed the religious content of Jung's 1494 vernacular work, but the treatment is cursory and there is no comparison to the Latin work. Sudhoff, *Deutsche Medizinische Inkunabeln*, 180.

38 Hamm, *The Reformation of Faith*, 50–87. On sin and sickness, see: Wolf von Siebenthal, *Krankheit als Folge der Sünde: Eine medizinhistorische Untersuchung* (Hanover: Schmorl & von Seefeld, 1950).

39 Jung, *Ein außerrvelt loblich tractat…*, sig. A4v.

40 Ibid., sig. A5r.

41 Jung may be arguing against the fifteenth-century Italian physician Antonio Guaineri, who believed that, because plague poisons worked through occult powers, prayers to saints or relics worn on the body were effective in warding off poisons. Lynn Thorndike, *A History of Magic and Experimental Science* Vol. IV, *Fourteenth and Fifteenth Centuries* (New York: Columbia University Press, 1934), 226.

42 Jung, *Ein außerrvelt loblich tractat,* sigs. A5r–v. I follow Sudhoff interpretation of this passage, that Jung is commenting on practices in the past. Sudhoff, *Deutsche Medizinische Inkunabeln*, 180.
43 Jung, *Tractatulus perutilis de pestilentia*, sig. B1v.
44 Jung, *Ein außerrvelt loblich tractat*, sig. A8v.
45 Ibid., sig. A6r.
46 Ibid., sig. A5v.
47 Ortolf von Baierland, *Arzneibuch* (Nuremberg: Anton Koberger, 1477), fol. 1r. Numerous examples of the use of Ecclesiasticus appear in the medieval Latin manuscripts for plague, as surveyed by Karl Sudhoff. Earlier plague pamphlets state that God gives the means to regain health, but do not present as sophisticated an argument for academic medicine as Jung.
48 *Ein Warhaftige Ertzney vñ Schatz des lebens wider die schwere vñ schnelle sucht der pestilentz. bweret von vil doctoren der ertzney* (Leipzig: Wolfgang Stöckel, 1517) and *Ein warhaftige ertzney und Schatz des lebens wider die schwere uñ schnelle sucht der pestilenty. bewert uō uil doctoren der ertzney* (Erfurt: Matthes Maler, ca. 1517).
49 *Hie vohet sich an der schatz des lebens vor inne man findt eyne warafftige arcteney wider die schwree vnde snelle sucht der pestilentzie. Bewert von vil doctoren in der arczeney* (Erfurt: 1493). Hans Folz, *Itc- von d pestilencz ein hübsch nüczlich vñ kurcz begriffes tractetlin getrukt im m cccc vñ in dem lxxxii iare hans folcz.* See the transcription in: Hans Folz, *Die Reimpaarsprüche*, Ed. Hanns Fischer (Munich: C. H. Beck, 1961), 429–437. The Erfurt text also seems to have been reprinted in 1494 as well. See Sudhoff's description of the 1494 incunable: Sudhoff, *Deutsche Medizinische Inkunabeln*, 178–179.
50 *Ein Warhaftige Ertzney vñ Schatz des lebens*, sig. A2r.
51 Ibid., sig. A2r.
52 Ibid., sigs. A2r–v.
53 Ibid, sig. A2r.
54 Ibid., sigs. A3v–4r.
55 Among Folz's many verse compositions is a plague text, appearing also in 1482.
56 Manfred Stürzbecher, "The Physici in German-Speaking Countries from the Middle-Age to the Enlightenment," in *The Town and State Physician in Europe from the Middle Ages to the Present*, Ed. Andrew W. Russell (Wolfenbüttel: Herzog August Bibliothek, 1979): 123–129.
57 *Ein Warhaftige Ertzney vñ Schatz des lebens*, sigs. A4v–B1r.
58 Ibid., sig. B4r.
59 Ibid., sigs. B2r–v
60 Ibid., sig. A4r.
61 Ibid., sig. B4v.
62 Hamm, *The Reformation of Faith*, 11–22.
63 For a large collection of late medieval plague iconography, see: Paul Heitz, Ed., *Pestblätter des XV. Jahrhunderts* (Strassburg: Heitz & Mündel, 1901).
64 *Vil menschen weren der pestelencz frey…* (Augsburg, ca. 1472). *Ein nutzlichs regiment fur die kranckheyt der pestilentz* (Nuremberg, ca. 1500). The Augsburg ca. 1472 and Nuremberg ca. 1500 prints are reproduced in Heinrich Dormeier, "'Ein geystliche ertzeney fur die grausam erschrecklich pestilentz': Schutzpatrone und frommer Abwehrzauber gegen die Pest," in *Das große Sterben: Seuchen mache Geschichte*, Eds. Hans Wilderotter and Michael Dorrmann (Berlin: Jovis,

1995): 54–93, 62–65. Note: the Bavarian State Library dates the Nuremberg text to ca. 1520. See call number: Einbl. I, 54.

65 Hans Folz, *Item ein fast köstlicher spruch von der pestilencz und anfenglich von den zeichen die ein künfftige pestilencz beteuten* (Nuremberg, 1482), fol. 2v.

66 Robert Jütte, *Ärzte, Heiler und Patienten: Medizinischer Alltag in der frühen Neuzeit* (Munich: Artemis & Winkler Verlag, 1991), 139. We can also presume that popular classes did not favor the sometimes strict dietary regimen that physicians typically imposed on their patients, since the lower social classes had fewer resources to alter their diet.

67 Woodcut, Nuremberg: Dürer School, ca. 1505. Reproduced in Esser, *Pest, Heilangst und Frömmigkeit*, image 52, 463.

68 Robert W. Scribner, "Cosmic Order and Daily Life: Sacred and Secular in Pre-Industrial German Society," in *Religion and Society in Early Modern Europe 1500–1800*, Ed. Kaspar von Greyerz (London: George Allen & Unwin, 1984): 17–32, 25.

69 Andree Hayum, *The Isenheim Altarpiece: God's Medicine and the Painter's Vision* (Princeton, NJ: Princeton University Press, 1989): 21–28.

70 *Ein warhaftige ertzney und Schatz des lebens wider die schwere uñ schnelle sucht der pestilenty. bewert uō uil doctoren der ertzney* (Erfurt: Matthes Maler, ca. 1517). Note that the date the Staatsbibliothek Regensburg gives (ca. 1560) cannot be correct, considering when the Leipzig editions appeared (1517), and considering that saints disappeared from title pages after 1530. Matthes Maler printed at the Black Horn in Erfurt between 1511 and 1525 and his last print appeared in 1536. Johannes Biereye, *Erfurt in seinen berühmten Persönlichkeiten* (Erfurt: Stenger, 1937), 413.

71 Conrad Schelling, *Eyn kurtz Regiment von dem Hochgelerten meister Conradt Schelling von Heidelberg doctor der Artzeny / vnd vnsers gnedigstē herñ Pfaltzgrauē kůrfürstē etc. lyb arzet / zu Eren vñ gefallen sein fůrstlichen gnaden...* (1502), sig. A2r.

72 Conrad Schelling, *Ein kurtz Regiment von dem hochgelerten meister Conradt Schelling von Heidelberg doctor der artzeny / vnd vnsers gnedigsten herrn Pfaltzgrauen kurfür sten rc. lib artzet / zů Eren vñ gefallen sein fürstlichen gnaden...* (Heidelberg, 1501).

73 Karl Sudhoff, "Pestschriften aus den ersten 150 Jahren nach der Epidemie des 'schwarzen Todes' 1348," *Archiv für Geschichte der Medizin* 5 (1912): 332–396, 355; and 6 (1913): 313–379, 313.

74 Hans Martin von Effra, "Christus als Arzt," in *Reallexikon zur deutschen Kunstgeschichte*, Vol. III, Eds. Ernst Gall and L. H. Heydenreich (Stuttgart: Alfred Druckenmueller, 1953): 639–643. On the use in the art commissioned by Pope Leo X, see: Hayum, *The Isenheim Altarpiece*, 37–38.

75 *Eyn Geistlich Regiment fürzůkom-en vnd zůvertreiben den Onheilsamen vnnd Gifftigen gepresten der Pestilentz leib vñ Sel vñ den Ewigē tot. Noch dem volgt ein gemein Regimēt iñ zeit der Pestilentz sich zů gebrauchē* (Oppenheym, 1511).

76 There is no discussion of divine anger in the text, but mere references that plague may come from evil pleasures and deeds or from God's orders (*gottes verhēckniß*): ibid., sig. A4v.

77 Ibid., sig. A4r.

78 Ibid., sig. A4v.

79 Ibid., sig. A2r.

80 While Fritz Krafft is incorrect in his assessment that authors before the seventeenth century did not describe Jesus specifically as an "Apotecker," his evidence shows at least that this term was rare before the seventeenth century, when it appeared as a motif in art. Fritz Krafft, *"Die Artznei kommt vom Hernn, und der Apoteker bereitet sie" biblische Rechtfertigung der Apotekerkunst im Protestantismus: Apoteken-Auslucht in Lemgo und Pharmako-Theologie* (Stuttgart: Wissenschaftliche Verlagsgesellschaft, 1999), 49–52.

81 For a similar reflection about how the apparent unpredictability of God was an important inspiration for cultural innovation: Esser, *Pest, Heilangst und Frömmigkeit*, 320.

82 Simon Pistoris, *Ein kurtz schon unnd gar trostlich regiment widder die sweren vñ erchreckliche̅ kranckheit der pestilentz. Durch den achtbaren hochgelarte̅ herren Simon pistoris doctor yn der artzney eylend begriffen / vnd dem Erbaren Rate zcu Leiptzick yn seynem wegzyehen zugeschryben vnd gelassen.* (Leipzig: Martin Landsberg, 1506); and Simon Pistoris, *Ein kurtz schon und gar trostliche regiment wider die schweren vnd erschrecklichen krancheyt der pestilentz. Durch den achtbaren hochgelarte̅ herre̅ Simone̅ Pistoris Doctorem in der artzney eylendt begriffen vnd tzu den andern mal vor andert dem Erbare̅ Rate tzu Leyptzck in seynez weg zyehen tzugeschrieben vñ gelassen.* (Leipzig: Martin Landesperg, 1517).

83 *Ein Neüw geordent Regime̅t / wyder den tödtlichen gebresten der Pestelentz. Auß viln bewerte̅ schriffte̅ / gemeinem volck zů uffhalt des lebens / iñ Reymen (vmb kürtz wille̅) zůsammen gesetzt / volgt hyernach* (Oppenheim, 1519).

84 One possible exception to this list is Martin Steinpeiss's 1515 tract, which ends with a prayer to God that states "Herr du bist gerecht: vnd dein gericht is gerecht," although in context it seems that Steinpeiss is talking about God's judgment of Steinpeiss's malevolent enemies, not of Germans in general. Martin Stainpeiss, *Ain hailsame ertzney: mit ierem zwesatz: zu behuetten wider den lauff der Pestelentz: aus bewertten geschriften der Ertzt: angezaigt durch Martinu̅ Stainpeiss von Wienn: lerer der ertzney: zw haill vnnd nutzperkait allen menschen* (Vienna, 1515), sig. B4r.

85 Heinrich Stromer's texts appeared in Leipzig in 1516 and 1517, and Simon Pistoris's was reissued in 1517. Leipzig experienced Pest from 1505–07 and again from 1518–20. Seyfarth, *Das Hospital zu St. Georg*, Vol. I, 35.

86 Balthasar Lothwiger, *Eyn kurtz nutzbar Regiment und Rath vor die schweren vñ erschrecklichen kranckheit der Pestile̅tz: Einem Erbarn Rathe tzu Halle vnd Jnwonern do selbist gunstlich tzugeeygent: durch den Achtbarn Hern Balthasar Lothwiger Doctorem vffs kortzte begriffen* (Leipzig: Wolfgang Stöckel, 1516), sig. A2r.

87 Ibid.

2 The German medicine of Johann Vochs

Medical and cultural reform on the eve of the Reformation

The sixteenth century began with great worry for German physicians. After the unsettling appearance of the French Disease in 1496, a widespread plague broke out in 1506, striking Cologne, Augsburg, Leipzig, and other major cities. Viewed as a clear expression of divine wrath, this sequence of afflictions moved some German scholars to reflect on the imperfections of their time. One obscure physician from Cologne, Johann Vochs, responded to these plagues by writing an unusual treatise that sharply criticizes contemporary medicine, religion, and the international drug trade. Seeking to protect Germans from harmful foreign ideas and economic interests, Vochs introduced a new "German" approach to northern bodies that undercut the standard plague advice and the traditional pharmacopeia of the time. Somewhat paradoxically, Vochs supported his ideas about German medicine with Hippocrates's teachings on locality and environment, using them to challenge physicians' systemic neglect of the particular characteristics of northern Europe. Vochs's new thought on healing Germans is also notable for its equal use of both personal experience and ancient theory in the production of new medical knowledge. This chapter investigates Vochs's vision for a specifically "German" medicine at the intersection of new and worrisome epidemics, the new patriotism of the German Renaissance, and German discontent with Italian scholars and merchants on the eve of the Reformation.

In 1507 Johann Vochs set out to correct the serious flaws burdening his homeland with his Latin treatise *On the Pestilence of the Present Year and Its Cure*.[1] Dedicated to one of the most influential German princes, the Elector Frederick the Wise of Saxony, this text offers a striking expression of German hopes and ambitions at the start of the sixteenth century. At its heart is an attack on the foreign scholars and merchants who seemed to be the real plague to the health, wealth, and thought of Germans. To liberate Germans from a perceived oppression by Italians and others, Vochs promoted medicine from native sources as proper treatments for German bodies, while also rejecting slavish devotion to medical texts that did not consider northern Europe. These reforms offered Germans a way to lessen their dependence on the foreign drug trade as well as the medical teachings of the Mediterranean world. Most important for the history of medicine and science is that Vochs's ideas encouraged German physicians to place greater weight on their own experience, since the bodies and *materia medica* of northern Europe were best known through experience. What resulted from Vochs's new medical localism was an important bending of the universal assumptions and propositions that had long dominated academic medicine and its responses to the plague.

History seems to have forgotten Vochs, despite the lasting impact of his medical localism on physicians, humanists, and botanists well into the Reformation era.[2] Although interest in indigenous medicine has medieval roots, Vochs stands at the forefront of its sixteenth-century renaissance. The history of German medical localism typically begins in the 1520s or 1530s with the achievements of some of the most prominent figures of early modern medicine and botany, including Paracelsus, Otto Brunfels, Hieronymus Bock, and Leonhart Fuchs. Missing from this history, however, is the man who seems to have first formulated this new and powerful concept of locality and first demonstrated its advantages. The case of Johann Vochs revises the current historical narrative that portrays Paracelsus as the founder of a German indigenous medicine, part of a long-standing historical bias that depicts Paracelsus as a lone reformer.[3] The call for a more "German" medicine is clearly older than Paracelsus's thought and was certainly not the product of one unique genius. German medical localism flourished among various scholars amidst the cultural strife of the early sixteenth century. Vochs's story reveals a history of this movement that does not prioritize Paracelsus and his so-called "Paracelsians."

This chapter seeks to explain the various ideas and motives behind Vochs's broad reform, and seeks to place Vochs at the forefront of the creation and promotion of a new indigenous medicine in northern Europe. It argues that a constellation of factors particular to the early sixteenth century inspired Vochs's turn to a German indigenous medicine and set the conditions for it to flourish more broadly. They include a burgeoning cultural patriotism among German scholars and politicians during the Northern Renaissance, new appreciation for personal experience and the Hippocratic idea of locality, and new attention to the issue of who profited from the trade in *materia medica* with the Middle East and Asia. In the rise of a German indigenous medicine in the decades before the Reformation one sees the growing confidence and willingness of German scholars to challenge intellectual traditions and economic norms, as well as the growing cultural chasm between northern and southern Europe.

Ultimately, the origins of this new localism lie within the new German cultural patriotism that thrived during the Renaissance. Within an intellectual context that began to prioritize things German, Vochs developed his new medical localism as a cultural, economic, and political attack on foreign interests within the Holy Roman Empire. Indeed, Vochs's medical reform is just one part of a larger desire to reform both the Roman Church and the Holy Roman Empire. After examining his thoughts on church and state, this chapter explores Vochs's medical ideas, including his thought on the relationship between personal experience and textual authority. The final section traces Vochs's legacy into the mid-sixteenth century. For the attention he called to medical localism and personal experience, Vochs's reforms hold special significance for the development of a more empirical science and medicine in northern Europe.

A new German identity and the Renaissance discovery of northern Europe

The German Renaissance at the end of the fifteenth century enlightens the origin of Vochs's particularly German medicine, as well as his calls to reform the Church and Holy Roman Empire. A new sort of German cultural patriotism animates Vochs's thought, apparent in his stated mission to inspire the youth of "Germania" to fight the "darkness of ignorance" for the "health of the republic."[4] Such attention to things German, including even an imaginary German "republic," colored the priorities of a broad set of elites after circa 1490. In one telling example from politics, the imperial delegates at the Diet of Cologne in 1512 formalized the empire's new name as the "Holy Roman Empire of the German Nation," despite the empire's diverse peoples and heritage.[5] In intellectual matters, the burgeoning German patriotism inspired German scholars to investigate northern Europe itself, including especially the subjects that ancient thinkers had neglected. No less than a Renaissance discovery of northern Europe resulted during this broader "Age of Exploration," as scholars prioritized the study of German lands and peoples for the first time.

German scholars first turned to ancient texts in their effort to build new knowledge of northern Europe. Although scholars of all sorts were a part of this effort, German humanists in particular were at the head of this intellectual current, which grew into a broad effort to define German cultural identity, past and present. Vochs's use of the terms "Germania" and "republic of Germania" evoked contemporary interest in Tacitus's *Germania*, an ancient Roman text about northern Europe that was rediscovered at Hersfeld Abbey, near Fulda, in 1455. This text was of great interest to German humanists since it provided them with new and positive accounts of the deep German past. Tacitus's *Germania* was a key source of inspiration for Conrad Celtis and Jakob Wimpfeling as they launched the cooperative project *Germania Illustrata*. This project sought to build a new and illustrious history of German lands, modeled on similar works by Italian humanists, specifically Flavio Biondo's 1453 history of the Italian peninsula.

Despite initial inspiration from Italian scholarship, the new attention to things German bore an anti-Italian edge, as German scholars sought to outgrow the shadow cast by the achievements of the Italian Renaissance. Part of this shadow included what humanists Celtis and Wimpfeling viewed as Italians' unfair opinions of Germans and northern Europe in general. Drawing on attitudes prevalent since antiquity, Italian humanists were prone to look down on northern Europe as the home of brutes, savages, and drunkards. But by the end of the fifteenth century German scholars began to view their own intellectual accomplishments as true rivals to that of the south and were eager to counter Italian claims of inferiority.[6]

As a leading German humanist in the effort to define a German cultural identity, Conrad Celtis is important for understanding Vochs's concerns and priorities. Vochs and Celtis seem to share three major goals: promoting a German patriotism in opposition to Italian influence and achievements; striving for moral reform within the Church as a "religious enlightenment"; and paying more attention to the natural details of German lands.[7] In a 1492 address to the University of Ingolstadt, Celtis urged study of the history and nature of German lands:

> Consider it shameful for yourselves to be unfamiliar with the histories of the Greeks and Latins. Consider it beyond all shame to be unfamiliar with the situation, the stars, the rivers, the mountains, the antiquities, and the nations of our region and land.[8]

This speech also bore an anti-Italian edge, reflecting the tension among German humanists between admiration for the Italian Renaissance and hostility to Italians' cultural influence in northern Europe. Celtis may also have inspired Vochs's appeal to the youth of Germania to fight for their homeland. Celtis stated: "Take up again, Oh German men, that old spirit of yours with which you so many times were a terror and specter to the Romans!"[9] The German men who responded to Celtis's call included some of the great humanists of the day: Beatus Rhenanus, Joannes Aventinus, and Hartmann Schedel, in addition to Wimpfeling.

Vochs was not a distinguished humanist of the time, however, and may not even fit within a loose definition of humanism.[10] Unfortunately, very little information exists about his life. All that is known about Vochs comes from his plague text, which is his sole publication.[11] The title page of his text identifies him as a doctor of arts and medicine.[12] Like many aspiring physicians and scholars, Vochs studied or worked for a time in Italian lands as a young man. In Vochs's case, this was "greater Greece" or southern Italian lands, where his teachers included Butio de Trincis and Mattheus de Sulmona, both obscure physicians or surgeons. After these formative years, Vochs returned north to practice medicine in Cologne for nearly forty years, as he states in his 1507 text.[13] This timeframe would likely place Vochs's birth during the 1440s.

Study in Italian lands, however, does not make the humanist. Vochs's work shows little sign of the hallmarks of humanism – a love of the eloquence of ancient authors or the adoption of new thinking from leading scholars of the Italian Renaissance. Largely absent in Vochs's work are references to contemporary Italian humanists Niccolo Leoniceno (1428–1524), Marsilio Ficino (1433–1499), and Giovanni Pico della Mirandola (1463–1494), who all advanced new insights into nature and medicine.[14] And despite a fondness for Hippocrates, as explored below, Vochs did not adhere to the strict Hellenism of some medical humanists. Vochs's text draws on Avicenna and medieval Arab physicians as readily as ancient Greeks. Moreover, Vochs's Latin often departs from classical forms favored by humanists, and has been described as "incomprehensible" and "barbaric" by one eighteenth-century commentator.[15]

But, if Vochs was not a humanist, he nonetheless shared some of their sentiments and methods, much like the later reformer Martin Luther. Indeed, Vochs even cultivated ties to humanist physicians, apparent in the dedication of his text, in which he states that he intended for Martin Mellerstadt (Martin Pollich) to examine his work before passing it on to the Elector Frederick the Wise.[16] Vochs's intent to reform culture and society more broadly also seem to follow the ambitious projects of some humanists. Even though most of his plague text focuses on rooting out errors in medicine, Vochs's broader vision echoes humanists' concerns about injustice within Church, state, and society. In the opening chapter of his plague text, Vochs depicts society as diseased through its religious and political leaders, effectively blaming them for the divine punishments of pestilence and French Disease. Since sin is the primary cause of the current plagues, Vochs points to the leaders of church and state as guilty of the greatest sins in German lands, offering what one nineteenth-century commentator described as "the most bitter complaints about the oppression of the people."[17]

Vochs first examines the justice systems of the Holy Roman Empire and laments that greater justice exists among the Turks and French. Vochs states that German courts are more likely to condemn those who appeal for justice to higher powers, thus needlessly creating paupers, orphans, and widows. Although the poor can in theory appeal to the German king or the Pope for ultimate justice, payments and expenses keep this from happening. Vochs criticizes church courts in particular, depicting them as extorting money from Germans while their clerical leaders yearn to be absent from their posts. In sum, Vochs sees "nothing of justice" in German lands and laments that "all are confused and without order" in society.[18] Vochs ends his harangue by condemning secular princes' wars as particularly unjust, and especially the murderous war in the days of Charles the Bold of Burgundy that depopulated German lands.[19]

In line with late medieval anticlericalism, Vochs saves his most severe criticism for the clergy itself. Two years before Erasmus wrote his *Praise of Folly*, Vochs attacked the wealth, luxury, and lusts of churchmen, condemning the clergy as a whole as desperately flawed – "a monstrosity redeemed by no virtue, loaded with faults and mighty only in libido."[20] As he describes the clergy's craven lust for money and women, Vochs cites the words of Constantine: "Today poison is sprinkled through the Church."

Foreshadowing Protestant concerns, Vochs calls for the revival of Julian law (*lex Julia*) to solve the problem of a sexually promiscuous clergy, referring to Roman laws from the reign of Augustus that criminalized adultery and encouraged marriage. Although adultery seems to be the glory of the clergy, Vochs reminds them that their true glory is reading the scriptures.[21] Through such criticism Vochs suggests that a reform of church and state would liberate Germania from special divine punishments, allowing it to thrive again. In sum, Vochs not only criticized German institutions at the time but also proposed reforms on the eve of the Reformation. In this way, Vochs shared much with contemporary humanists, including new attention to things German and the injustice of the time.

German locality and indigenous medicine as reform

If it was humanists who promoted a love of things German and suspicion of things Italian, it was Vochs who extended such concerns to medicine. Vochs's text does not dwell on the reform of church and state, but soon introduces a multifaceted reform of medicine designed to protect the health and wealth of Germans. His medical thought has two main thrusts: the promotion of locality as the key to understanding German bodies and their appropriate treatments; and attacks on potentially harmful medicines and the foreigners who sell them. This group of dangerous medicines includes a wide set of exotic ingredients as well as recent alchemical inventions, which Vochs viewed with great suspicion. Most importantly, in developing a more German perspective on medicine, Vochs drew on the thought of Hippocrates, thereby returning to the source of Western medicine in order to criticize the medicine of his own time.

Vochs's unusual local approach to the plague appears at the very start of his text, in his dedication to the Elector Frederick the Wise. Here Vochs begins with the idea that plagues are inherently difficult to treat because they are punishments from God. In this vein, Vochs believes that not all plagues are alike, and thus denies that there can be a universal remedy. Reflecting upon the staggering number of remedies in physicians' plague texts, and drawing upon his own experience from his forty-year career, Vochs observes that some remedies work better in some places than others. At this point Vochs appeals to the particular qualities of localities in order to explain the differences in sicknesses and treatments:

> [S]ince particular places of states and territories have properties from waters, from mountains and minerals, from blowing winds, from flat ground, depths and heights. And for that reason the inhabitants are disposed to this and that sickness.[22]

This sort of environmental explanation has deep roots in Western medicine, finding early expression in Hippocrates's foundational text, *Airs, Waters and*

Places, of circa 400 BC.[23] Yet the application of a local and environmental perspective to plague was unusual in plague texts produced after 1348, since physicians' explanations typically remained on a universal and divine level.[24] Probably because this is a prefatory section, Vochs does not cite Hippocrates or any learned authority for his environmental approach, although his interest in Hippocrates becomes clear later. And worth mentioning here, but explored further in Chapter 5, is that Vochs offers an unusual explanation of the plague's causes that focuses on water in the environment, rather than the more traditional focus on air among Galenic physicians.[25]

Vochs returns to the subject of locality when he later discusses the dangers of "pestilence pills," which were compounded antidotal pills that many physicians recommend in their plague tracts. Here Vochs introduces his larger argument on the particular nature of German bodies, combined with an attack on imported medicines that threaten the health of such bodies. Vochs targets the pestilence pills of Rufus of Ephesus, a Greek physician of the first century AD, as well as the pills developed more recently by Antonio Guaineri, a fifteenth-century Italian medical professor at the University of Pavia. The heart of Vochs's attack centers on the ingredients of aloe, myrrh, and saffron, as well as the confusing multitude of ingredients in such compounded products. Here Vochs begins a medical argument that recurs throughout the text as he rejects or amends much contemporary plague medicine. The main problem is that some of the ingredients found in traditional plague medicines are neither suited to German lands nor appropriate for German bodies, which often have an abundance of phlegm, the wet and cold humor. Vochs contends that, while plague results from a corruption of this abundant phlegm in Germans, substances such as aloe purge more readily the yellow bile (also known as choler, the warm and dry humor), and thus do little to restore the body's humoral balance.[26]

Vochs provides more theoretical explanations for his regional and environmental approach in a later section devoted to preserving the body from plague. Here Vochs introduces a set of rules for treating with German bodies, the first of which offers the broadest theoretical vision:

> The first rule: the bodies of the Germans are best suited for maximum humidity, and are kept in good shape in humid circumstances. For each thing is well kept in a place which is most natural to itself and is nurtured by foods with the same make-up of which it consists from creation.[27]

Broadening this logic from foods to medicines, Vochs cites Hippocrates that "medicine needs to be given according to the region, time and age."[28] Vochs embraces the Hippocratic notion that a person's physical qualities and humoral make-up differ according to region or geography, and further develops ideas about the differences between northern and southern Europe. Vochs states that, just as the northern regions of Europe are colder and more humid, German bodies are colder and more humid than the bodies of Italians and Frenchmen (*Italos, Gallos*). In complexional terms, this makes German bodies prone to having an abundance of phlegm, the cold and wet humor, as well as blood, the warm and moist humor. An abundance of yellow bile (choler), the hot and dry humor, therefore does not harm German bodies in the same way that it does for Italians and Frenchmen. Thus, since many plague medicines from southern lands are focused on balancing the choler in the body, they do no good for German bodies.

Vochs's particular view of German bodies undercut the traditional pharmacopeia of Western medicine, not to mention the contemporary trade in *materia medica* with the eastern Mediterranean, Middle East, and distant Asia. In his six rules for protecting German bodies, Vochs again warns against saffron and myrrh, and adds a new warning about camphor.[29] Vochs does not reject all imported medicines, however, but encourages caution in any case, since there could be severe consequences for people who accept blindly the medical products and advice of foreigners. Vochs warns that inappropriate medicines can kill or bring madness, noting especially the misuse of saffron.[30] Here Vochs turns against other common exotics, such as "bolus" and terra sigillata, a mineral mined on the Greek island of Lemnos.[31] Vochs explains that these medicines only multiply the dry and cold humors in bodies that should, rather, remain more humid by nature. The imbalance caused by such medicines can be dangerous, since it traps the body's humidities, thereby creating obstructions that could lead to pestilential putrefaction.[32] In this way, the use of bolus and terra sigillata can even bring about pestilential sicknesses, rather than prevent them. At this point Vochs warns against following the medical "sophists" who recommend terra sigillata, such as the ninth-century Arabic physician Mesue, identified here as John Damascene.[33]

Going beyond theoretical discussions, Vochs extends his attack to the contemporary trade of spices and medicines, targeting especially the foreign merchants (*exteros*) who import dangerous products. Vochs depicts these merchants as driven to German lands by a "greedy and raging thirst" when rumors of plague begin to swirl. Once they arrive and see the desperate mood, they raise the prices of their products, knowing well that the rustic German masses place great faith in pestilence pills and exotics.[34] Due to their numerous abuses, Vochs urges Emperor Maximilian I to issue an edict against foreign merchants, who drain the vigor of Germany with their wild lust for profit. Vochs argues that an imperial ban on saffron, cinnamon, cubeb pepper, the "wood of death" (*ligno quasi mortuo*), and other exotic products would benefit German bodies and pocketbooks. To emphasize his point, Vochs states that pestilence pills should be thrown out of the window, rather than put into bodies, due to their harmful effects. And, in a telling comment on popular medical belief, Vochs deplores the common assumption that German lands are sterile of healing plants, apparent in the many who chase after medicines from India, Arabia, and the Red Sea for even the slightest sickness or wound.[35]

After attacking dangerous exotics, Vochs transitions to the promotion of native German medicines. Most strikingly, Vochs even goes so far as to develop his own version of theriac, drawing on "our German plants" rather than those "from the forests of India and Arabia."[36] Such a move to Germanize theriac is significant since this remedy was among the most prestigious medicines of ancient and medieval Europe. Theriac had been famous for its antidotal powers since the first century AD, when Greek physicians first compounded it from a long list of ingredients. Some physicians regarded theriac as a universal panacea for poisons and after 1348 favored it in the fight against pestilential poisons. By the early sixteenth century, however, Vochs and other physicians noticed that this drug no longer measured up to ancient accounts of its miraculous healing powers. This inspired a variety of attempts to recover the power of the ancient theriac, whether by seeking the authentic recipe in ancient sources or experimenting with new recipes. Historian Richard Palmer has described the sixteenth-century "race" in Italy to recover or invent a powerful theriac, even viewing it as driving a "quiet revolution" in knowledge about medical simples.[37] While many of Palmer's examples come from mid-sixteenth-century Italian lands, Vochs's case reveals an earlier preoccupation with this antidote in northern Europe.

Vochs hails his own creation as a "theriac of the poor," since it draws primarily on less expensive, native ingredients. Here he seems to reach out to common people, who were perhaps the most vulnerable to knavish merchants peddling inappropriate medicines. Lest his audience doubt that his theriac measures up to the expensive imports, Vochs appeals to his own experience and claims that his theriac is at least as good as the ancient theriac of Andromachus and may be better, "which you would know from certain and true examples." This was no small claim, since the theriac of Andromachus was the original theriac, dating to the first century AD. Theriac resulted from this Greek physicians' efforts to improve mithridatum, an older compound antidote, by adding viper flesh and increasing the opium dose.[38] Vochs continued the evolution of this antidote, however, by developing a version that does not need to be aged for twelve years, does not use opium and its sleep of oblivion, and avoids the mistakes that can occur when using snake parts as ingredients, such as confusing the head and tail.[39] Most importantly, Vochs reveals the recipe for his theriac, which calls for a long list of botanical ingredients, including sage, gentian, betonica, pimpinella (anise), and absinth, among others. While most of the ingredients are at home in northern Europe, red coral appears as well, indicating that the recipe was not intended to be exclusively of native extraction.[40] In a nod to the special significance of this recipe, an early modern reader noted it with the Latin annotation "Tyraca pau." in the copy held at the Stadtbibliothek Trier. This is a likely reference to the "theriac of the poor," and is one of the relatively few annotations in the book.[41] As explored below, this "theriac of the poor" drew much interest from physicians during the sixteenth century and became known as the "German theriac."

To support his new promotion of native German medicines, Vochs does not cite any precedent, much less the long tradition of indigenous medicine that existed in northern Europe during the Middle Ages. A brief review of this tradition, however, reveals that Vochs added a variety of elements to these medieval medical texts, whether he was aware of them or not. For example, one of the oldest medical texts of German-speaking Europe, the Lorsch Medical Codex of circa 796, promotes native plants as cheaper replacements for exotic imports. Its author does not deny the medical value of such imports, however, as does Vochs.[42] Reliance on native medicinal plants presumably thrived within the practical, monastery-based medicine of northern Europe during the Middle Ages. Traces of this medical world exist in the manuscripts that became important channels for recording and spreading information on German *materia medica*. The shift from manuscript to print in the late fifteenth century brought new attention to German plants as well, as seen in the *Herbarius Moguntinus* (1484), which devoted seventy-five percent of its 150 chapters to plants that grew wild in German lands.[43] But, unlike Vochs, the author of the *Herbarius Moguntinus* does not recognize the text's own focus on indigenous plants, much less develop political or economic arguments in favor of native products. Rather than ideas about indigeneity or German identity, one finds references to Avicenna and Arnald de Villanova in this text's introduction.[44] Therefore, in comparison to German medical texts of earlier centuries, Vochs's emphasis on German identity and locality appears to be new. During a time of new German self-awareness and expanding geographical horizons, Vochs did much to invent the notion of the indigenous.[45]

It is surprising that Vochs incorporated a new emphasis on things German in his text, given that nearly all medical texts written before 1507 were universal in outlook. The greatest works of medicine, botany, and natural history aimed to collect natural knowledge from all corners of the known world. Some of the most common German botanical and medical works of the late Middle Ages, such as the *Gart der Gesundheit* and *Ortus Sanitatis*, also do not single out native herbs for praise. In the first German vernacular herbal, the *Gart der Gesundheit* of 1485, the editor, Bernhard von Breidenbach, notes after a pilgrimage to the Holy Land the "many precious herbs that do not grow in these German lands."[46] Moreover, a universal outlook characterized the entire medical profession. In the late Middle Ages German physicians often trained at Italian universities, where they immersed themselves in the texts of the ancient Mediterranean, even though such texts often lacked specific knowledge of northern Europe. This international outlook appeared less attractive to some in the early sixteenth century, however, amid the concerns of the time.

In justifying his attempt to create a new theriac of local extraction, Vochs presses his attack on foreign merchants further. Vochs seems to resent that the merchants of Venice and Genoa have a near-monopoly on the production and trade in theriac. First he singles out abuses by the theriac merchants of Venice and Genoa, such as the likelihood of falsification among the dealers of rare, exotic medicines. Vochs also associates theriac with the vilest sorts of popular salesmen, who resort to theatrical trials in the marketplace to deceive their unwitting audience:

> This antidote is sold indiscriminately, dispensed promiscuously, and even created by the vilest idiots. The salesmen even swallow whole serpents, newts, and spiders. And in this trial [*proba*] the vulgar people, who lack a guide, stand there and are satisfied that the truth is shown.[47]

In this rhetorical move, Vochs reduces the well-established trade in one of the most esteemed contemporary medicines to the lowliest stratum of the medical marketplace.[48]

Such concerns about the exclusive theriac trade reflect broader concerns about merchant monopolies in the spice and drug trade within the Holy Roman Empire during the early sixteenth century. In this respect, Vochs's text is an important antecedent to what historians have called the *Monopolstreit*, in which the regulation of merchant monopolies occupied debates at imperial diets through the 1530s. German princes feared the growing wealth and influence of foreign merchants as well as the upstart German merchant families who aligned with them and collected fabulous profits from their exclusive contracts. One cause for new attention to whom was profiting from the spice and drug trade was the rapid rise of Portugal after 1498, when its new sea route to India revolutionized the trade. In targeting foreign monopolies and the king of Portugal, the rhetoric of the *Monopolstreit* brought to imperial politics new arguments that foreign merchants were stripping Germany bare of precious money.[49] Judging by the fact that Vochs dedicated his text to Elector Frederick the Wise of Saxony, Vochs seems to have sought common cause with the German princes in this emerging fight. In this way, Vochs's plague text of 1507 anticipated both the political and religious struggles that occupied the Holy Roman Empire in the coming revolutionary decades.

Experience in medicine: Vochs's attack on sophistry and alchemy

Alongside his surprising statements on local and foreign medicines, Vochs makes equally surprising statements on medical traditions of learning ("medical sophistry") as well as alchemy. Both topics reflect Vochs's larger effort to raise the status of experience in the production of medical knowledge, which places him near the forefront of this broader transformation in early modern medicine and science. As seen above, Vochs's thought allowed him to reject or ignore much recent thought on plague, while he focused rather on more local treatments, often known through personal experience.

Thus Vochs explains that his text omits the ideas of many doctors precisely because they lack knowledge gained through personal experience:

> [F]ew physicians are found who practice in many plagues or in great cities. And for this reason they are able to write or teach nothing about their own experience, but glorify the writings of others.

This pro-experience statement combines with his criticism of physicians' over-reliance on philosophy, as Vochs cites the words of the twelfth-century Andalusian physician Avenzoar (Ibn Zuhr): "[Y]ou will be certain that the discipline (*scientia*) of medicine is not to be performed perfectly unless you have long practice of many years and long experience and in no way with sophisticated logical reasoning."[50] Vochs views a medicine that is practical and active as the proper end of intellectual inquiry, implicitly condemning philosophizing for its own sake.[51]

Vochs finds that medicating German bodies requires trusting experience as much as ancient textual authorities, grounded as they were in the *materia medica* of the Mediterranean and beyond. After he encourages his readers to throw away the much-esteemed "pestilence pills" of Rufus, Vochs mourns that few follow his advice, since the ancient authorities remain entrenched in peoples' minds: "[T]hey walk around on the feet of Rufus and others." At this point Vochs makes experience an equal partner in the production of medical knowledge: "I however want to make no one a god, but as with Galen, I believe something of no writing unless I will see a trial (*experientiam*)."[52] Vochs's use of an ancient authority such as Galen to fight blind acceptance of textual knowledge suggests a humanist's attack on the scholastic methods of the Middle Ages. Vochs wanted to bring his profession back to a standard of knowledge that blended reason, textual authority, and personal experience, which presumably reigned among ancient figures such as Galen. In this production of knowledge, personal experience could even trump textual authority, especially when mating ancient medical theory with the conditions of northern Europe. On the whole, Vochs's thought was not a rejection of traditional academic medicine but, rather, a renewal of experience in the attempt to fashion a new medicine that was focused on German bodies.

Vochs's appreciation of experience was not out of place among the leading medical thinkers of the time. At the turn of the sixteenth century medical humanists throughout Europe began to question and supplement ancient knowledge based on their own experience with nature and ancient texts. At this time Italian humanists worked to remove the influence of medieval Arabic commentators on Greek texts, which they saw as corrupting classical thought. Some even found errors in ancient texts, such as Niccolo Leoniceno, who corrected Pliny's *Natural History* based on his personal experience (*experientia*) with healing plants.[53] The medical humanists of northern Europe carried this approach further, finding much work in describing and classifying local plants that were unknown to the ancients. Within a northern European context, personal experience became as important as ever to physicians in the production of knowledge.

Vochs's nuanced thought on experience in medicine is also revealed in his thought on alchemy, which shows an openness to the discovery of new medicines through experimentation, but also incredulity regarding the biggest claims of alchemical theory. Alchemy deserves close attention, since the subject was emerging at the end of the fifteenth century as an important, but disputed, frontier of medical innovation. Since the Black Death of the fourteenth century, alchemy had been slowly changing plague advice as physicians and laypeople alike took notice of alchemy's claims to access miraculous healing powers.[54] The work of alchemists encouraged greater appreciation for experience within medicine, and in this regard was similar to the new medical thought of figures such as Vochs and Leoniceno. The two disciplines were separated by an institutional and intellectual chasm, however, since university medical faculties did not teach alchemy, and humanists were often critical of alchemy's claims to success.

Behind much of the alchemy in German plague texts of Vochs's era was the work of the Pavian medical professor Antonio Guaineri (? – ca. 1446).[55] Guaineri left a lasting impression on German physicians through his double treatise on plague and poisons of circa 1440, which introduced alchemical products to plague medicine. In his plague text, physicians could find detailed information on alchemical products, methods and instruments, including *aqua vitae*, *aqua ardens*, alembics, baths of Mary, distillation, coction, and sublimation.[56] Guaineri had personal ties to alchemists and was an early pioneer in his attempts to integrate their findings and products into learned medicine. He is famous for claiming that it was possible to make the panacea known as potable gold (*aurum potabile*), based on the testimony of two trustworthy alchemists.[57] Most importantly, Guaineri's alchemical thought was a major source of inspiration for various German physicians, including Ulrich Ellenbog and Caspar Kegler, as explored in depth in Chapter 4.[58] Ellenbog, the city physician of Memmingen, incorporated a complex alchemical recipe into his plague pamphlet of circa 1485. This recipe called for distilling herbs, gold, and alcohol in multiple steps, resulting in a water described as the "very best" of his recipes. It possessed an "inexpressible power and virtue" that penetrated immediately to defend the heart from plague's poison.[59] Guaineri's influence here is likely, since Ellenbog counted among his students at the University of Pavia.[60]

Vochs shared contemporary interest in alchemy, including its promise to create new medicines through experience and divine power. His esteem for alchemy was reflected in his belief that all physicians, including even Hippocrates (!), had relied on alchemical discoveries in the hunt for new remedies:

> You, said Mesue, go to the alchemists and confer with them. No one in their right mind contends how much this action is profitable for

> medicine. And, certainly, I think – and my opinion is close to the truth – that our parent Hippocrates and all the others have used this device in their secret actions. For I have seen wondrous cures and actions, which even restored a man from death to life in a moment. In the same way, they amputate the head and the tail from a snake, and join them again to the body.[61]

This statement connecting Hippocrates to the alchemical tradition is surprising, since most contemporary physicians would presume that alchemy did not exist in the time of Hippocrates. It is also surprising due to the institutional and intellectual divide in Vochs's era, which kept ancient Greek medicine separate from the alchemical or Hermetic traditions. Vochs assumes, however, that alchemy has always been available as a source of innovation. Reflecting further on the history of medical experimentation, Vochs describes the invention of theriac as resulting from a similar process of divine inspiration and experimentation, citing Avicenna for support.[62] Following the precedent of Hippocrates, Avicenna, and Guaineri, Vochs's invention of his own "theriac of the poor" makes sense within a worldview in which God causes the plague but also inspires new experimentation to cure it.

But, like many learned physicians, Vochs did not necessarily accept the alchemists' grandest claims, much less the alchemical products that were multiplying around him in the early sixteenth century. Vochs dismisses as unhelpful Raymund Lull's grand work on making *aqua vitae*, while the work of John of Rupescissa appears to be riddled with errors. Only after rejecting these alchemical masters does Vochs turn against Guaineri for his more recent alchemical recommendations for plague. Vochs rejects Guaineri's work, as well as that of other "investigators" (*inquisitores*) and "potion-makers" (*distillatores*), for its errors and inconstancy. Vochs shows much knowledge of alchemical techniques as he points out technical errors in Guaineri's writings on *aqua vitae*. At a general level, Vochs views alchemists' search for omnipotent cures as misguided and the ultimate cause of their failure. On a practical level, Vochs maligns alchemy's impact, since medical men are inexperienced at following complex alchemical recipes, thus resulting in medicines of death. The strongest condemnation of *aqua vitae* comes as Vochs argues that the "water of life" is contrary to human nature as a "water of death."[63] In a similar way, Vochs rejects Guaineri's thoughts on potable gold.[64]

Alchemical experimentation often lacked credibility among learned physicians in the early sixteenth century because it was based on ideas external to classical Hippocratic–Galenic medicine. To many physicians it seemed to lack the principles and rationality that guided their own discipline, while its practitioners seemed to rush from experiment to experiment with their heads in smoke. A minority of physicians in the early sixteenth century, including Vochs, would agree that alchemical experimentation resulted in discoveries that may be useful in particular cases, but the empirical and case-specific knowledge that it generated paled before the universal knowledge taken to lie at the heart of Hippocratic–Galenic medicine. While Vochs's openness to some aspects of alchemy may be surprising for the time, his attacks on its practitioners is fairly typical. It was common for humanists to target the errors, ignorance, and greed of alchemists and astrologers rather than dismiss these disciplines altogether.[65]

The indigenous medicine movement after Vochs

Vochs's text appeared only twice in print, once in Magdeburg in 1507 and again in Cologne in 1537, when the medical professor Johann Dryander edited and reissued the text. But, despite its relative obscurity in the early sixteenth century, Vochs's text may have had a considerable impact on its time. The case of its impact is certainly much clearer after Dryander reissued the work in 1537. In any case, Vochs's writing touched on deep concerns that other prominent German authors had. In the decades after Vochs's text appeared, attacks on foreign merchants and medicines proliferated as the Reformation deepened the growing cultural divide between northern and southern Europe. By the 1520s the various physicians, humanists, and theologians who were attacking exotics and/or promoting indigenous medicine began to resemble a disparate movement. In the first decade of the Reformation social and political concern for Germania intensified, along with anti-Roman sentiment and hopes for Church reform. The work of the humanist Ulrich van Hutten illustrates this fusion of political and religious issues best. In his 1519 text *Fever*, Hutten connects the preference for foreign spices with a soft and un-German lifestyle, embodied in a fictitious church prelate who had recently returned from Rome. Here the luxury of Rome is portrayed as dangerous to the soul, contrasted with the authentic simplicity of the Germans. In 1524 Martin Luther also joined the attack on the spice trade as part of his broader reform of Christian life and society. In terms similar to Vochs, Luther even sought to rid the land of exotic spices and all such useless luxuries, which he saw as only draining wealth from the country to the benefit of foreign, Catholic interests.[66] Thus, the propagandists of the emerging Protestant Reformation strengthened moral arguments for local medicines by attacking the corrupting influence of foreign luxuries. Among their creative contributions was the addition of anti-papal rhetoric to these older themes.

Due to a lack of histories on the origins of German medical localism, it is common to mistake Paracelsus as the originator of this trend. Paracelsus wrote his famous work on the topic, the *Herbarius*, during the mid- or later 1520s, however, and only after the texts and statements by Vochs, Hutten, and Luther.[67] In his *Herbarius*, Paracelsus attacks foreign imports and praises the medical products of German lands, but not in a way that was very original at the time. The texts by Vochs and Paracelsus overlap on their praise of German medicines, as well as attacks on the foreign drug trade, knavish Italians, and German ignorance. Paracelsus's strongest praise of German medicines comes near the start of the *Herbarius*, in words that seem to echo Vochs at times:

> There are in Germany so many more and better medicines than are to be found in Arabia, Chaldea, Persia and Greece that it would be more reasonable for the people of such places to get their medicines from us Germans... Indeed these medicines are so good, that neither Italy, France, nor any other realm can boast of better ones.[68]

Although Paracelsus draws a contrast between native and foreign medicines that would have been familiar to Vochs, Paracelsus's statement of German superiority within world medicine certainly went beyond Vochs's German pride. Despite this difference, Vochs would have likely cheered Paracelsus's statement of medical localism: "Each land, to be sure, gives birth to its own special kinds of sickness, its own medicine, and its own physician."[69] Vochs would also agree with the anti-Italian tone as Paracelsus continues:

> That this has not come to light for such a long time is the fault of Italy, the mother of ignorance and inexperience. For the Italians saw to it that the Germans thought nothing of their own plants, but took everything from Italy itself or from beyond the sea. This they realized was to their own advantage...[70]

Paracelsus continues in much the same way as Vochs, targeting merchants of exotic medicines as well as the books of southern Europe that know nothing of German medicines.

Considering the overlapping content between the works of Vochs and Paracelsus, one could say that Vochs anticipated, or perhaps even influenced, the thought of Paracelsus. One can speculate whether the two had met during Paracelsus's travels or if Paracelsus had encountered Vochs's text before he wrote his own. But, despite some overlap between the texts, Vochs's work goes well beyond that of Paracelsus by developing a medical philosophy aimed at explaining and treating German bodies. Paracelsus's *Herbarius*, by comparison, is a simple review of a handful of herbs and minerals, not all of which are of local origin, since red coral, terra sigillata, and bolus armenus make notable appearances. Paracelsus also does not develop his ideas about medical localism to the extent that Vochs does. Furthermore, Paracelsus's *Herbarius* remained unpublished until 1568, thereby diminishing its historical impact in comparison to Vochs's text.

The full flourishing of interest in German indigenous medicine came in the 1530s with Otto Brunfels and Hieronymus Bock, hailed among the German fathers of modern botany. There is no evidence that these early botanists knew of Vochs's work, and yet they stood together in promoting a radically new appreciation of native *materia medica*. Brunfels first published his *Herbarum vivae eicones* (*Living Images of Herbs*) in 1530, while Bock published his *New Kreütter Buch* in 1539. Each work carefully separates native and foreign plants and pays particular attention to German medical simples. Brunfels also expressed dislike for "alien medicines" in favor of the local.[71] These works are generally regarded as the start of serious efforts to relate the plants of northern Europe to the botanical writings of antiquity.

The new interest in native healing plants was also not limited to German lands in the sixteenth century. The French medical humanist Symphorien Champier published in 1533 his text *Hortus Gallicus, pro Gallis in Gallia scriptus*, which aimed to teach Frenchmen how to heal their sicknesses with French remedies.[72] In a century that witnessed the large-scale importation of many new plants and medicines from lands afar, the distinction between local and foreign became more current among scholars and activists. Over the course of the sixteenth century, then, the distinction between local and foreign grew sharper and inspired new interest in indigenous plants. Further research is necessary to establish whether the new appreciation for the indigenous began in German lands or if Vochs and Hutten had predecessors or counterparts elsewhere in transalpine Europe.

Vochs's text was certainly a part of later discussions of local and foreign medicines during the sixteenth century. His text enjoyed a renaissance in 1537 when the Marburg medical professor Johann Dryander deemed it worthy of a new edition, thus renewing the call for German princes to act against harmful exotics. Dryander reprinted it in a more readable form and included his own commentary in an introduction. Here Dryander hails Vochs's work in fighting alchemists and others who miserably extort money from Germans.[73] A similarly enthusiastic reception came from the Leipzig physician Johann Reusch, who included many of Vochs's ideas in his 1539 vernacular plague treatise, including the key idea that German lands have many precious simples that are better suited for the German people than Indian and Arabian medicines. Echoing Vochs's concerns, Reusch uses these ideas to fight the power of Genoese merchants and alchemists who cheat the country. Reusch also reprinted the recipe of Vochs's "theriac of the poor," rebranding it as the "German theriac."[74] Furthermore, the famous author Walther Hermann Ryff included Vochs's "German theriac" in his 1542 book on confected medicines, doubtlessly reaching a broad audience.[75] One of the last references to Vochs's "German theriac" in a plague text came from the Brandenburg physician Valentin Trutiger in 1563.[76]

Conclusion

Vochs's story reveals a coming of age for northern Europe, as a chorus of scholars, beginning with Vochs, began to argue for Germany's own *materia medica* as better medicine for native people than the imports from afar. This idea represents a bending of the universal culture, if not the universal philosophy, that underlay learned medicine and cultural views of the plague.

The turn to a German indigenous medicine allowed Vochs to champion three significant reforms at once, all aimed at improving the health, wealth, and autonomy of Germans. First, it justified attacks on foreign merchants, who were seen as extracting precious money from Germans in exchange for useless products. Second, since a German indigenous medicine was inherently antithetical to contemporary learned traditions, it allowed him to ignore works of scholastic medicine, many of them from French and Italian scholars. Vochs was happy to do so, since he saw little point to the learned medical disputations of his time and condemned sophistry in medical matters. Finally, it allowed him to remind his peers that experience is an equal partner with philosophy in the production of medical knowledge, since many German herbs and medicines were unknown to the ancients and therefore could not be known through text-based learned authority. Vochs sought a more practical and socially accessible medical practice that drew as much on personal experience as Hippocratic and Galenic principles. In sum, Vochs spurred the broader quest for new medicines in the sixteenth century by encouraging physicians to explore and experiment in the natural world in the hopes of recovering the power of ancient healers.

Vochs's broader historical significance as a critic who anticipated the Reformation is just as striking. His attention to the social and economic issues surrounding his "theriac of the poor" fits the trend of German humanists joining princes and churchmen in urging broad reforms in various aspects of life by the early sixteenth century. Many parallels exist between the origins of Vochs's reform of medicine and the emerging reform of religion. Concerns about the loss of money, the perceived lack of respect for northern Europe, and the perceived loss of moral authority lie behind each reforming effort. Stories of innocent Germans being fleeced of their money by greedy Italians also constituted a prominent criticism of the Roman Church in the decades before the Reformation. In this way, historians should recognize the extent that the broader social, cultural, and economic concerns of the early sixteenth century penetrated various aspects of life, including medicine. A fuller exploration of how the Protestant Reformation affected healing traditions in the coming decades follows in Chapter 3.

Notes

1 Johann Vochs, *De pestilentia Anni p[raese]ntis et ei[us] cura* (Magdeburg, 1507). Listed in the VD16 as V 2021.

2 Today's neglect of Vochs contrasts with the interest of nineteenth-century historians, who focused on Vochs's unusual explanation of the origins of the French Disease (a result of bad food) or his bizarre statement that the printing press was invented first in Cologne and thereafter spread to Mainz. Fr. J. Behrend, Ed., *Archiv für Syphilis und Hautkrankheiten*, Vol. I (Berlin: August Hirschwald, 1846), 57. Friedrich Everhard von Mering & Ludwig Reischert, *Zur Geschichte*

der Stadt Köln am Rhein: Von ihrer Gründung bis zur Gegenwart, Vol. I (Cologne: Johann Wilhelm Dietz, 1838), 292.

3 Even the best histories of medical localism in northern Europe begin their story with Paracelsus: Alix Cooper, *Inventing the Indigenous: Local Knowledge and Natural History in Early Modern Europe* (Cambridge: Cambridge University Press, 2007); Andrew Wear, "The Early Modern Debate about Foreign Drugs: Localism versus Universalism in Medicine," *The Lancet* 354 (1999): 149–151; Martha Baldwin, "Danish Medicines for the Danes and the Defense of Indigenous Medicines," in *Reading the Book of Nature: The Other Side of the Scientific Revolution*, Eds. Allen G. Debus and Michael T. Walton (Kirksville, MO: Sixteenth Century Journal Publishers, 1998): 163–180.

4 Vochs, *De pestilentia*, sig. H7r.

5 Michael Stolleis, "Public Law and Patriotism in the Holy Roman Empire," in *Infinite Boundaries: Order, Disorder and Reorder in Early Modern German Culture*, Ed. Max Reinhart (Kirksville, MO: Sixteenth Century Journal Publishers, 1998): 11–33.

6 Christine Johnson, *The German Discovery of the World: Renaissance Encounters with the Strange and Marvelous* (Charlottesville, VA: University of Virginia Press, 2008).

7 Lewis W. Spitz, *The Religious Renaissance of the German Humanists* (Cambridge, MA: Harvard University Press, 1963), 83; James Overfield, "Germany," in *The Renaissance in National Context*, Eds. Roy Porter and Mikulas Teich (Cambridge: Cambridge University Press, 1992): 92–122, esp. 92–93, 108–109.

8 Also given in: David J. Collins, *Reforming Saints: Saints' Lives and Their Authors in Germany, 1470–1530* (Oxford: Oxford University Press, 2008), quotation at 75.

9 Spitz, *The Religious Renaissance*, 85–86.

10 For a deep exploration of how Italian humanists defined themselves: Patrick Baker, *Italian Renaissance Humanism in the Mirror* (Cambridge: Cambridge University Press, 2015).

11 The collapse and destruction of the Cologne city archive in 2009 has limited biographical research. More information may come to light if parts of the archive's holdings are restored. Entries on Vochs in biographical dictionaries are brief and incomplete. Jöcher (AGL Vol. 4, 1751), *Biographisch Lexikon der hervorragende Ärtze aller Zeiten und Volker*, 2nd Edn., Vol. 5, 1934 (517).

12 Vochs, *De pestilentia,* title page.

13 Vochs states that he practiced medicine in southern Italy ("magna Graecia"), and mentions King Alfonso IV of Sicily and King Ferdinand, who came to the throne in 1458: Vochs, *De pestilentia*, sig. H7r.

14 Vochs did refer to Marsilio Ficino once, but only to point out his erroneous understanding of human blood and to scold him for disregarding Galen: ibid., sigs. C2v–3r.

15 Christoph Girtanner, *Abhandlung über die venerischen Krankheit*, Vol. II (Göttingen: Johann Christian Dieterich, 1793), 37.

16 Vochs, *De pestilentia,* sigs. A2v–3r. Martin Mellerstadt, or Martin Pollich von Mellerstadt, was the first rector of the University of Wittenberg, founded in 1502. In the early sixteenth century Mellerstadt was known for battling the scholastic physician Simon Pistoris over interpretations of the French Disease: Jon Arrizabalaga, John Henderson, and Roger French, *The Great Pox: The French*

Disease in Renaissance Europe (New Haven, CT: Yale University Press, 1997), 90–97.

17 H. Maeser, *Historisch-pathologische Untersuchungen: Als Beiträge zur Geschichte der Volkskrankheiten*, Vol. II (Dresden: Verlag von Gerhard Fleischer, 1841), 6.

18 Vochs, *De pestilentia*, sigs. A4r–5r.

19 Ibid., sigs. A5v–6r.

20 Ibid., sig. A5r.

21 Ibid., sig. A5r.

22 Ibid., sigs. A2r–v.

23 For a brief introduction to the basic ideas of ancient Western medicine, including environmentalism: Mary Lindemann, *Medicine and Society in Early Modern Europe* (Cambridge: Cambridge University Press, 2010), 13–17.

24 Ann G. Carmichael, "Universal and Particular: The Language of Plague, 1348–1500," in *Pestilential Complexities: Understanding Medieval Plague*, *Medical History*, Ed. Vivian Nutton (London: Wellcome Trust Centre, 2008): 17–52.

25 Vochs, *De pestilentia*, sig. B3r.

26 Ibid., sigs. B5r–v.

27 Ibid., sig. E1r.

28 Ibid., sig. E1r.

29 He also warns against using sugar in medical confections as a substitute for opiates: ibid., sigs. E1v–2r.

30 Ibid., sig. B6v.

31 "Bolus" here probably refers to bolus armenicus, a medicinal dirt/mineral collected from Armenia or the Levant.

32 Ibid., sigs. E1r–v.

33 John Damascene is one name for John Mesue, an Arabic physician of the ninth century: Cornelius O'Boyle, *The Art of Medicine: Medical Teaching at the University of Paris* (Leiden: Brill, 1998), 114.

34 Vochs, *De pestilentia*, sig. B6v.

35 Ibid., sigs. B6v–C1r.

36 Ibid., sig. F6r.

37 Richard Palmer, "Pharmacy in the Republic of Venice in the Sixteenth Century," in *The Medical Renaissance of the Sixteenth Century*, Eds. A. Wear, R. K. French, and I. M. Lonie (Cambridge: Cambridge University Press, 1985): 108–110.

38 Christiane Nockels Fabbri, "Treating Medieval Plague: The Wonderful Virtues of Theriac," *Early Science and Medicine* 12 (2007): 247–283.

39 Vochs, *De pestilentia*, sigs. F6r–v (36r–v).

40 Ibid., sigs. F6r–v.

41 Stadtbibliothek Trier, Signatur Hs 2539: 2 an, sig. F6r.

42 Gundolf Keil, Ed., *Das Lorscher Arzneibuch*, Vol. II, Trans Ulrich Stoll and Gundolf Keil (Stuttgart: Wissenschaftliche Verlagsgesellschaft, 1989), 8–11, 25.

43 Brigitte Baumann and Helmut Baumann, *Die Mainzer Kräuterbuch-Inkunabeln: Herbarius Moguntinus, Gart der Gesundheit, Hortus Sanitatis* (Stuttgart: Anton Hiersemann, 2010), 102. Baumann and Baumann seem to support the idea that Johann Wonnecke von Cube is the author of both the *Gart der Gesundheit* and the *Herbarius Moguntinus*: 99.

44 *Herbarius Moguntinus* (or) *[R]ogatu plurimo[rum] inopu[m] num[m]o[rum] egentiu[m] appotecas refuta[n]tiu[m] occasione illa, q[uia] necessaria ibide[m] ad*

corp[us] egru[m] specta[n]tia su[n]t cara simplicia et composita… (Mainz: Peter Schöffer, 1484), first page.

45 This history of Vochs supplements Alix Cooper's fine study of indigeneity among Paracelsus and seventeenth-century figures: Cooper, *Inventing the Indigenous.*

46 Baumann and Baumann, *Die Mainzer Kräuterbuch-Inkunabeln*, 137–138. Agnes Arber, *Herbals, Their Origin and Evolution: A Chapter in the History of Botany, 1470–1670*, 2nd Edn. (Cambridge: Cambridge University Press, 1938), 20–37.

47 Vochs, *De pestilentia*, sig. F6r.

48 For a description of other theatrical experiments using antidotes, see: Thomas Holste, *Der Theriakkrämer: Ein Beitrag zur Frühgeschichte der Arzneimittelwerbung* (Pattensen: Horst Wellm Verlag, 1977), 77–81.

49 Johnson, *The German Discovery*, 132–140.

50 Vochs, *De pestilentia*, sig. F5r.

51 Ibid., sigs. F5r–v.

52 Ibid., sig. C1r.

53 Christoph Friedrich and Wolf-Dieter Müller-Jahncke, *Rudolf Schmitz: Geschichte der Pharmazie*, Vol. II, *Von der Frühen Neuzeit bis zur Gegenwart* (Eschborn: Govi Verlag, 2005), 96–97.

54 German interest in alchemy swelled along with the number of alchemical texts made available through print in the late fifteenth and early sixteenth centuries. Rudolf Hirsch, "The Invention of Printing and the Diffusion of Alchemical and Chemical Knowledge," *Chymia* 3 (1950): 115–141, esp. 118–119. Hirsch finds that German printers led the production of alchemical texts in the period between 1501 and 1536.

55 Guaineri taught at the University of Pavia beginning in 1412, became physician to the Duke of Savoy in 1427, and died sometime after 1446. Danielle Jacquart, "Theory, Everyday Practice, and Three Fifteenth-Century Physicians," *Osiris* 2nd series 6 (1990): 140–160, at 141.

56 Antonio Guaineri, [*De peste; de venenis*] (Venice: Reynaldus de Novimagio, 1487?).

57 Jacquart, "Theory, Everyday Practice," 153–154; Karl Sudhoff, "Pestschriften aus den ersten 150 Jahren nach der Epidemie des 'schwarzen Todes' 1348" 17, *Archiv für Geschichte der Medizin* 16 (1925): 77–188, 117–118; Lynn Thorndike, *A History of Magic and Experimental Science*, Vol. IV, *Fourteenth and Fifteenth Centuries* (New York: Columbia University Press, 1934), 230–231.

58 Guaineri's *Practica* appears as the alchemical reference work in Caspar Kegler's 1529 pamphlet and one of the few works cited there. Rather than describing the process of producing aqua vitae, Kegler refers his readers for more explicit directions to the printed "Practica Guanerij." Caspar Kegler, *Eyn Nutzlichs vnd trostlichs Regiment…* (Leipzig: Valten Schumann, 1529), fol. 19r. Two works with this title appeared in the Kegler family library: "practica Guernerij" and "practica Guainerij." Stadtarchiv Leipzig (SAL), Richterstube Inventarien und Hilfsbuch, 1547–1549, fols. 3v–4r.

59 [Ulrich Ellenbog], *Hie nach volget ein gut regimēt und ordnūg vnd bewert p-servativa vnd ler. wie man sich wider dē geprechen der pestilentz aufhalten vnd bewaren sol* (Eichstätt: Michael Reyser, ca. 1485–90), fols. 31–33.

60 Ulrich Ellenbog, *Von Den Gifftigen Besen Tempffen und Reuchen*, Eds. Franz Koelsch and Friedrich Zoepfl (Munich: Verlag der Münchner Drucke, 1927), fol.

VI. For a more detailed biography, see: Anton Breher, *Der Memminger Stadtarzt Ulrich Ellenbog und seine Pestschriften* (Kempten: Oechelhäuser, 1942).

61 Vochs, *De pestilentia*, sig. D2r.

62 Ibid., sigs. C6r–v.

63 Ibid., sigs. D1r–2v.

64 Ibid., sig. D4r.

65 Spitz, *The Religious Renaissance*, 93 (speaking specifically here about Celtis and Ficino on astrology).

66 Johnson, *The German Discovery*, 144–145.

67 Bruce T. Moran, "The Herbarius of Paracelsus," *Pharmacy in History* 39 (1993): 99–128, date of composition at 101.

68 Ibid., 104.

69 Ibid.

70 Ibid.

71 Cooper, *Inventing the Indigenous*, 35.

72 Ibid., 36.

73 Johann Dryander, Ed., *Opusculum praeclarum de omni Pestilentia, sive sit ab aere corrupto, sive ab aquis putridis, aut a cavaderibus: & de diuturna peste morbi Gallici...* (Cologne, 1537), sigs. Aa3r, Aa4r–v.

74 Part salesman, Reusch added that this powerful native medicine was on sale from the "careful" apothecary of Leipzig, Michael Hoffmann. Johann Reusch, *Regiment Doctor Johan Reüschen Wie sich zur zeit der Pestilentz zu halten sey / Die einwoner der Stadt Leiptzigk / vornemlich belangendt* (Leyptzigk: Nickel Schmidt, 1539), sigs. B5r–6r.

75 Walther Hermann Ryff, *Warhafftige / künstliche / gerechte vnderweisung vnnd anzeygung Alle Latwergen / Confect / Conseruen / einbeytzungen vnd einmachungen / von mancherley früchten / blůmen / kreütern vnnd wurtzeln / sampt andern künstlichen vnd anmütigen stucken / wie solche in den Apotecken gemacht* (1542), sig. lxxxvb.

76 Valentin Trutiger, *Regiment. Wider die Pestilentz in dieser gefehrlichne zeit / wie sich die gemeine bürgerschafft der löblichen vnd Churfürstlichen / beider Art / vnd Newenstadt Brandbenburg / vnd andere etc. in solcher zeit verhalten sollen* (Wittenberg: Veit Creutzer, 1563), sig. C4v.

3 The reformation of healing

Plague, physicians, and Protestantism in the 1520s

The 1520s were a decade of shocking events and rapid change in German-speaking lands. Although this decade is best known for the Protestant Reformation's sudden rise, its cultural ferment was richer than the standard historical narratives of spiritual passions and political rifts. The Reformation's first decade was filled with other tumultuous and fearsome events as German society suffered widespread plagues, popular insurrection, foreign invasion, and even astrologers' predictions of a catastrophic flood.[1] The biblical proportions of these afflictions were not lost on contemporary observers, as some looked for the end of the world.[2] The next two chapters examine how this unusual conjunction of portending catastrophes during the 1520s created the context for important medical, religious, and cultural innovations.

This chapter sheds new light on the early history of the Protestant Reformation by exploring the intersection of plagues, physicians, and religious reformers within German vernacular literature of the 1520s. Despite recent work on the medical and disease context of the Reformation, most histories of the Reformation have not integrated these topics into their narratives.[3] This chapter, however, argues that plague and medicine (in both spiritual and natural forms) belong at the center of Reformation history, since their story provides important insights into the Reformation's agents, appeal, and cultural impact. In the story outlined here, physicians, clerics, and printers began a broad reform of healing by 1521 that targeted both spiritual and natural medicine. This movement was as important to its plagued era as it is overlooked today. Although historians can trace this reform of healing in various medical and religious texts, vernacular plague literature was a key locus of reform. These sources provide unparalleled access to contemporary advice on both spiritual and natural health, revealing how plague and the Reformation affected each other.

Despite the near-absence of epidemics in Reformation history, plagues new and old played key roles in the movement's early events and cultural context. In 1520 a plague that had ravaged cities along the Rhine began to spread further inland, reaching Nuremberg in that year and other major cities by 1521. If not for this plague, the famous Diet of Worms of 1521 would have been the Diet of Nuremberg. As it was, the recently excommunicated Martin Luther had to travel further to appear before Emperor Charles V and answer for his writings. This plague persisted in central Germany until 1527, just before a new and puzzling epidemic arrived in 1529.[4] Dubbed the English Sweating Sickness, this novel epidemic added to the fears of new and mysterious sicknesses that had been growing since the French Disease appeared in Europe around 1495.

This succession of plagues and upheavals created a moment in which medieval healing traditions became particularly malleable, opening the door to high-minded and self-promoting innovators alike. These reformers began to reimagine the spiritual and natural medicines of the late Middle Ages in the hopes of finding more powerful sources of healing for their plagued era. In other words, the cultural and disease context of the 1520s inspired a broad reform of healing, led first by physicians and their printers and soon joined by Protestant clerics, including Martin Luther and Urbanus Rhegius. Even though this loose collection of reforming physicians and clerics may not have shared all of the same priorities, their cause was most effective where their interests overlapped. Physicians and reforming clerics found common cause in omitting saints from healing traditions and in promoting natural medicine as a divinely ordained source of aid.

To be clear, not all reforms pursued by physicians and clerics during this decade were inspired by evangelical (Protestant) ideas. While evangelical reformers, including both physicians and clerics, sought to establish channels of healing that they viewed as more biblical and proper, some physicians likely sought these reforms out of worldly motives alone. Stronger praise for natural medicine and its practitioners combined with a new silence on the healing powers of saints. These twin developments served to bolster physicians' social authority, which was far from secure at the time. Physicians and other medical workers of the sixteenth century had much to gain as they attempted to place their "mandate and power to heal on a plane with religion."[5] Thus one cannot attribute the broad reform of healing after 1520 to Protestantism alone, despite its primary role as a driver of change. Defining this broad reform of healing and the role of Protestantism within it are the major goals of this chapter.

The chapter begins by surveying the decline of the saints in printed plague literature amidst an atmosphere of religious dispute between 1519 and 1521. It then moves chronologically to examine the diversity of reformers at the Reformation's onset in 1521. Early activists included physicians such as the radical Alexander Seitz and Johann Copp, who spoke as prophets of fearsome divine punishments as they criticized the Roman Church. Early reformers also include Ambrosius Jung of Augsburg, who changed his advice on the confession of sins out of evangelical inspiration as early as 1521, and thereby initiated a Protestant reform of spiritual medicine of enduring importance. Only later in the 1520s did a distinctly Lutheran position emerge as Martin Luther embraced the new rhetoric of the reform of healing while also attacking false evangelical views and their proponents. By 1530 this diverse collection of reformers established new approaches to healing that would guide German medical culture for the rest of the sixteenth century.

From saints to natural medicine: the first signs of reform

The Reformation's impact on healing was apparent to observers in the sixteenth century. Contemporary historian Johannes Manlius attributed the following saying to Heinrich Stromer von Auerbach (ca. 1476–1542), dean of the medical faculty at the University of Leipzig:

> The great man, the Doctor of Auerbach, said that the restoration of the Gospel [i.e., the Reformation] has been harmful to all artists and craftsmen, except for medical practitioners... It has benefitted them since, after the saints' healing power declined, people fled in turn to the medical practitioners.[6]

Here Stromer offers a compelling view that the Reformation aided the cause of natural medicine when the movement rejected saintly healing.[7] The fact that this passage appears alongside pious statements from Martin Luther and Philip Melanchthon suggests that Stromer's observation rang true to later Lutheran observers such as Manlius. While Stromer's statement has a tinge of self-promotion, his observation nonetheless matches one of the biggest changes in German plague literature during the first half of the sixteenth century. Natural medicine and its practitioners gained new prominence as saints disappeared from text and image, representing an important chapter in physicians' attempts to expand their influence within German cities.

Despite physicians' long-standing worldly ambitions, the emerging Protestant movement began an intense phase in the reform of healing, first targeting saints. By the early 1520s evangelical preachers were promoting the idea that humans should have unmediated access to divine grace, thereby condemning the mediating role of the medieval Church as man-made and inferior to biblical models. Attacks on the cult of the saints grew fierce, as preachers denounced saints' roles as intercessors with God, while the more radical preached against statues and images as blasphemous idols.[8] Plague authors participated in this cultural turn against the saints, beginning as early as 1519, whether from a religious or professional motive. In the following decade physicians and their printers across German lands omitted saints in both word and image, replacing them in many cases with a new emphasis on faith and moral improvement. Some physicians certainly made these changes as a result of having embraced evangelical reforms, although the lack of evidence makes it impossible to ascertain the role of religious reform in most cases. What is surprising is that the turn against the saints was nearly universal in plague literature by 1521. At this moment the evangelical movement was in its infancy, relatively leaderless and undefined, yet driving a lasting change in German plague publication.

The first indication of a changing spiritual tone in plague writing comes in the 1519 pamphlet by the Swiss humanist and reformer Joachim von Watt (Vadianus, 1484–1551). This work is notable for its lack of saintly intercessors and for its decidedly biblical rhetoric on sin, faith, and moral reform during plague.[9] Although such biblical themes were by no means innovative, their appearance contrasts with the typical spiritual advice of German pamphlets from the two preceding decades. More typical in 1519 was the plague pamphlet by the physician Sixtus Kolbenschlag, which does not mention sin or repentance but seeks mercy in appeals to God and Sts. Sebastian and Roch.[10] Also important is that Vadianus emphasizes the saving power of divine grace, as he recommends that all Christians place God before their eyes and surrender themselves to the protection of his grace. Humanism and the emerging religious reform were likely sources of inspiration for Vadianus's new tone, since at the time he was an enthusiast of recent biblical scholarship and was immersed in Luther's thought. Earlier in 1519 Vadianus had attended the Leipzig Disputation and afterwards traveled to Wittenberg, having warmed to Luther's cause like many young humanists.[11]

The shift away from saints is also evident in one image used in Vadianus's 1519 pamphlet (Figure 3.1). Where one might expect the picture of a saint in an earlier print, Vadianus offers a picture of the bloodletting man. This diagram instructs the reader on where to draw blood to help the body combat the plague's poisons. More specifically, if a bubo or swelling (indicated by dots on the diagram) appears near the shoulder, the surgeon must draw blood from the hand, as the diagram shows a line connecting the bubo to the site of bloodletting. Such medical illustrations aided the pamphlet's appeal as an instructive manual and represent a subtle shift. Like Vadianus's subtle shift in the spiritual tone, this shift in imagery might not appear significant on its own. It was, however, the first shift in a long-term trend away from religious images and towards naturalistic ones in the coming decades.

Similarities between the bloodletting man and late medieval depictions of St. Sebastian reveal how subtle this shift in imagery could be, masking the greater cultural change that lies behind the differences. Note the many similarities between Figures 1.2 and 3.1, for example. Whereas images of saints lent spiritual meaning to the viewer's own suffering and may have served as channels of healing through spiritual contemplation, the new bloodletting man depicts ways that humans can limit or end suffering through their own actions. Whereas one was a portal to supernatural powers, the other aimed for worldly, "how-to" information. In this way, plague treatises of the 1520s participated in a broader publication trend, in which authors and printers developed the market for vernacular and practical literature on various topics, seemingly leaving saints behind. One

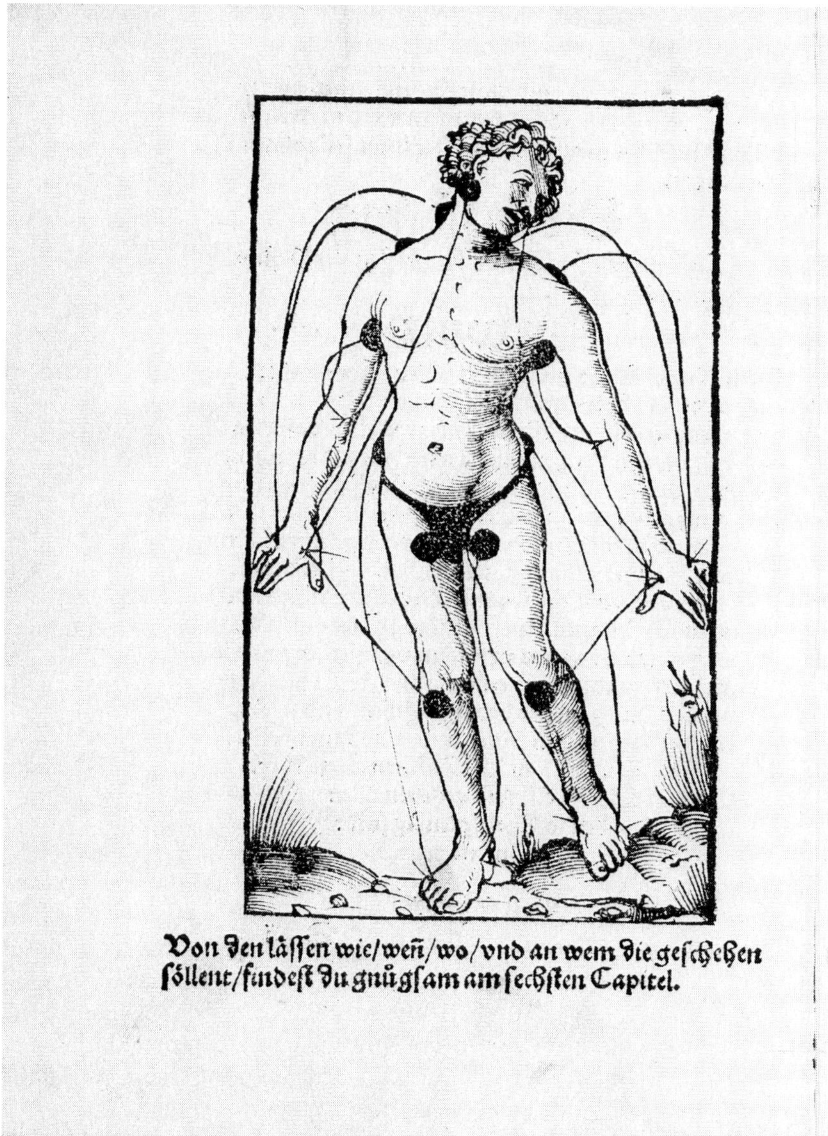

Figure 3.1 The bloodletting man

Joachim von Watt, *Ein kurtz und trüwlich underricht…* (Basel: Adam Petri, 1519), D3r.

Herzog August Bibliothek, Wolfenbüttel

Call number: N. 96.4° Helmst. (7) (reproduced with permission)

broad study of print in Strasbourg found that by 1530 the publication of "scientific" books surpassed the publication of religious works, and that they remained more numerous throughout the entire sixteenth century.[12] In this way, the Reformation contributed to a turning point for printed technical and medical literature in German-speaking lands. The case of the bloodletting man indicates that sometimes the gains of worldly information came at the expense of the late medieval spiritual world. Furthermore, this cultural shift is epitomized in Vadianus's justification of natural medicine, placed prominently in his text: "God helps those who help and care for themselves."[13] The cultural ethos of physicians and printers was suffused with human action. In the decades after 1519 the bloodletting man appeared as saints declined, and appeared most often in plague pamphlets from Augsburg, Nuremberg, and Regensburg – all centers of evangelical reform and vernacular print.[14]

Vadianus marks the start of a broader trend in plague literature, as German physicians and anonymous authors revived interest in preaching moral reform in the 1520s, as they added more discussion of sin, repentance, and divine punishment. City leaders may have encouraged this trend in the attempts to promote social stability as plagues became widespread. The opening sentence of a single-leaf broadside from Nuremberg exemplifies the change under way in 1520: "The almighty God punishes us humans angrily on account of our sins with the imposition of the *Pestilentz*..." Saints had not yet lost their presence in all plague prints, however, since this broadside recommends turning to Sts. Mary, Sebastian, and Roch in addition to Jesus for protection.[15] Appearing at the start of a decade of religious change, this was the last plague print from Nuremberg to mention saints.

Indicative of Nuremberg's future was a different pamphlet of 1520, a fourteen-page work by an anonymous author.[16] This pamphlet became the model for future Nuremberg civic pamphlets, reissued by the city council multiple times starting in 1533.[17] Although its medical advice is standard for the time, the lengthy spiritual advice that opens the pamphlet is noteworthy. Here the author encourages the audience to conquer fears through faith in God and the use of naturalistic medicine. Notably, it is silent on the topic of saintly healing. Healing begins through reconciliation with God, as the "real and true doctor of soul and body" from whom one receives the "medicine of salvation." One interesting passage praises the advantages of a stoical faith:

> He who places his trust in God with a properly ordered faith will be able to accept joy and sorrow, happiness and difficulty, health and sickness, death and life exactly the same, and can carry everything that happens in life as joyous and acceptable. Since the fear of death does not completely scare him, he is able to speak to God with a steadfast heart and spirit: In you I live, in you I die, I am yours dead and alive.[18]

Such a shift away from saintly protection and towards an emphasis on faith in God matches the basic priorities of the new evangelical spiritual healing that began to thrive in this decade.

By 1521 the decline of the saints in vernacular plague treatises was nearly universal as the genre boomed along with vernacular print in general. More importantly, this decline would prove to be utter and permanent in most German print centers. In this first great wave of vernacular plague publication in 1521, only two out of sixteen plague treatises by physicians mention a saint. But even in these cases the saint's role is muted or disputed. At the end of his pamphlet, Johannes Klainmüller of Augsburg simply commends his service and work to God "and his highest queen Maria."[19] More tellingly, Alexander Seitz of Munich mentions the Virgin Mary, but minimizes her protection of Munich in favor of a strikingly physical and local explanation of plague's origins.[20] Soon thereafter Seitz fled Munich under duress, as explored below.

The saints' sudden disappearance is surprising, given that the sixteen plague treatises examined from 1521 were printed in geographically diverse cities, including Munich, Ingolstadt, Vienna, Schwaz, Augsburg, Leipzig, and Erfurt. But the trend was not limited to new texts written in 1521. When printers reissued older texts, they also purged them of references to saints, such as the pamphlet by Ulrich Rülein von Calw, the physician of Freiberg in Saxony. Like many contemporary pamphlets, Rülein's original of 1507 provides an illustration of St. Sebastian on its cover, does not moralize the plague's cause, and ends with the terse statement "God is recommended and St. Sebastian."[21] Rülein's revised pamphlet of 1521 omits the illustration and reference to St. Sebastian, however, offering instead the more biblical statement that God's anger brings the current *Pestilentz*.[22] Saints would not return to plague literature in any significant way until after the Council of Trent, when a small number of Bavarian authors revived them.[23]

How can one explain the saints' rapid decline in plague treatises? It is unlikely that nearly all of the physician authors in 1521 suddenly embraced the new evangelical attacks on the saints, although some individuals likely did. Physicians such as Vadianus were ready for the evangelical preaching on saints, since humanists such as Erasmus had long criticized aspects of the cult of the saints. As the historian David Collins has pointed out, Luther's criticism of the veneration of saints "was strongest on points that other churchmen had already articulated." But a more likely explanation of the scope and duration of the saints' decline was the sense of uncertainty among northern European scholars concerning the status of saintly intercession. This uncertainty persisted until the Roman Church defended and reaffirmed saintly intercession at the Council of Trent.[24] Practical reasons also likely drove the saints' broad decline among physicians, since saints and sacramentals represented some degree of competition within the social world of healing. In just one example, a 1497 vernacular miracle book that promoted the Marian pilgrimage to Altötting, Bavaria, described the Virgin Mary as a doctor above all doctors due to her exceptional healing powers.[25] But perhaps decisive in this broad decline of the saints were the commercial considerations for physicians and printers amidst the new climate of religious controversy. In a competitive marketplace for healers and books, physicians and printers likely chose silence on the topic lest they offend the broad audience that they targeted.

The revolt and activism of 1521

The year 1521 saw much more than the rapid decline of the saints, also seeing the rise of activist physicians who used their plague literature to join the larger revolt that was shaking the highest levels of Church and empire. Plague literature offered these reformers a way to shape the prevailing sentiments and to respond to the events of 1521, the most dramatic of which was Luther's unremitting revolt against the papacy. After Luther refused to recant his positions before Emperor Charles V at the Diet of Worms in May 1521, the fracture of Western Christendom began in earnest. Luther and other preachers may have inspired some physicians to write, but many seem to have acted independently to address their own religious, political, and social grievances. Although the physicians Alexander Seitz, Johann Copp, and Ambrosius Jung appear in few histories of the Reformation, these obscure men deserve to be included in this broader history, since they too pursued reforms within their communities as learned laymen and civic officials. Their participation in reform demonstrates the growing importance of city physicians in civic cultural debates, as well as the impulse that epidemics gave to reforming efforts.

One important factor in the growth of physicians' activism in 1521 was the growth of vernacular print, which enabled authors to imagine a new and broader audience. The sixteen vernacular plague treatises that streamed off presses in 1521 were likely following the commercial success of religious pamphlets as well as responding to reader demand amidst the widespread epidemics of that year. As new print shops realized the profitability of vernacular sermons by new celebrities such as Luther, they rushed to market other vernacular products aimed at a broad audience. Such products included astrological writings as well as plague literature. Although plague pamphlets addressed to the "common man" date from 1473, the Reformation era was their heyday. Plague literature also became more popular in format during the 1520s, paralleling the evangelical effort to reach the "common man" by making information more accessible.[26]

The writings by the physicians Alexander Seitz (1470– ca. 1545) and Johann Copp (ca. 1490–1558) offer glimpses into how reformers shaped the fears and convictions of circa 1521 through plague and astrological literature. Sensing that dramatic times had gripped German lands, these activists predicted stunning events, such as a massive divine flood and the fall of the

Roman Church. Seitz and Copp were among a group of German physicians and astrologers who warned of a chastening flood in a series of pamphlets written between 1520 and 1525.[27] Seitz forecast the destruction for early 1524 with unusual and frightening specificity:

> [These conjunctions] will bring from the natural course of the heavens… so much lightning, thunder, hail as well as cloud-bursting rain upon mountain and valley that castle and city will be destroyed and the people will fearfully scream, howl, spoil and suffer more than is horrible to hear, let alone tolerate.[28]

By publicizing this extreme prediction, Seitz sought a great moral conversion from his audience in order to halt the coming divine flood, much like the biblical Ninevites, whom he cites as an example. In this Bible passage, God sends the prophet Jonah to the city Nineveh to preach that God will destroy the city in forty days unless the Ninevites repent.[29]

Both Seitz and Copp, the city physicians of Munich and Erfurt, respectively, saw themselves as prophets in the manner of Jonah as they wrote in 1521. To this end they embraced the new opportunities of vernacular print. Seitz's flood pamphlet was just one of three works that he composed on the approaching flood, each of which targeted different audiences. In 1521 Seitz popularized his original twenty-nine-chapter treatise on the subject as a short pamphlet addressed to the common man. Seitz also courted the most popular audience in 1521, according to one visitor at the Diet of Worms, who spotted him selling his flood prognostication to the crowds in "large illustrated letters" (*grossen gemalten brieffen*). The witness described Seitz's broadsides as forecasting "frightening and horrible things, also giving a great flood not seen since the time of Noah." At the Diet of Worms, concerns about the coming flood reached a broader European stage, as international visitors took notice and spread the news in their home countries.[30]

The radical views of Seitz and Copp extended to their plague pamphlets of 1521 as well. These works are special for their direct attacks on the Roman Church, not seen in plague treatises since Johann Vochs's 1507 text. Seitz directed his attack at religious orders, specifically the Beghards and Beguines, while holding up the secular laity as more Christian than the religious. As the city physician of Munich this was a daring move, since the town's religious orders were well established and influential. Seitz charged the Beghards and Beguines with neglecting their divine duty to care for the sick, portraying them as living immoderate and slothful lives. While they lived off the needy by begging food and charging rents, their chattering prayers did not help their fellow men with their earthly burdens. In contrast, Seitz believed that the prayers of pious, true, industrious people brought greater divine pleasure, while these orders were "truly not the brotherhood to which Christ called us."[31]

The most striking aspect of Copp's plague pamphlet is his patriotic attack on the Roman Church, which recalls Vochs's perceived struggle between Germans and Italians. In his prescriptions for diet during the plague, Copp assails the Church's dietary rules as unchristian and particularly unfair to Germans:

> Thus the Romans have made so many laws for us poor Germans and have also created the rule that we must eat fish at certain times (whichever times please them) if we actually want to avoid hunger. I think this is a good and useful law for fishermen, but I hope that God may for once give us the grace with which we can open our eyes and adhere to Christ's laws, in which he places his soul before us, rather than adhere alone to the laws of those who desire the wool and the milk from us poor lambs…[32]

Copp, instead, wants Germans to eat whatever benefits their health, and cites Matthew 15:11 for support: "[I]t is not what enters one's mouth that defiles the soul, but what comes out of the mouth." Two important strategies for attacking the medieval Church deserve comment here, since they were common among the pamphleteers of the early Reformation. Copp weakens the authority of the Roman Church by appealing to divine law, rather than the Church's laws, which he portrays as greedy and rooted in devious human nature. And, much like various German humanists of the time, Copp frames the conflict as one between two nations, Romans and Germans, rather than a conflict within a unified Church.

Copp finishes his criticism of the Church in a prophetic manner by praying that a verse from Matthew 15 may soon come to pass, that "every plant my heavenly Father has not planted will be uprooted." Striking a foreboding tone, Copp adds that this time is not distant.[33] Copp also notes that his outspoken nature on the subject has attracted the attention of the Church, which would like to condemn him as a heretic. But he remained recalcitrant, justifying his views as in accord with divine laws, much like Luther at the Diet of Worms in that same year.[34] Interestingly enough, this passage is the only section annotated in the copy at the Augsburg Staat- und Stadtsbibliothek, indicating that Copp's words attracted attention in their day.[35] Furthermore, the final words in his pamphlet offer a simple evangelical view of salvation based on faith: "Praise, Honor, and Thanks to God the Almighty, who created and redeemed us and promised eternal life to those who believe and are baptized."[36]

Seitz and Copp clearly identified with the evangelical reform of their time. Shortly after 1521 Seitz left Bavaria, and during the 1520s he sought protection among the more tolerant cities of Strasbourg, Zurich, and Basel, where he developed wildly independent religious views.[37] As he wrote in 1521 Copp addressed Erfurt just after the city had greeted Luther on his way to the Diet of Worms and experienced the turbulent "parson storm"

(*Pfaffensturm*) revolt that pressed the city council for greater religious freedoms.[38] Furthermore, Copp's contemporary astrological pamphlets dispel any doubt that he harbored evangelical convictions in 1521. Even before he wrote on plague, in 1520 Copp had dedicated his astrological pamphlet to Martin Luther, in which he predicts the fall of the "Babylonian" Church in the coming year.[39] In later astrological publications for the years 1523 and 1524, Copp speaks of God's kingdom on earth in apocalyptic terms, attacks monasticism and pilgrimage, and states that the restoration of the pure Gospel has begun.[40]

The activism of Seitz and Copp was unusual within contemporary plague treatises, even during the turbulent year of 1521. Spiritual advice occupies significantly less space in the 1521 pamphlets by the imperial physicians Nikolaus Pol, Johann Salius, and Georg Tannstetter (1482–1535), even though these works were also short and addressed to a broad audience.[41] Imperial patronage, or the lack thereof, seems to have made a considerable difference in how these authors wrote on the plague. The imperial physicians served their Habsburg patrons by encouraging stability in society as they did not predict coming cataclysms or the Apocalypse, nor did they criticize the Roman Church. The tone of their writing is also less personal in nature, lacking the references to personal experience that were typical among physicians who were pushing for change in medicine, religion, and society during the sixteenth century.

Seitz's agenda extended beyond spiritual issues and into natural medicine and was noteworthy for its personal character. Besides his prediction of the divine flood, Seitz wrote pamphlets on plague and bloodletting in 1521 that argue for medical reforms. Seitz's attack on the practice of bleeding plague victims blends personal observation with scholarly learning, much like other medical reformers of the time. He states clearly that bloodletting has cost innumerable lives and defends his unorthodox view by citing words reminiscent of Luther in 1521: "[T]he characteristic of a free conscience is to fear no one concerning the truth."[42] Seitz wanted physicians to recognize the complexities of bloodletting, pointing out the nuanced views of Avicenna, Mesue, and Gentilis, who advocated bloodletting only when the blood was poisoned.[43] To support his case Seitz relates his own experience. Among recent patients at the monastery of Scheffelar, ten that had blood drawn soon died, while the one person left alone soon recovered. Seitz also states that, when plague broke out in his own home, he saved six people without bloodletting, while the one he bled soon died.[44]

Seitz's plague pamphlet of 1521 similarly contains unusual medical thought based on personal experience. Most strikingly, he offers a local and physical explanation of the plague's origins within Munich that comes at the expense of popular religious belief. Addressing the problem of why more people from St. Peter's parish were dying of plague compared to the parish of Our Lady's Church (*Frauenkirche*), Seitz discards the popular explanation that the Virgin Mary gives special protection to her own parish. While Seitz believes that both parishes enjoy Mary's equal love and mercy, he seeks the answer in the physical purity of these two neighborhoods. Seitz blames the prevailing winds for differences in purity, since the most dangerous midday wind strikes the houses of St. Peter's parish, while the other parish receives the healthy midnight wind. Seitz also connects cleanliness and plague protection by explaining that the alleys of Our Lady's parish are much nicer, lighter, and cleaner. Seitz notes that he observed this connection in his earlier work in the Swiss Aargau, where he witnessed more plague deaths in the dirtier rural villages compared to the cleaner town of Baden.[45] Such thoughts represent an interesting "local" reflection on plague's origins that breaks the conventions of a genre given to discussing scholarly authorities rather than local circumstances.

Seitz's plague pamphlet of 1521 also departs from many contemporary plague pamphlets in its intense effort to justify medicine. Even though physicians had long been concerned with justifying the use of natural medicine to a broad audience, Seitz takes the standard rhetoric to a new and extreme level. As was common at the time, Seitz cites Ecclesiasticus 38 to demonstrate the divine foundation of medicine and physicians: choosing to take medicine honors God, while not taking medicine shortens one's life. Seitz takes the reasoning further, however, to state that those who do not take medicine commit suicide, since no one has the right to shorten one's life.[46] This was an extreme position and marks the first time it appeared in German plague literature, although it gained prominence later after Martin Luther embraced it in his popular plague sermon of 1527, as discussed below.

In sum, Seitz and Copp contributed to the turbulence of their time as self-styled prophets and acted as reformers in their own right. The case of Seitz, moreover, confirms the persona of a reformer in this volatile era, first encountered in Johann Vochs. As medicine and healing began to change along with its cultural context, men such as Seitz and Vochs pursued reforms in both medicine and religion.

The Protestant reform of "spiritual medicine"

The omission of saints and sacramentals from late medieval spiritual medicine was just the beginning of a specifically Protestant reform movement. In the decades after 1520 Protestant physicians and clerics began to reimagine other aspects of "spiritual medicine." These efforts brought new emphasis on faith and trust in God or Jesus and attempted to redefine the process of confession as a direct interaction between penitent and God. The new evangelical "spiritual medicine" was useful as a new and purportedly better plague treatment and also as a way to attract converts. In this regard it became central to the popularization of evangelical religious reforms, forming the foundation of much devotional literature in later decades, apparent in the work of the physician Ambrosius Jung and the cleric Urbanus Rhegius. Their stories provide an early history of Protestant spiritual medicine, which has been well studied heretofore only among later English Calvinists.[47]

The plague pamphlets of the Augsburg physician Ambrosius Jung (1471–1548) provide a detailed glimpse into how this reform of spiritual medicine unfolded in the Reformation's first decades. Jung first published two plague pamphlets in 1494, one in Latin and one in German, and later revised this German work in 1521 and 1535.[48] His first vernacular pamphlet portrays himself as a pious young doctor interested in his community's spiritual and medical health, certainly an effort to impress his patrons, the bishop, and the cathedral chapter of Augsburg. Jung's genuine interest in spiritual issues is borne out over the decades, however, as he revised his formula of "spiritual medicine" in light of contemporary religious reforms. The revisions of 1521 and 1535 reveal Jung as an independent reformer, attempting to change local piety even before local preachers. Jung's pamphlets were also among the more successful in the early history of the plague genre, as his 1521 work was reprinted five times with minor revisions in Augsburg, Strasbourg, and Innsbruck up to 1563.[49]

As one might expect, Jung's "spiritual medicine" in 1494 contained the standard elements of traditional piety. When plague is near, Jung encouraged his readers to seek a "spiritual medicine" (*geystliche artzney*) from the spiritual fathers of the Holy Scriptures and confessor priests. The spiritual medicine here is confession for all who have "wounded themselves deeply" with sin:

> Then repent by first turning yourself to God with a repentant heart, with a remorseful expression of confession and complete acts of atonement and penance with the intention thereafter of keeping the commandments of God. Perhaps the Almighty God sees the thought and good will of your heart and forgives you, but do not deceive Him. You err. But as far as you are righteous, you will find mercy.[50]

These statements are traditional in form and theology considering their emphasis on good works, such as the act of confession and the performance of penance, as well as the explicit role of the confessor priest. Divine forgiveness also seems to be conditional, dependent upon proper performance. Jung revised this key passage in 1521 and again in 1535, however, revealing a continuing process of reform:

> 1521: As the Almighty God grips a person with this sickness / he must react as a Christian / turn to Him with the entire heart / and seek His most-healing medicine / true regret and confession / and take with the highest desire of the heart / His precious body / in which lies the throwing off and forgiveness of all sins / and the eternal life / and give yourself over entirely to His mercy and grace.[51]

> 1535: As the Almighty God grips a person with this sickness / he must react as a Christian / turn to Him with the entire heart / and seek His most-healing medicine / true regret and recognition of one's sins / with the bitterness of his heart / he must turn himself over to the good will of the Lord / and Christ his savior with a firm faith / since He died for your sins / and rose again for your justification / and trust the Lord of the Gospel / that your sins are forgiven.[52]

The new elements in Jung's 1521 instructions for confession reveal that he was taking part in broader religious reform efforts in Augsburg. Although the standard formula appears, that one must turn to God with true regret, give confession (*beicht*), and lead a repentant life, the priestly confessor is notably absent. Confession becomes instead a direct interaction with God, part of a process to prepare for receiving the Eucharist. In his revisions of 1535, Jung omits the reference to the Eucharist and dropped the very term "confession" in favor of "recognition of one's sins" (*bekantnuß seiner sünd*), while including new references to faith and trust in God. Jung here seems to be endorsing the view that the process of receiving forgiveness is an internal and spiritual process, independent of external acts and sacraments. Faith also plays a key role in this process rather than acts of atonement. Brief comparison to a more traditional plague pamphlet from Augsburg illustrates how far Jung's advice had come. The 1531 edition of a plague pamphlet by the Spanish physician Luis von Lobera does not mention divine punishment, sin, or confession but, rather, promotes gaining divine favor through divine services such as fasting, prayer, and alms giving. And, much like Ambrosius Jung's pamphlet of 1494, divine mercy comes if the works are pleasing to God and is not a simple matter of trust and faith, as in Jung's 1535 formulation.[53]

Jung reformed his "spiritual medicine" while also revising other parts of his pamphlets according to evangelical views. He opens his 1521 text with the heading "Jhesus Maria" whereas the opening of 1494 calls upon the Trinity, Virgin Mary, and heavenly host. Jung also replaces references to saints in his 1494 preface with a new description of an angry God in 1521, softened, however, by the image of Jesus as a "supernatural doctor" who can heal in body and soul.[54] In 1535 Jung doubles the preaching in his introduction and replaces "Jhesus Maria" at the opening with the evangelical "Christ Jesus our Justice." In this longer introduction, Jung dwells on the inability of humans to perfect their own nature and offers Christ as the solution in characteristically Lutheran language: if humans are to be freed from the punishments of an angry God, "it must happen through our sole mediator and seat of grace (*gnadenstůhl*), Jesus Christ, to whom we have open admittance, who also bears every burden with us."[55] Use of the term "seat of grace" (*gnadenstůhl*) suggests that Jung drew from Martin Luther's 1532 "Sermon on the Sum of the Christian Life," who famously used this term to contrast between the judgment and mercy functions of Christ. Jung's overall message emphasizes the mercy of God, since God means only to discipline his children by sending the *Pestilentz*. By accompanying this punishment with his healing word, Jung states that God acts like a "true Doctor, who will not allow people to spoil in great danger."[56]

Jung's revisions hold much in common with trends among Augsburg's reforming preachers.[57] In 1521 the Augsburg cathedral preacher Urbanus Rhegius also began to publicize his ideas on how to confess one's sins daily, published in a seven-page vernacular pamphlet. While Rhegius is careful in this pamphlet not to deny the role of the confessor priest or auricular confession, his intent is to strengthen a sinner's direct relationship with God. For Rhegius, the biblical King David becomes the model of the penitent, as a man who achieved a great reversal of fortune when he sought forgiveness from God. Rhegius proposes some words that a person can say daily to confess to God, although he acknowledges that one can say any words one chooses. Much like Jung, Rhegius describes true penitence as a "healing medicine" and God as a true doctor of sinners.[58] Both Jung and Rhegius led the reforming trend in Augsburg in 1521, since emphasis on the repentance of King David and descriptions of God/Christ as a doctor became dominant themes in later Protestant plague literature.

Although a direct connection between Jung and Rhegius in 1521 is unclear, they were reacting to the same conditions on the eve of the Reformation in which the meaning and form of confession were up for debate. The reform of confession was of great interest to the laity in particular, and physicians were no exception. Historian Miriam Chrisman explains that the lack of clerical action on confession in the early years of the German Reformation prompted the laity to act themselves. Her work demonstrates that nobles, male and female, worked to abolish auricular confession to a priest in favor of confession to a fellow layperson or directly to God. The fact that Ambrosius Jung omitted the role of the confessor priest from his directions for confession in 1521, while Rhegius did not, also conforms to Chrisman's interpretation: "The reformers wrote on the question, the laity acted."[59]

Jung and Rhegius were also friends as well as allies within Augsburg civic politics. When Rhegius married Anna Weißbrugger in Augsburg in 1525, Jung marched behind the bride and groom in the wedding procession, following Augsburg's mayor Ulrich Rechlinger, local evangelical preachers, and other dignitaries.[60] This ceremony was an act of defiance to traditional religious teachings and Catholic political forces within the city. Although it is difficult to categorize Jung into one of the emerging Protestant camps, it is clear that he moved among the Protestant clerical and political elites of his day. Jung was also a friend of the Strasbourg reformer Martin Bucer and has been described as a Zwinglian activist by some historians.[61]

Specifically Protestant voices appeared in plague and religious devotional literature from Augsburg by the end of the 1520s. Most important for the evangelical reform of "spiritual medicine" in the German Reformation was

Urbanus Rhegius's 1529 work *Spiritual Medicine for Healthy and Sick during These Dangerous Times*.[62] This sixty-two page pamphlet propagandizes Protestant spiritual healing, promoting the idea that healing and salvation come through an intense direct relationship with God. Here Rhegius describes his work as spreading spiritual medicine for spiritual comfort, as prepared from Christ's pharmacy, the Holy Scriptures.[63] Since it was marketed self-consciously during threatening times to a broad audience, it bears many similarities to vernacular plague pamphlets and certainly was inspired by the same atmosphere of religious tension and fear of divine punishment. While Rhegius's "spiritual medicine" appears as various evangelical teachings and practices that ease fears, repentance and confession play a central role in the work. Echoing his 1521 pamphlet on daily confession, Rhegius states that sinners who repent and turn to God can have forgiveness daily. Rhegius believed that, when a sinner turns to God in repentance, his/her sickness or punishment either stops or otherwise serves to better his/her relationship with God.[64] This demonstrates the great pastoral role that Protestant reformers envisioned for sickness and medicine in this decade.[65] Much advice also comforts sinners fearing death and Hell. Arguing against saintly intercession, Rhegius states that God alone is a person's helper in need and that sinners stand alone in the hands of God.[66]

Rhegius's 1529 work on spiritual medicine is of great importance to the history of the Reformation since it became a best-selling devotional text. It was reprinted an extraordinary ninety times in ten languages over the next century, spreading Protestant "spiritual medicine" far and wide in Europe.[67] Thus, the reform of "spiritual medicine" became an integral part of the Protestant Reformation, and "spiritual medicine" itself became an important tool for evangelizing among Europe's vernacular audiences. One can say that Rhegius – and Jung to a lesser extent – made "spiritual medicine" into a Protestant program of persuasion for this plagued era.

The Protestant Reformation and natural medicine

The Protestant Reformation's impact on healing extended beyond spiritual medicine and even affected attitudes about natural medicine. While physicians began a broad reform in the 1520s, Protestant clerics supported their agenda while also seeking to advance their own interests. Martin Luther's thought in particular reveals Protestants' new embrace of natural medicine by the later 1520s, as Protestant leaders sought to reform life and society more broadly. Following the rejection of saints and sacramentals as avenues of divine healing, Luther intensified contemporary praise of earthly medicine as divine and necessary. With his new rhetoric Luther embraced physicians' unfolding reform of healing and sought to guide it in the face of two emergent concerns in the later 1520s: fears that "faith alone" encouraged medical passivity, and the effort to find biblically sanctioned avenues of divine healing that could replace saints and sacramentals within Protestant culture.

Luther's plague sermon of 1527 is well known as one of the most reprinted plague texts of the sixteenth century, as well as for its discussion of the ethical issues surrounding whether one should flee the plague. Against medieval precedent, Luther recommended that Christians remain in their communities during a plague in order to show their trust in God, although he also justified flight to some extent as well. Another important break with medieval precedent was Luther's rejection of the notion that a general poisoning of the atmosphere caused the Wittenberg plague of 1527, as explored further in Chapter 5. Luther believed, rather, that its origin lay entirely in the level of local filth.[68] Luther's pamphlet of 1527 was among the most reprinted plague texts of the time, appearing in nine editions in its first year and at least thirty total printings up to 1631.[69] As a result, Luther became one of the era's leading voices on plague.

Just as important for the German reform of healing was that Luther's plague sermon of 1527 embraced the decade's new and stronger praise for physicians and natural medicine. Its unusually strong justification of natural medicine has only recently drawn attention.[70] Like many authors before him, Luther gave the standard justification of medicine from Ecclesiasticus 38, that God created medicines for the benefit of humans and that the prudent do not neglect them. What makes Luther's position special, however, is his embrace of the more extreme view, first seen in Alexander Seitz's 1521 plague treatise, that equates the neglect of medicine with suicide. In Luther's view, he who neglects medicine murders himself, just like a person who neglects food, drink, clothes, and shelter.[71]

Luther's threat of grave sin for those who neglect medicine is the heart of a broader attack on Christian resistance to natural medicine, which some feared had grown in response to Protestant reforms. A small minority of the new Protestant preachers began to proclaim that "true" Christians do not use natural medicine but rely on faith alone during sickness. In a 1532 record from his Table Talk, Luther mentions that his Wittenberg rival Andreas Karlstadt (1486–1541) was preaching exactly this. The issue arose when the mayor of Wittenberg sought Luther's opinion on the subject, having heard of Karlstadt's views.[72] Given his plague advice of 1527, Luther had long disdained this resistance to natural medicine and therefore encouraged earthly action. Luther believed that the logic of faith alone could endanger physical health when extended to medical matters.

The force of Luther's defense of natural medicine indicates that he was concerned about much more than divergent preachers, and was also fighting other beliefs that may have strengthened resistance to natural medicine. Recent converts to the evangelical teachings may have believed that their new and "pure" Christianity promised greater protection from the divine punishment of plague, thus making natural medicine unnecessary. And the new Protestant emphasis on the power of God as well as mankind's powerlessness in matters of salvation may have encouraged more traditional forms of fatalism – that God has predetermined the end of a person's life, which human action cannot alter. For Luther, however, the divine command to use natural medicine outweighed all of these other considerations.

Although Luther was very friendly to natural medicine and its practitioners, his broader thought on healing and medicine was rooted in spiritual concerns. Luther viewed life as a continual struggle against the Devil, sin, and sickness, for which only Christian faith offered an ultimate solution.[73] Like many theologians, Luther prioritized the health of the soul over the health of the body and believed that spiritual healing had to precede bodily healing. What was new to Luther's thought, however, was his theology of faith alone and the implications he developed from this idea. He believed that only Christ could heal the root cause of sickness, which was sin, thus supporting his arguments against the cult of the saints. Luther was also fond of using medical metaphors to express his spirituality, describing even the Word of God as a "medicine" used by Christ to sustain the health of his people.[74]

More important for the Protestant reform of healing was Luther's idea that natural medicine contains the Word of God, the most potent force on earth for Protestants. For Luther, pills or medicinal herbs work when the Word of God binds to them in a miraculous way. This belief is an extension of Luther's view of divine agency in the physical world, which holds that God works in the world through external media, such as the physical elements of the sacraments, through the spoken words of a preacher, or through creation itself. Luther recognized little separation between primary and secondary causes on earth since he viewed God to be present in creation. Although God's presence is obscured to the human senses and reason, a person can recognize divine presence in creation through faith.[75] Thus Luther judged natural medicine to be a worthy and necessary means of divine healing power.

A fundamental motive in Luther's praise of natural medicine may have also been strategic in nature. In the attempt to build a new Protestant piety that had social depth, it was important to find proper replacements for saints and sacramentals. In the absence of these tangible aids of spiritual consolation that were so important within late medieval piety, Protestant piety may have seemed spare and otherworldly to many. Luther himself admitted the difficulties of believing that one could gain salvation by "faith alone" for those accustomed to contributing to their own salvation through their own earthly actions.[76] Luther then may have viewed natural medicine, suffused with divine power, as it were, to be an appropriate replacement for saints and sacramentals in the new piety. Natural medicine could be both physical and divine, but, unlike saintly intercession, had the advantage of direct biblical justification.

The Protestant embrace of natural medicine also blended well with the self-help ethics underpinning practical and technical literature, which experienced rapid growth in the sixteenth century. Luther and his followers sought an active laity that did not shy from helping themselves to the divine gift of medicine. Although Luther praised physicians as administrators of

God's healing creation, he believed that anyone can administer these divine healing gifts, including healers of the lower medical orders and self-healers. Alongside Luther's response to Karlstadt in 1532 is an interesting reflection on the failures of physicians and the successes of lay healers:

> Healing comes from the application of nature derived from books, even as knowledge of law is not from books but is drawn from nature. It is remarkable that a prince is sure to find effective the medicines which he administers to himself but finds ineffective what his physician prescribes. So both electors have eye drops which help when they take them, no matter whether their affliction is caused by heat or cold, but a physician would not dare prescribe the drops.[77]

Here Luther chides physicians for their over-reliance on book learning and specifically the Greek theories of heat and cold. Luther implies that, if one wants to experience divine healing, one must turn to God's creation itself rather than ancient books.

The reform of healing in popular print and images

The Protestant reform of healing reached audiences far and wide not only in vernacular plague literature but also in other medical and religious texts and images. Luther's attack on resistance to natural medicine became a new priority among other authors seeking to bolster the cause of natural medicine. Luther's words appeared in one of the most popular general medical pamphlets of the era, the *Pharmacy for the Common Man*, produced in Augsburg around 1529. This anonymous work compiles recipes from previous books by Hieronymus Brunschwig and Michael Puff von Schrick, but stands out for the unusual three-page sermon that opens the text. This preface echoes Luther's efforts to justify medicine as a necessary divine art and draws a close comparison between medicine and the Word of God:

> The medical arts are the most precious, most useful, and most necessary thing that has come to earth and will ever come to earth. Like the worthy, healing Word of God that is given and spread within the world and fully comforts, edifies, and satisfies blind, fearful, and quaking hearts and consciences with the help of the Holy Spirit, medicine most potently protects and graciously saves the sick, weak souls from eternal death, from the depravity and ill-intent of the Devil, and from hellish pain.[78]

Much like Luther's message, earthly medicine here not only fights sickness but also aids the soul in the supernatural struggle against the Devil. Someone who experiences God's healing power is likely to have a strong faith that can resist the Devil.

The most telling link between the *Pharmacy for the Common Man* and Luther's medical thought is the former's attack on resistance to natural medicine that the author sees among Protestants and the wealthy. The author states that people have the wrong sense of the evangelical message when they ignore the admonitions of pastors and spiritual leaders to visit the doctors (*ärzte*) but, rather, insist that God will heal them without medicine. Although these people think they have a good evangelical view, the author believes it is blasphemous to wait for spiritual healing while neglecting God's gift of earthly medicine. Suggesting that the wealthy refuse to see doctors out of stinginess, the author uses particularly strong language to denounce greed: "You can refuse the medicine that God offers to help you… and Mammon, who is your god, can also let you die in the Devil's name."[79]

The evangelical preface of the *Pharmacy for the Common Man* appeared many times in contemporary printed media, lasting well into the seventeenth century. Many, if not all, of the pamphlet's eighteen editions listed in the VD16 contain this preface, including texts produced between circa 1529 and 1564 in the cities of Augsburg, Nuremberg, Erfurt, Vienna, Leipzig, and Marburg.[80] The preface also appears among later versions of the text in the seventeenth century, including an Erfurt print of 1619.[81] Much of the *Pharmacy*'s content, including the preface, was also reprinted under different titles into the seventeenth century, thus spreading the message even further.[82]

The key themes of the broad reform of healing – the decline of the saints and the increasing prominence of natural medicine – are also apparent in changes made to the images used in this text and other medical literature of the time. Among the most remarkable expressions of Protestants' new medical ethic is the title page woodcut that appears on the early Augsburg editions of the *Pharmacy for the Common Man* (Figure 3.2). This woodcut celebrates the most autonomous form of medical self-help by depicting a common man and woman cultivating herbs in the countryside. God appears in the sky commanding or blessing the work carried out below. In a possible artistic portrayal of Luther's idea that effective medicines contain the Word of God, the artist uses Sirach/Ecclesiasticus 38 as a border: "The Lord brought forth medicine from the earth, and the wise man does not neglect it."[83] This image appeared on the original edition from Heinrich Stainer's press in Augsburg circa 1529, as well as the later edition of circa 1530. Augsburg printers reused the image to adorn other general medical works intended for the common man and poor country folk until at least 1549.[84]

This image differs dramatically from the standard late medieval images of saints, which were intended for spiritual contemplation. Here the focus is on earthly life, drawn naturalistically enough to recognize a city in the distance and authentic herbs in the foreground. A Protestant theme of spiritual equality is also present in the inclusion of both a common man and woman with a commanding God. Most striking, however, is the artist's emphasis on

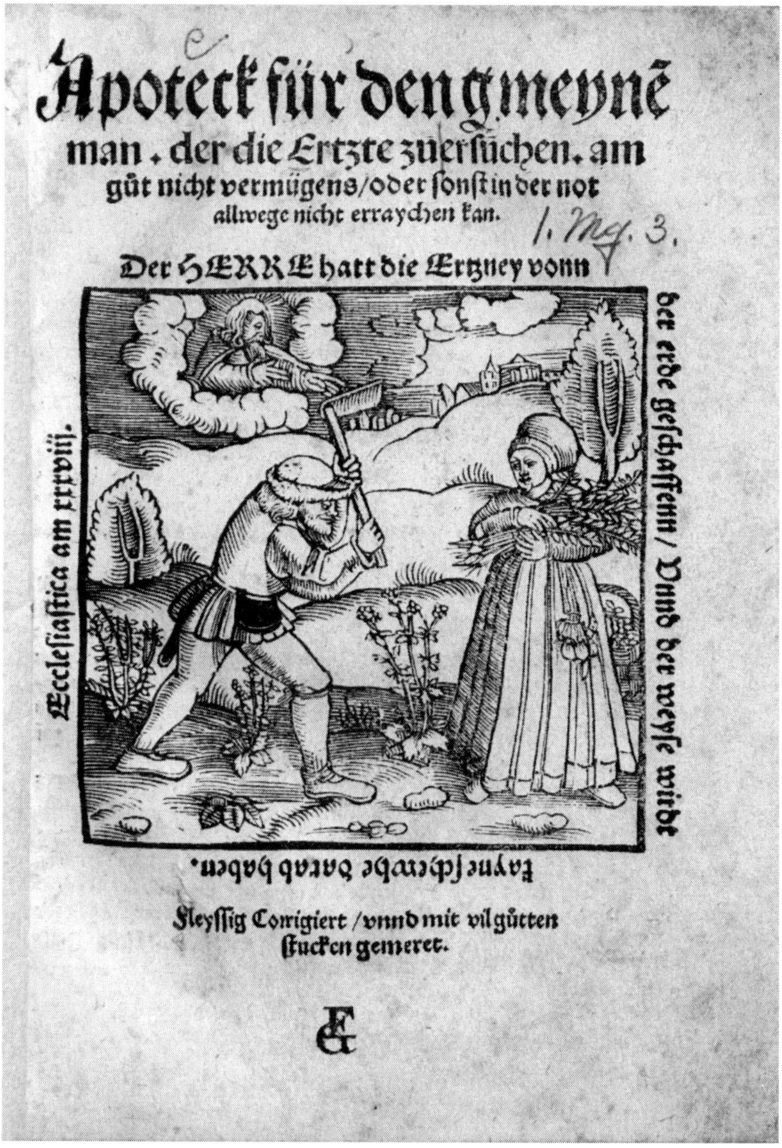
Apoteck für den gmeynē
man. der die Ertzte zu ersüchen. am
güt nicht vermügens/oder sonst in der not
allwege nicht erraychen kan.
Der HERRE hatt die Ertzney vonn
der erde geschaffenn/ Vnnd der weyse wirdt
kayne scheühe darab haben.
Ecclesiastica am xxxviij.
Fleyssig Corrigiert/vnnd mit vil gütten
stucken gemeret.

Figure 3.2 The divine origin of medicine
Title page illustration: *Apoteck für den gmeynē man* (Augsburg?: Stainer?, 1530?)
Boston Medical Library in the Francis A. Countway Library of Medicine
Call number: Rare Books 1.Mg.3 (reproduced with permission)

the activity of harvesting the medicinal plants. Protestant themes appear in the man and woman's direct access to the divine healing powers of the earth, in contrast to late medieval works that focused on the figures that mediate healing to humans. As seen in Chapter 1, Culmacher's image of circa 1495 (Figure 1.1) gives a level of spiritual helpers between earth and God that included saints and the Virgin Mary. Furthermore, in this 1529 image God is no longer linked to the angel of death but, rather, to the medicinal plants as the agents of life.

The image's emphasis on the common man and woman also fits the pamphlet's title and medical content. The title advertises aid for the common man who cannot afford medicine or who cannot reach a doctor in time. The *Pharmacy for the Common Man* was also among the most user-friendly and "popular" pamphlets of the era, since its recipes offer simple medicines made by boiling and distilling and due to its translation of the Latin notation used by physicians and pharmacists. For example, the author explains that the "Recipe" or "R." that starts many recipes means "take," that one "dragma" is equivalent in weight to one quintlin, and so forth.[85] Such explanations were an important bridge between the medical culture of learned professionals and that of home medicine.

One other title page image of circa 1530 depicts the general shift away from saints and towards natural medicine, although it is difficult to tie it directly to a specifically Protestant message (Figure 3.3). In this Constance edition of Caspar Kegler's plague pamphlet, the artist reworks the traditional image from Culmacher's pamphlet of circa 1495 (Figure 1.1), amounting to a fundamental change in the method of plague protection.[86] Although the Kegler image mirrors the format of the Culmacher image, the artist replaces all references to spiritual medicine with forms of natural medicine. The Eucharist, prayer, and the saints disappear in favor of herbs, medicines, and medical tools. The saints themselves become two physicians, who stand ready with swords and medicine to resist the scourge of God. Their foreign dress suggests that they are physicians from eastern lands, perhaps Andromachus and Mithridates offering their ancient antidotes of theriac and mithridate, or perhaps even Sts. Cosmas and Damian holding medicine and a urine flask. If the artist did draw upon the iconography of Sts. Cosmas and Damian to make this image, the removal of their halos emphasizes their roles as physicians rather than saints. This omission would make sense amid the decline of the saints during the 1520s, as explored above. In any case, the artist depicts these men as powerful, since the shapes of their vessels match the vessels that resist the sword of the angel of death.[87] This image contrasts with the earlier editions of Kegler's plague pamphlet that appeared in Leipzig in 1521 and 1529, which feature images of St. Christopher and St. Veronica, respectively (Figure 3.4). The last vernacular plague treatise to feature an image of a saint was the 1530 Regensburg edition of Kegler's work, which retained the 1529 image of St. Veronica with the *sudarium* of Christ.[88]

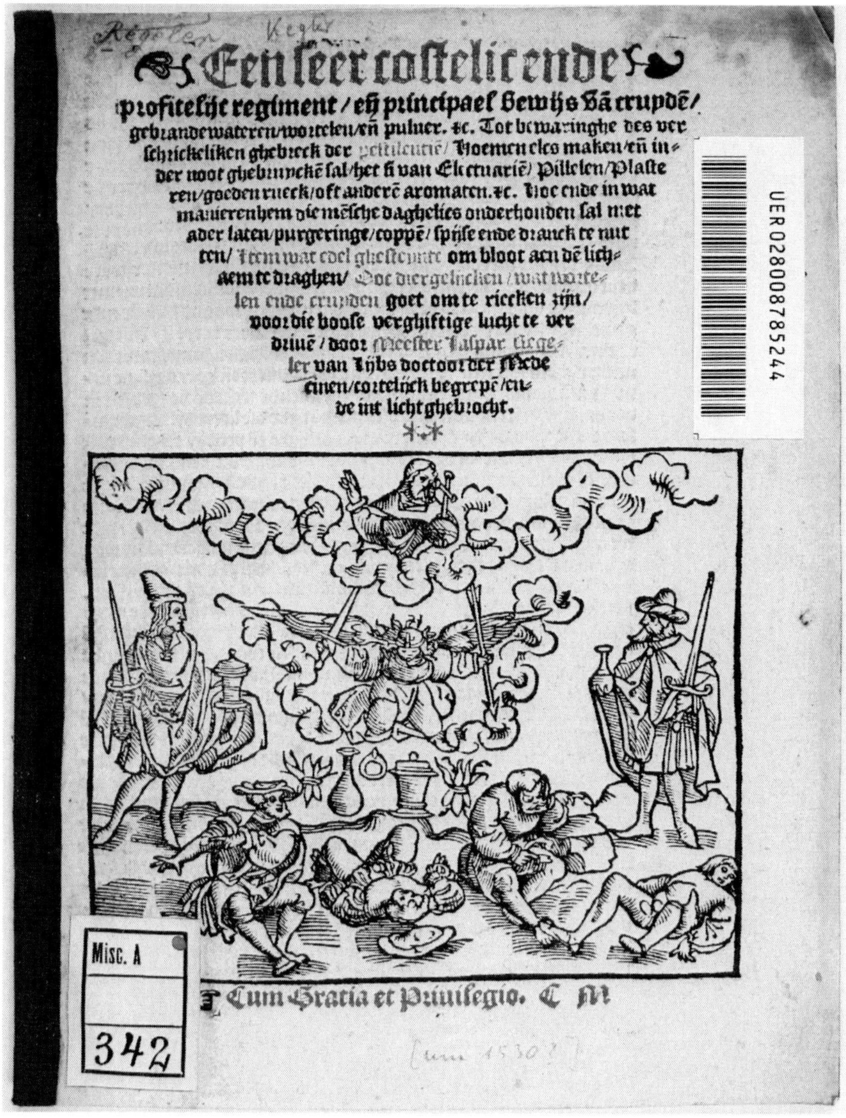

Figure 3.3 Medicine as defense against the divine scourge
Title page illustration: Caspar Kegler, *Een seer costelic ende profitelije regiment...* (Constance: Johann Haselberck, ca. 1530)
University Library Erlangen-Nürnberg
Call number: H00 / Misc.A 342 (reproduced with permission)

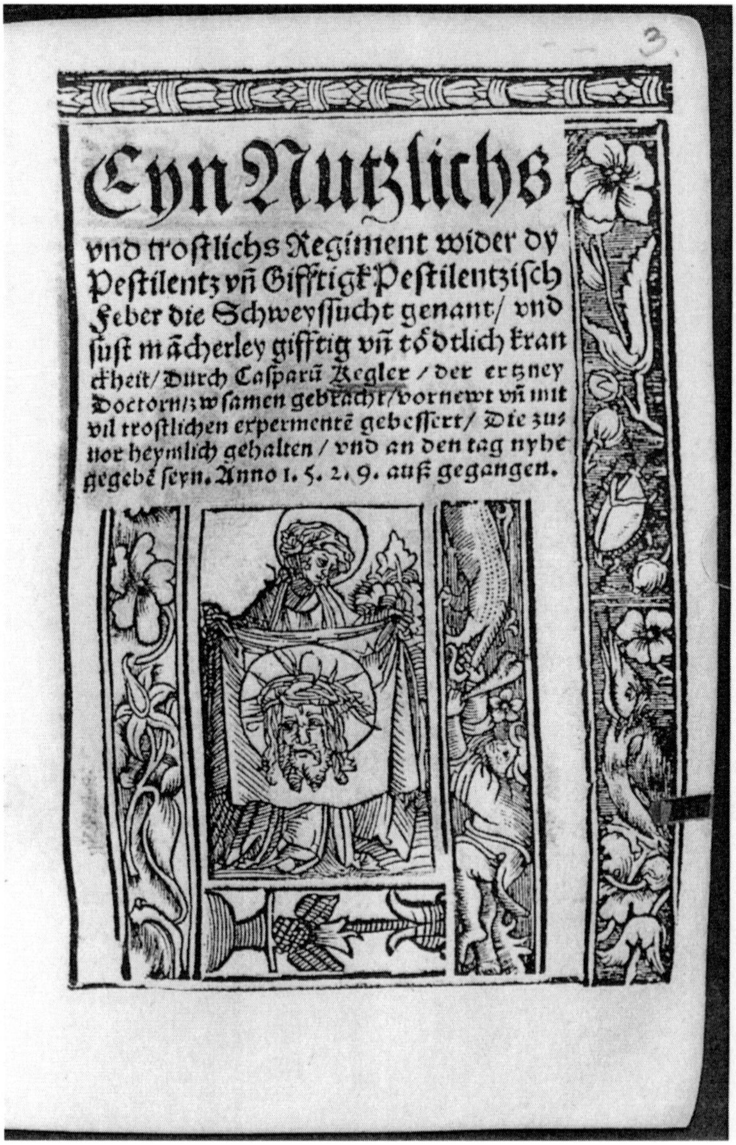
Eyn Nutzlichs
vnd trostlichs Regiment wider dy
Pestilentz vñ Gifftigk Pestilentzisch
Feber die Schweyssucht genant/ vnd
sust mãcherley gifftig vñ tödtlich kran
ckheit/ Durch Casparũ Kegler / der ertzney
Doctorn/ zusamen gebracht/ vornewt vñ mit
vil trostlichen expermentẽ gebessert/ Die zu
uor heymlich gehalten / vnd an den tag nyhe
gegebẽ seyn. Anno 1.5.2.9. auß gegangen.

Figure 3.4 St. Veronica and Jesus (*sudarium*)

Title page illustration: Caspar Kegler, *Eyn Nutzlichs vnd trostlichs Regiment…* (Leipzig: Valten Schumann, 1529)

Bayerischer Staatsbibliothek München

Call number: Res/ Path 98 #Beibd.3 (reproduced with permission)

Upon first inspection, the Constance illustration's emphasis on ancient medicines of pagan pedigree may strike the modern viewer as a secularization or naturalization of the plague response. In light of contemporary preaching on the divine power of natural medicine, however, we can surmise that common opinion understood that divine or perhaps magical power enables the medicines to resist the angel of death.[89] Moreover, there was a long tradition of physicians since Avicenna that described the miraculous healing power of theriac and other medicines in divine terms. In this image it is up to the plagued humans to take up and use the elements of God's creation so that God can protect them from the angel of punishment and death. While this depiction of natural medicine is not necessarily Lutheran, or even Protestant, it depicts nonetheless how natural medicine gained prominence through the decline of the saints. In this reworking of the late medieval image nature retains divine healing powers and is therefore not a secularization of healing.

Conclusion

Epidemics affecting German lands between 1519 and 1530 heightened fears about physical health just as new preaching heightened concerns about the moral authority and teachings of the traditional Church. It is no surprise, then, that some physicians responded to both concerns in their vernacular plague literature. In this atmosphere, healing itself became an important front for reformers' new agendas, since this topic touched equally on body, soul, and society. While physicians seem to have been happy to omit saints from their texts and to incorporate stronger justifications of natural medicine, others took their reforms further to participate in the unfolding Protestant Reformation. The new evangelical preaching played a primary role in bringing about this broad reform of healing through its attack on saints and through its reformers' savvy use of vernacular print. Yet this Protestant reform of healing also fit the worldly motives of university-trained physicians as they sought greater social authority. Thus, through an overlapping of interests, physicians and evangelical reformers brought about a reform of late medieval healing, natural and spiritual, during the 1520s. Chapter 5 explores how this reform shaped spiritual and natural medicine in profound ways later in the sixteenth century.

Notes

1 Beyond proliferating epidemics, this unusual conjunction of events included the German Peasants' War of 1524–25, the sack of Rome by imperial forces in 1527, and the Ottoman siege of Vienna in 1529. On flood predictions: Heike Talkenberger, *Sintflut: Prophetie und Zeitgeschehen in Texten und Holzschnitten astrologischer Flugschriften 1488–1528* (Tübingen: Niemeyer, 1990).

2 Andrew Cunningham and Ole Peter Grell, *The Four Horsemen of the Apocalypse: Religion, War, Famine and Death in Reformation Europe* (Cambridge: Cambridge University Press, 2000). See also Caspar Kegler's use of an apocalyptic tone in Chapter 4 below.

3 Even the most wide-ranging collections of articles on Reformation history overlook physicians, medicine/healing, and disease: R. Po-chia Hsia, Ed., *A Companion to the Reformation World* (Malden, MA: Blackwell, 2004). New attempts to survey the Reformation also do not mention these topics: Euan Cameron, *The European Reformation*, 2nd Edn (Oxford: Oxford University Press, 2012); Lee Palmer Wandel, *The Reformation: Towards a New History* (Cambridge: Cambridge University Press, 2011). This neglect comes despite recent work on medicine and the Reformation: Jürgen Helm and Annette Winkelmann, Eds., *Religious Confessions and the Sciences in the Sixteenth Century* (Leiden: Brill, 2001); Ole Peter Grell and Andrew Cunningham, Eds., *Medicine and the Reformation* (London: Routledge, 1993).

4 John L. Flood, "'Safer on the Battlefield than in the City': England, the 'Sweating Sickness', and the Continent," *Renaissance Studies* 17 (2003): 147–176; Otto Clemen, "Zur Literatur über den englischen Schweiß von 1529," *Archiv für Geschichte der Medizin* 15 (1923): 85–97.

5 Steven Ozment, *Magdalena and Balthasar* (New Haven, CT: Yale University Press, 1989), 125.

6 "Doctor Aurbachius optimus vir, dicebat instaurationem Euangelij fuisse detrimentosam omnibus artificibus, exceptis medicis. Omnes enim pictores, statuarij, aurifices conqueruntur se valde esurire. Medicis vero prodest, quia postquam sancti desiderunt curare morbos, iterum ad medicos homines confugiunt." Johannes Manlius, *LOCORVM communium collectanea: A IOHANNE MANLIO per multos annos, tum ex Lectionibus D. PHILIPPI MELANCHTONIS, tum ex aliorum doctissimorum virorum relationibus excerpta, & nuper in odinem ab eodem redacta, iamque postremum recognita.* (1572), fol. 70. Johannes Manlius lived in the second half of the sixteenth century and was a historian and adviser of Emperor Maximilian II. Christian Gottlieb Jöcher, *Christian Gottlieb Jöchers Allgemeines Gelehrten-Lexicon*, Vol. III (Hildesheim: Georg Olms, 1961), 114–115.

7 Otto Clemen interpreted this saying as coming from Heinrich Stromer, "Zur Lebensgeschichte Heinrich Stromers von Auerbach," *Neues Archiv für sächsische Geschichte* 24 (1903): 100–110, 108. It is possible, however, that this "Doctor Aurbachius" is the lesser-known Sebastian Roth von Auerbach (ca. 1492–1555). Although these two were not related, both men were medical professors at the University of Leipzig and were proponents of the Reformation. On Roth, see: Jöcher, *Christian Jöchers Allgemeines Gelehrten-Lexicon*, Vol. III, 2250.

8 On the turn against the saints in the early Reformation, see: Carlos Eire, *War against the Idols: The Reformation of Worship from Erasmus to Calvin* (Cambridge: Cambridge University Press, 1986); Carol Piper Heming, *Protestants and the Cult of the Saints in German-Speaking Europe, 1517–1531* (Kirksville, MO: Truman State University Press, 2003); and Bridget Heal, "Images of the Virgin Mary and Marian Devotion in Protestant Nuremberg," in *Religion and Superstition in Reformation Europe*, Eds. Helen Parish and William G. Naphy (Manchester: Manchester University Press, 2002): 25–46.

9 Joachim von Watt/Vadianus, *Ein kurtz und trüwlich underricht / wider die sorgklich kranckeyt der Pestilētz / nach aller notturfft vnd ordnung so in söllichem fal / betracht uñ gehaltē werden mag: neulich ußgan gen / uñ zů nutz gemeyner Lantschafft der eydgenoschafft zůsamen bracht im xv. hundert vnd xix. Jar* (Basel: Adam Petri, 1519).

10 Sixtus Kolbenschlag, *Ein nutzbarlichs Regiment von Doctor Sixten Kolbenschlag von Mergathem wider die pestilentz zů bewaren und Ihenen die do mit begriffen hilff zů reichen* (Nuremberg: Fryderichen Peypus, 1519), fol. 11. Very little is known about Kolbenschlag's life.

11 Johannes Ninck, *Arzt und Reformator Vadian: Ein Charakterbild aus großer Zeit* (St. Gallen: Buchhandlung der Evangelischen Gesellschaft St. Gallens, 1936), 68–78, at 70.

12 Miriam Usher Chrisman, *Lay Culture, Learned Culture: Books and Social Change in Strasbourg, 1480–1599* (New Haven, CT: Yale University Press, 1982), 170–182.

13 Von Watt/Vadianus, sig. B2r.

14 See also *Regiment wider die Pestilentz* (Nuremberg: Fryderich Beypuß, 1520); and Marcus Deas Veringer, *Ein Kurtz nützlichs Regiment / Wie sich ein egklicher vor der Pestilentz bewaren / vnd der selben entpfliehen / auch mit hilff des Allmechtigen Gottes / seines leibs gesundthait / erhalten soll...* (Augsburg: Heynrich Stainer, 1533); as well as Achilles P. Gasser, *Ainfeltiger vñ gegrünter bericht / wie menigklich sich in Pestilentzischem vbergang / mit artznyen / vnd anderer lybs not / halten / bewaren / vnd genören soll...* (Nuremberg: Johann Petreius, 1544). After 1555 the image appeared in various plague publications from Regensburg.

15 *Regiment wider die Pestilentz*. This single-leaf broadside is reprinted in Hans Wilderotter and Michael Dorrmann, Eds., *Das große Sterben: Seuchen machen Geschichte* (Berlin: Jovis, 1995), 124.

16 *Ein kurtz Regiment auß vil treffenlichen zůsamen geprachten tractaten verstendiger artzt gezogen / wie sich zu zeitē der pestilentz zuhalten sey* (Nuremberg: Friedrich Peypus, 1520).

17 *Ein kurtz Regiment wie sich zu zeiten der Pestilentz zu halten sey* (Nuremberg: Johann Petreium, 1533).

18 *Ein kurtz Regiment auß vil treffenlichen zůsamen geprachten tractaten...*, sig. A2r.

19 Johannes Klainmüller, *Ain hymlischen unn Natürlichen anzaygung diser sterblichenleüff mit ainem nutzlichen und trostlichen regiment wie sich des Mensch hallten soll / mit aderlassen Ertzneyen / unn gutter regierung / zü Eren ainer gantzen gemain der kayserlichen Stat Augspurg geordnet durch Doctore Johannes Klainmüller od Walhopter* (Augsburg: Hans Schönsperger, 1521), sig. C4r.

20 Peter Ukena, Ed., *Alexander Seitz: Sämtliche Schriften*, 2 Vols. (Berlin: Walter de Gruyter, 1975), Vol. I, 167–168.

21 Ulrich Rülein von Calw, *Ein kurtz regiment vor die pestelentz / dem Erbarn Radt zcu Freyberg / durch den achtbaren höchgelarten Herren Udalricum von kalw Doctorem yn der Ertztey / zcu geschryben* (Leipzig: Martin Landsperg, 1507), sig. C5r. An alternative spelling of "von Calw" is "von Kalbe."

22 Ulrich Rülein von Calw, *Ein underweysūg wie mann sich tzu der tzeit der pestilentz halten sol. Allen einwoneren der stat Freybergk tzu gut yn einn kurtze*

summe gebracht (Leipzig: Valent Schumann, 1521), sig. A4r. The 1521 text is only seven pages long, reduced from twenty-nine pages in the 1507 work. For a facsimile: Wilhelm Pieper, *Ulrich Rülein von Calw und sein Bergbüchlein: Mit Urtext-Faksimile und Übertragnung des Bergbüchleins von etwa 1500 und Faksimile der Pestschrift von 1521* (Berlin: Akademie Verlag, 1955).

23 Erik Anton Heinrichs, "The Plague Cure: Physicians, Clerics and the Reform of Healing in Germany, 1473–1650," Ph.D. dissertation, Harvard University, 2009, 225–267.

24 David J. Collins, *Reforming Saints: Saints' Lives and Their Authors in Germany, 1470–1530* (Oxford: Oxford University Press, 2008), 10–12, quotation at 131.

25 Peter Assion, "Geistliche und weltliche Heilkunst in Konkurrenz," in *Bayerisches Jahrbuch für Volkskunde 1976/77* (Würzburg: Kommissionsverlag Karl Hart, 1978), 7–23, esp. 10–16.

26 Robert W. Scribner and C. Scott Dixon, *The German Reformation*, 2nd Edn (Basingstoke, UK: Palgrave Macmillan, 2003), 20–21.

27 Historian Heike Talkenberger concluded that flood pamphlets comprise a special category of astrological literature due to the drama of the forecasted misfortunes, the references to the End Times, the authors' pleas for repentance and the direct appeals to the common man: Talkenberger, *Sintflut: Prophetie und Zeitgeschehen*, 154, 303.

28 Ukena, *Alexander Seitz: Sämtliche Schriften*, Vol. II, 64. See also Talkenberger, *Sintflut: Prophetie und Zeitgeschehen*, 185.

29 Jonah, 3:1–5 (NRSV).

30 Talkenberger, *Sintflut: Prophetie und Zeitgeschehen*, 185–190.

31 Ibid., 161–162.

32 Johann Copp, *Ein nutzlich Regiment wie man sich halten sol das man gesunden leyb behalt / vñ sunderlich vor die pestilentz / zu gut allen Christen vnnd nemlich denn eynwondern der löblichē statt Erffordt / durch Joannē Copp vō Lantspurg Doctorem mit höchstem fleyß gemacht* (Erfurt: Matthes Maler, 1521), fol. 11r. This tract was written on August 31, 1521.

33 Ibid., fol. 11r.

34 Ibid., fol. 11v.

35 Augsburg Staats- und Stadtbibliothek, call number: 4 Med 226.

36 Ibid., fol. 24r.

37 Karl Schottenloher, *Doktor Alexander Seitz und seine Schriften: Ein Kleinbild aus dem Münchner Ärtzeleben des XVI. Jahrhunderts* (Munich: Verlag der Münchner Drucke, 1925), 14–15; Gottlieb Linder, "Doktor Alexander Sytz: Ein Lebensbild aus der Reformationszeit," *Zeitschrift für Allgemeine Geschichte, Kultur-, Literatur-, u. Kunstgeschichte* 3 (1886): 228–232.

38 Robert W. Scribner, "Civic Unity and Reformation in Erfurt," *Past and Present* 66 (1975): 29–60, esp. 39–40.

39 Talkenberger, *Sintflut: Prophetie und Zeitgeschehen*, 225. This pamphlet proved popular, appearing in six editions between 1521 and 1523 in various cities across Germany.

40 Ibid., 227–228.

41 Nikolaus Pol, *Vndericht Nicoly pol d erzney docters i halt wie sich d gemain man im lauff des sterbens zu Insprugg des 1521 jars / bewarn sol…* (Schwatz: Joseph Piernsieder, 1521); Johannes Salius (Hans Saltzman), *Ein nutzliche ordnung vnd regiment wider die Pestilentz durch Doctor Hansen Saltzman von Steir / des*

Durchleichtigisten Fuersten vnnd herren herrn Ferdinanden Ertzhertzogen von Osterreych. c. Leybartzt. dem gemainenn man zw nutz furchtperlich gemacht... (Vienna: Johannes Singriener, 1521); Georg Tannstetter, *Regiment für den lauff der Pestilentz durch Georgē Tañstetter von Rain der siben freyen künst vnnd Ertzney doctor: kurtzlich beschriben Anno. 1521* (1521).

42 Seitz attributes this saying to Macrobius: Ukena, *Alexander Seitz: Sämtliche Schriften*, Vol. I, 192.

43 Ibid., 193.

44 Ibid., 194.

45 Alexander Seitz, *Ain schöner Tractat von dem Saturnischē gschoß der Pestilentz mit ettlichen klügen fragstucken / dariñ der vn gelert man sich irret / zü gferlichem abbruch seins lebens / ee zeit / alles durch den hochgelerten philosophum Alexander Seitzen von Marckbach Doctor zü München, auß menschlicher lieb trewlich beschriben / vnd verantwurt* (1521). See also: Ukena, *Alexander Seitz: Sämtliche Schriften*, Vol. I, 167–168; Schottenloher, *Doktor Alexander Seitz*, 14.

46 Ibid., 158–159.

47 David N. Harley, "Spiritual Physic, Providence, and English Medicine, 1560–1640," in Grell and Cunningham, *Medicine and the Reformation*: 101–135.

48 Ambrosius Jung, *Ein außerrvelt loblich tractat vñ regiment in dem schwären zeit der pestilentz...* (Augsburg: Hans Schönsperger, 1494); Ambrosius Jung, *Tractatulus perutilis de pestilentia ex diuersis auctoribus aggregatus...* (Augsburg: Hans Schönsperger, 1494).

49 For all Jung editions, see: Heinrichs, "The Plague Cure," appendix 3.

50 Jung, *Ein außerrvelt loblich tractat*, sig. A5r.

51 Ambrosius Jung, *Ain nutzliche trostliche vnd kurtze vnderrichtung / wie man sich in disen schwären leüffen der pestilentz halten sol / durch Doctor Ambrosium Jungen / statartzt zu Augspurg / dem gemainen mañ zů hilff vnd gůttem / der nit andern beystand hat / verordnet* (1521), sigs. B1v–2r.

52 Ambrosius Jung, *Ain nutzliche trostliche vnd kurtze vnderrichtung / wie man sich in disen schwären leüffen der Pestilentz haltē soll / durch Ambrosium Jungen / der Artzney Doctor zů Augsburg / dem gemainen mann zů hilff vnd gůtem / der nit andern beystand hat / verordnet. MDXXXV* (Augsburg: Philipp Vlhart, 1535), sig. B3r.

53 Luis (Abulensis) von Lobera, *Ein nutzlich Regiment der gesundtheyt / Genant das Vanquete / oder Gastmal der Edlen diener von der Complexion / Eigenschafft / Schad / vnd nutz allerley Speyß / Trancks / vñ von allem / darmit sich der mensch in gesundtheyt enthelt / Mit sampt einem kurtzen Regiment / Wye man sich in der Pestilentz / Pestilentzischen fieber vnnd Schweyß halten soll* (Augsburg: Heynrich Steyner, 1531), fol. 76.

54 Jung, *Ain nutzliche trostliche*, 1521, sigs. A2r–v.

55 "[M]ůß es durch vnseren ainigen mitler vnd gnadenstůhl Jesum Christum geschehen / zů dem wir dann vnnseren freyen zůgang haben / der auch alles mittleyden mit vns tragen ist..." Jung, *Ain nutzliche trostliche*, 1535, sigs. A2r–v.

56 "[T]rewer Artzet / der den so inn grosser kranckhait nit verderben will lassen." Ibid., sig. A2v. The emphasis on the word of God, which Jung also states is now proclaimed purely in many places, is a further indication of Jung's commitment to the evangelical cause.

57 Important predecessors in the reform of confession included the writing of Martin Luther, as well as Erasmus's new Greek Bible. Carlos Eire, "Early Modern

Catholic Piety in Translation," in *Cultural Translation in Early Modern Europe*, Eds. Peter Burke and R. Po-chia Hsia (Cambridge: Cambridge University Press, 2007): 83–100, at 88.

58 "[M]itt der hailsam-en ertzney warer penitentz." Urbanus Rhegius, *Underricht Wie ain Christenmensch got seinem herren teglich beichten soll Doctoris Urbani Regij Thůmpredigers zů Augspurg rc. M.D.XXI* (Augsburg: Silvanum Ottmar, 1521), sigs. A3r–4r.

59 Miriam Chrisman, *Conflicting Visions of Reform: German Lay Propaganda Pamphlets, 1519–1530* (Atlantic Highlands, NJ: Humanities Press, 1996), 94–98.

60 This information comes from the Augsburg chronicle: Clemens Sender, *Die Chroniken der deutschen Städte vom 14. bis ins 16. Jahrhundert*, Vol. XXIII (Leipzig: Verlag von S. Hirzel, 1894), 177–178.

61 Biographers connect Jung firmly to the Protestant Reformation. Josef Fleischmann and Peter Assion describe Jung as a "stiff-necked" follower of Zwingli who worked to make Augsburg Zwinglian: Josef Fleischmann, "Die Ärztefamilie Jung," *Lebensbilder aus dem Bayerischen Schwaben* 4 (1955): 14–43; Peter Assion, "Ambrosius Jung," in *Die deutsche Literatur des Mittelalters, Verfasserlexikon*, Vol. IV, Ed. Kurt Ruh (Berlin: Walter de Gruyter, 1983): 905–907. Yet another source depicts Jung as a follower of Luther: "Ambrosius Jung," in *Deutsches Biographisches Archiv*, Microfiche Edn., Ed. Bernhard Fabian (Munich: K G Saur Verlag, 1982).

62 Here I cite the 1530 version: Urbanus Rhegius, *Geystlich ärtzney für gesund vnd krancken zů disen gefärlichen zeyten gemert vnd gebessert* (Augsburg: Alexander Weyssenhorn, 1530).

63 Ibid., sig. D7r.

64 Ibid., sig. A5v.

65 Mitchell Lewis Hammond, "Medicine and Pastoral Care for the Dying in Protestant Germany," in *Ways of Knowing: Ten Interdisciplinary Essays*, Ed. Mary Lindemann (Boston: Brill, 2004), 113–136.

66 Rhegius, *Geystlich ärtzney für gesund*, sig. A7r.

67 Scott H. Hendrix, "Urbanus Rhegius," in *Theologische Realenzyklopädie*, Vol. XXIX (Berlin: Walter de Gruyter, 1998): 155–156, 156. The original appeared in 1529 as Urbanus Rhegius, *Seelenn ärtzney für gesund vnd krancken zů disen gefärlichen zeyten…* (Alexander Weissenhorn, 1529). Some later editions of this work appeared along with the tract *Tröstung aus göttlicher Schrift* by Caspar Huberinus. Gunther Franz, *Huberinus-Rhegius-Holbein: Bibliographische und druckgeschichtliche Untersuchung der verbreitesten Trost- und Erbauungsschriften des 16. Jahrhunderts* (Nieuwkoop: B. De Graff, 1973), 97–144.

68 *D. Martin Luthers Werke: Kritische Gesammtausgabe*, Vol. XXIII, *Predigten und Schriften 1527* (Weimar: Böhlau, 1901), 369.

69 Ibid., 323–337.

70 Hammond, "Medicine and Pastoral Care." On Luther and plague, see also: Heinrich Dormeier, "Die Flucht vor der Pest als religiöses Problem," in *Laienfrommigkeit im späten Mittelalter*, Ed. Klaus Schreiner (Munich: R. Oldenburg Verlag, 1992): 331–397.

71 *D. Martin Luthers Werke*, Vol. XXIII, 365. Earlier in the text Luther also describes those who leave neighbors to face certain and grave danger in the same terms, as murderers (353). This reveals that the text overall has a rhetorical and ethical "edge" that is absent in other plague pamphlets.

72 *Luther's Works*, Vol. LIV, *Table Talk*, Eds. and Trans. Theodore G. Tappert and Helmut T. Lehmann (Philadelphia: Fortress Press, 1967), 53–54; Vivian Nutton, "Murders and Miracles: Lay Attitudes towards Medicine in Classical Antiquity," in *Patients and Practitioners: Lay Perceptions of Medicine in Pre-industrial Society*, Ed. Roy Porter (Cambridge: Cambridge University Press, 1985): 23–54, 50–51.

73 See the best survey of Luther and medicine in English: Carter Lindberg, "The Lutheran Tradition," in *Caring and Curing: Health and Medicine in the Western Religious Traditions*, Eds. Ronald L. Numbers and Darrel W. Amundsen (Baltimore: Johns Hopkins University Press, 1998): 173–203.

74 Johann Anselm Steiger, *Medizinische Theologie: Christus Medicus und Theologia Medicinalis bei Martin Luther und im Luthertum der Barockzeit* (Leiden: Brill, 2005), 20–21.

75 Ibid., 39–41. See also: Lindberg, "The Lutheran Tradition." Lindberg also emphasizes that Luther saw little separation between faith and medicine.

76 Martin Luther, "Sermon on the Sum of a Christian Life" (1532).

77 *Luther's Works*, Vol. LIV, 53–54.

78 *Apoteck für den gmeynē man. der die Ertzte zuersuchen. am gůt nict vermügens / oder sonst in der not allwege nicht erraychen kan* (Augsburg?: Heinrich Stainer?, 1529?), Aib–ii. The exact wording here is drawn from this ca. 1530 edition, although the very first in the publication history (see below) has this passage as well.

79 Ibid., sigs. A1v–2r.

80 *Verzeichnis der im deutschen Sprachbereich erschienenen Drucke des XVI. Jahrhunderts* (Stuttgart: Anton Hiersemann), B8680. The latest work of this title examined: *Apoteck für den gemeynen Mann / der die Artzte zuersůchen am gůt nicht vermag / oder sunst in der not allwegen nit erreychen kan. Fleissig Corrugieret / vnd mit vil gůten stücken gemehret* (Marburg: Kleeblat, 1560).

81 *Apoteck für den gemeinen Mann…* (Erfurt: Singe, 1619).

82 Hieronymus Brunschwig, *Haußarmen Schatz. Gute gebreuchliche vn- bewerte Artzneien / zu Allerhandt gebrechen des gantzen Leibs / Für den gemeinen Mann insonderheit / so die Apotecken nit erreychen / oder die Artzte zuersuchen am gut nicht vermag / gestellt vnd mit fleiß zusamen getragen / jetzt von newem in truck verfertigt* (Frankfurt, 1568).

83 *Apoteck für den gmeynē man* (Augsburg: Heinrich Stainer, ca. 1529), title page. See also: Sirach 38:4 (NRSV).

84 Hieronymus Brunschwig, *Hauß apoteck. Zu yeden leibs gebresten für den gemainen man[n] und dz arm Landvolck* (Augsburg: Heinrich Stainer, 1545); and Hieronymus Brunschwig, *Hauß Apoteck* (Augsburg: Zimmermann, 1549).

85 *Apoteck für den gmeynē man* (Augsburg, ca. 1530), fol. 13r.

86 The Culmacher image appeared twice more (1506 and 1517) on the title page of Simon Pistoris's plague pamphlet (Leipzig: Martin Landsberg). The "Constance" image graces the cover of this work: Caspar Kegler, *Een seer costelic ende profitelije regiment / ey- principael bewijs hā crupdē / gebrande waterern / worterlen / eñ puluer. ec. Tot bewaringhe des verschrickeliken ghebreck der pestilentiē…* (Constans: Johann Haselberck, ca. 1530). The Constance pamphlet is unusual as the only example of a German vernacular plague pamphlet translated into Dutch. It was printed in Constance by the itinerant bookseller Johann Haselberg, who apparently sought to peddle the book in the Netherlands.

87 Andromachus with theriac and Mithridates with mithridatum show up on the title page of one baroque plague pamphlet: Malachias Geiger, *Kurzer Underricht vnd Güetachten Wie mann sich bey ietzigen sterbens Läuffē Praeseruieren vnnd Da iemand inficiert würde Curieren solle Sambt Ainer Instruction für die Wündartzt vnd Warter auch anderen welche sich bey dergleichen Kranckhen brauchen lassen* (Munich, 1649).

88 Caspar Kegler, *Eyn Nutzlichs vñ tröstlichs Regiment wider die Pestilentz vnd gifftig Pestilētzisch Feber…* (Regensburg: Paulum Khol), 1530.

89 Johann Haselberg translated, edited, and printed this 1521 pamphlet in Constance, ca. 1530. Caspar Kegler, *Einn Regiment durch Doctorem Casparum Kegler gemacht Darinnen sich / vor der Erschrecklichē kranckheyt / der pestilentz / preseruiren / bewaren vnd enthalten…* (Leipzig: Valentinum Schuman, 1521), Aiii. On the difficulties of interpreting "common opinion" from Reformation propaganda, see: Robert W. Scribner, *For the Sake of Simple Folk: Popular Propaganda for the German Reformation* (Cambridge: Cambridge University Press, 1981), 1–13.

4 The plague cures of Caspar Kegler

Print, alchemy, and medical marketing, 1521–1607

Amid the plagues and upheavals of the 1520s, one entrepreneurial physician excelled at recognizing the era's new possibilities. Caspar Kegler (ca. 1461–1537) took self-promotion and commercial innovation to a new level as his vernacular plague treatise became one of the most reprinted of the sixteenth century.[1] This Leipzig medical professor became well known for inventing and advertising secret, alchemical plague cures in printed texts, including the famed "Doctor Caspar Kegler's Electuary." This cure was among the first of a new sort of brand-name medicine that began to thrive in early modern Europe. Kegler's life and work therefore shed light on how medicine changed during the broader economic, social, and technological changes of the sixteenth century. While many scholars look to the eighteenth-century "consumer revolution" for the growth of medical marketing in Europe, Kegler's story demonstrates that certain physicians brought commercial innovations to plague treatises by the 1520s and that these changes fostered a more empirical approach to healing among learned physicians.[2]

An investigation of "the highly learned and honorable Herr Caspar Kegler the medical doctor" is long overdue, since his biography is neither widely available nor complete, despite the popularity of his texts in the sixteenth century.[3] Printed editions of Kegler's 1521 pamphlet and its expanded version of 1529 rivaled the many editions of Martin Luther's plague sermon, as they appeared at least twenty-one times between 1521 and 1607, including in cities as far as Graz, Constance, and Königsberg.[4] Kegler's work allows a better understanding of the physician-alchemists who pre-date Paracelsus, whom historians portray too often as a "lone prophet" of reform or mistake as the first to introduce secret, alchemical medicines.[5] Paracelsus dominates the narrative of German medical history so thoroughly that the history of entrepreneurial physician-alchemists follows the activities of "Paracelsians," such as Leonhart Thurneysser zum Thurn (1530–1596).[6] Kegler's story provides earlier evidence of these pursuits among German physicians, however, and reveals the diversity of medical practitioners using alchemical ideas and techniques before the wide reception of Paracelsus's work.

More importantly, this chapter probes Kegler's cultural, intellectual, and commercial context for the various factors that inspired novel medicines and contributed to the man's celebrity. Important to these tasks is understanding the growing interest in distilled medicines and practical alchemy among professional healers and laypeople, new efforts to reach out to the German "common man" in vernacular print, and the social and cultural turbulence unleashed by persistent epidemics and the Protestant Reformation.[7] This chapter argues that close connections between commerce, alchemical experimentation, and attempts to bridge social and professional boundaries within Leipzig inspired Kegler's novel medicines and fostered his empirical approach to healing. Kegler's cures became famous because they offered novel solutions to the seemingly novel problems that Germans faced, and because they benefitted from the salesmanship of family members and support from Saxon nobles.

Kegler's case contributes to the history of brand-name medicines in Europe by highlighting the creative products of central European markets and by revealing the many people involved in the making of the brand-name cure, including a medical professor, his family, merchants, and printers. Whereas other accounts of brand-name novelties pursue later Italian figures, such as Leonardo Fioravanti (1518–1588), or focus on medical consumerism in England during the seventeenth and eighteenth centuries, various merchants were peddling "Doctor Caspar Kegler's Electuary" in cities north of the Alps by the mid-sixteenth century.[8] The thriving markets of central Europe bred commercial innovations, encouraged by the growing wealth among nobles and merchants, population expansion, and increasing confidence among the urban middle classes on worldly and spiritual issues. Although there was no "consumer society" in the sixteenth century on the order of that of later centuries, these changes represent an early social broadening of consumer culture, as the upper classes and "common man" alike sought to use the material world for their comfort and as entrepreneurs made products designed to appeal to their desires.[9] Kegler's early medical marketing prefigures many techniques that became common later, including the use of printed advertising and brand names, as well as attempts to manipulate consumers with new products that appealed to their hopes and fears.

If defined generally as the imaginative names that healers and merchants create to distinguish between products, brand names have existed in medical markets since antiquity. New to sixteenth-century markets, however, was the sudden growth of brand-name novelties, especially cures named after a claimed inventor, as entrepreneurs developed new ways to market their products.[10] Confidence in the new products swelled as entrepreneurs advertised in printed texts and apothecaries sold the novelties alongside the favored standbys of classical medicine: theriac and mithridate. Although some new medicines marketed in early modern Europe were genuinely novel, such as guaiacum and other botanicals imported from the New World, many were novel in name only, as their creators presumably made only insignificant changes to existing recipes.[11] Although it is impossible to assess the content of Kegler's secret electuary, it is most likely that Kegler's innovations were mainly commercial rather than medical in nature.

Kegler's commercial activities are significant, however, since his proprietary approach to his best cures represents a departure from medieval literature on experiments (*experimenta*) and secrets (*secreta*). Medieval physicians often shared compilations of their experiments and secrets with each other, forming recipe collections that became the basis of an ongoing and collaborative experimental tradition. Scholastic physicians found such recipes to be effective in practice, but were secrets in the sense that no one could explain their efficacy through logical reasoning or by appealing to authority.[12] Kegler's special recipes became proprietary secrets, however, that the Kegler family believed to belong to them and not to physicians or experimenters more generally. Alchemy played a role in these changing notions of secrecy and ownership, since the inventors of alchemical cures typically concealed essential details about their products, either to maintain the traditional secrecy of their field or out of commercial motive. Alchemists believed that their techniques accessed the immaterial and hidden powers of nature and thereby produced secret information.[13]

Attention to the commercial aims of physicians adds to an emerging understanding of the ways that commerce contributed to the transformation of science and medicine in the early modern period.[14] Historian Harold Cook has argued recently that the values of modern science arose first in the seventeenth century among Dutch merchants, for whom being clear, consistent, and non-theoretical was essential to gain commercial credibility.[15] Kegler's work, however, reveals a different relationship between commerce and the investigation of nature in an era of secrecy and burgeoning vernacular literature. Due to the scarcity of patents in Kegler's era, secrecy protected and even promoted experimentation with new medicines, while the vernacular form of Kegler's pamphlets encouraged a more practical approach to healing that emphasized efficacy and personal experience over theory and scholarship.[16] On this latter point, Kegler's case supports the view of historian William Eamon that the vernacular "how-to" literature of the sixteenth century shared attitudes and values that encouraged empirical investigations of nature.[17] Furthermore, Kegler's story as a physician who addressed a broad audience contributes to the work of other historians who have highlighted the scientific importance of sixteenth-century vernacular sources and non-academic figures. Sailors and merchants, authors of popular technical and medical books, male and female alchemists, and other experimenters in cities and courts across Europe now inform the picture of how empirical investigations of nature thrived during the sixteenth century.[18]

Commerce, plague, and medicine in Leipzig

As one of the great centers of trade, print, and scholarship in central Europe, Leipzig bred commercial innovation in the early sixteenth century. Home to renowned imperial markets as well as one of the oldest universities of the Holy Roman Empire, Leipzig drew merchants, scholars, and students from across the empire and beyond.[19] Caspar Kegler was one such student who sought his fortune in Leipzig as he arrived at the university in 1485.[20] Kegler found a city prospering both from the region's mining boom and its favorable location on the roads and waterways between Nuremberg and its trading partners to the east. Important to Leipzig's rise were the efforts of the dukes of Albertine Saxony, Albrecht III (1464–1500) and Georg I (1500–1539), who cultivated the city as the financial and commercial center of their lands.[21]

To understand how medicine changed through commercialization in the sixteenth century, one must enter the heart of this vibrant city and trace the wealth of its medical entrepreneurs. The center of Leipzig was the city hall and marketplace, ringed by the opulent homes of patricians and captains of commerce. Three times a year this central location held the imperial markets that raised the city's prestige and commercial stature above that of its neighbors. At this crossroads of central Europe, physicians and apothecaries benefitted from easy access to medicinal ingredients, including precious materials from foreign trade networks. In addition to a thriving trade in books, grain, cattle, and metals, Leipzig's markets were renowned for their imported spices and textiles, which gave the markets an exotic flair.[22] Among the wares were nutmeg, cinnamon, cloves, ginger, pepper, cardamom, bay leaf, myrrh, incense, figs, raisins, rice, mustard, sugar, honey, wine, brandy, saffron, caraway seed, tree oils, dyes, oak-leaf galls, and wine crystals. Those interested in chemical experimentation had easy access to silver, copper, and lead as well as compounds such as alum and vitriol.[23]

One opulent home adjacent to city hall belonged to the physician Heinrich Stromer von Auerbach (1482–1542), a prominent humanist, city councilor, and dean of the Leipzig medical faculty, whose life and work provide important contrasts to Kegler's own. Kegler and Stromer counted among the ambitious citizens who arrived in Leipzig as it blossomed and who then succeeded as entrepreneurs there.[24] While Kegler's main commercial interests fell within medicine, Stromer grew rich as a wine merchant and founder of Auerbach's Cellar, an institution of revelry immortalized centuries later by Johann Wolfgang von Goethe.[25] Kegler found fame, however, by creating and promoting his own medicines, and perhaps even selling them to the crowds that visited Leipzig's markets every year. Kegler owned a store at Leipzig's city hall, which presumably served as an outlet for his products.[26] A physician who prepared and sold medicines was somewhat unusual in the sixteenth century, but not unknown.[27] The sale of medicines was typically the sole domain of apothecaries in German towns, yet various Leipzig physicians seem to have had close ties to the trade. Leipzig's first appointed city physician, Georg Schiltel, married the daughter of the apothecary at the Lion Pharmacy and amassed such wealth in his career that he bought the knight's estate of Abtnaundorf.[28] Nearing the end of his career in 1529,

Kegler counted among Leipzig's wealthy citizens, owning two homes and a garden in addition to his shop.[29]

It is no surprise that sixteenth-century physicians sought income from various ventures since their profession had only a small and tenuous stake in the local medical market. Learned, university-trained physicians were relatively scarce in early modern cities in comparison to other healers.[30] Most importantly, many people did not necessarily need or desire the help of learned physicians, but more typically sought medical aid from barber-surgeons, bath attendants, herb sellers, and various unlicensed healers who explained sickness in more popular terms.[31] Plague, however, presented physicians with opportunities to demonstrate the usefulness of their learning and experience, and perhaps for this reason Kegler focused his professional career on plague. During his residence in Leipzig, plague-like epidemics struck the city in 1484–86, 1495, 1505–07, and 1518–20, while a mysterious pestilence known as the English Sweating Sickness appeared in 1529.[32] Writing just before this epidemic arrived in 1529, Kegler stated that he had served his beloved city for forty years and risked his life by remaining there during four epidemics.[33] As a medical student, Kegler distinguished himself for honorable service amidst plague, earning Leipzig citizenship and a remission of civic taxes in 1508.[34] After becoming a doctor of medicine in 1511, Kegler became the first physician to work regularly at Leipzig's St. Georg hospital, serving occasionally at its lazaretto (*Pestilentzhaus*).[35] Kegler also lectured at the University of Leipzig between 1523 and 1537 as a professor of medicine.[36] His 1521 and 1529 pamphlets established the reputation of his medicines among physicians, apothecaries, princes, and printers throughout German lands, and probably among the literate middle classes of German cities as well (Figure 3.4). Six printed editions appeared during his lifetime in Leipzig, Erfurt (1530), and Regensburg (1530), while a Dutch translation appeared in Constance (ca. 1530), the work of the printer and itinerant bookseller Johann Haselberg (Figure 3.3).[37]

Print and the making of Kegler's signature cures

Kegler's main innovation was the merging of two of Leipzig's important products – books and medicines – in an entrepreneurial way that seems at home within Leipzig's marketplace. The print shops that thrived in Leipzig by the end of the fifteenth century provided a new medium for local physicians to reach and influence a broad audience, especially regarding plague.[38] It became increasingly common for German physicians during Kegler's lifetime to publish vernacular literature in order to advise local people on preventing and curing the plague. The events of the early Reformation also prepared the ground for Kegler's pamphlets by expanding the market for printed literature and by altering the course of Leipzig's print industry. After imperial officials at the Diet of Worms denounced Luther in 1521, Duke Georg I of Albertine Saxony enforced the imperial ban on Luther's works immediately.

These events worked to Kegler's advantage, since Leipzig's printers sought immediate replacements for Luther's controversial and profitable works.[39] Sensing an opportunity, printers and physicians produced greater numbers of plague literature to fill this gap. Kegler's first edition of 1521 was among the very first vernacular plague works printed by Valentin Schumann, reflecting a sudden turn away from steady print runs of Luther's works.[40]

The rapid expansion of vernacular print had notable effects on medicine, demonstrating a phenomenon that historian Lisa Jardine describes as "the interrelatedness of cultural innovation and shrewd financial exploitation of a new market opportunity."[41] While Jardine was speaking of the commoditization of printed books in the late fifteenth century, a similar phenomenon occurred in Leipzig, as print opened new opportunities to entrepreneurs by speeding the social and geographical distribution of one physician's cures and ideas. A physician who could entice a broad audience could achieve much in this era while also changing the character of medicine itself. In the German vernacular, cures resembled less the medicines of the fourteenth and fifteenth centuries, but became more personal and proprietary, referring to contemporary physicians and individual experience rather than to a Greek or Roman heritage. A corollary of this trend was the appearance of medicines whose names emphasized their local and German roots, such as the Silesian terra sigillata, a German version of the classic Mediterranean "sealed earth."[42] The appearance of new medicines did not mean the sudden decline of the traditional medicines of antiquity, which hung on tenaciously into the eighteenth century. It did mean, however, that some physicians were beginning to supplement ancient knowledge and rely more heavily on their own experience and discoveries.

Kegler's printed pamphlets of 1521 and 1529 promoted his own electuary and aqua vitae alongside a great variety of recipes for preventing and curing plague. A distinctly personal character distinguishes Kegler's work from that of most contemporary physicians, witnessed in his possessive language while describing "his own" medicines.[43] Most strikingly, Kegler promotes his own special cures as the best medicines available, even greater than theriac and mithridate:

> Above all of these is my electuary, used early in the day on an empty stomach two peas in size. A person is protected for twenty-four hours with the help of God. Also smear an amount the size of two hemp seeds in the nostrils with the fingers pressing the nose shut. This prevents the brain from being poisoned for a day.[44]

The popularity of such a cure was presumably aided by the fact that it required just one simple treatment for all-day protection, and was limited in efficacy only by God's will, not by an individual's humoral make-up. Elsewhere in the text, his *aqua vitae* garners the highest praise among curative medicines:

> Take the following medicine as instructed and sweat. Take the powder, the onion water, my electuary or my aqua vitae, which is the most sure among the others and all medicines. I have experienced its effect as often as I have used it, unlike other powders, electuaries and others. Therefore I have always trusted it the most and have taken it myself when in need. I have also saved the lives of my wife, children and entire household many times using it with divine help.[45]

Here Kegler appeals to a practical audience by describing the tried-and-true efficacy of his medicine, instead of describing its ancient or scholarly pedigree as many contemporary physicians did. Kegler also attempts to win trust from his reader by describing the cure's use on his family, household, and own body.

Kegler's pamphlets attracted an audience among physicians, surgeons, merchants, and laypeople since he offered medicines and an approach to the body that appealed to popular expectations but remained for the most part within the bounds of Galenic-Hippocratic medicine. Brief comparison with Heinrich Stromer's plague literature, printed first in Leipzig in 1516, demonstrates Kegler's popularizing efforts. As one might expect of a prominent scholar, Stromer's writings follow the learned format of the late medieval plague treatise and demonstrate his mastery of classical scholarship. With his many learned citations, Stromer most likely sought to impress his illustrious patrons, including Elector Albrecht of Brandenburg, rather than produce a text that prioritized the interests of a broad, literate audience.[46] The recipes in Stromer's vernacular work appear often in Latin and offer few instructions, keeping the preparation of medicines to professional apothecaries and a Latinate audience. Finally, there are no alchemical medicines such as *aqua vitae* in Stromer's work, since these products were not a part of classical medicine. Kegler's work, on the other hand, emphasizes the new and empirical, focused on tried-and-true recipes rather than theoretical discussion, basing the authority of his cures on personal experience rather than ancient masters.[47] Moreover, the basic form of Kegler's 1521 pamphlet was more accessible to a lay audience, since his recipes appeared in German along with instructions for preparing most of them.

At a more fundamental level, the pamphlets by Stromer and Kegler differ in their approach to the body and sickness, as reflected in the basic structure of the texts. This difference is more in emphasis and format than in substance, but is important nonetheless. Stromer's advice follows closely the regulation of the six *res non naturales*, a basic framework for treatment in Galenic-Hippocratic medicine that required a person to moderate diet, exercise, and emotions, among other things. Although it was a fundamental part of learned ancient medicine, it was presumably not popular, since such a regimen required great discipline of diet and lifestyle. Studies suggest, rather, that many preferred the pills and treatments that required little effort and had immediate effects.[48] Furthermore, Stromer's lengthy suggestions for diet indicate that he was not writing for people who had limited dietary options, since he recommended foods that were not the traditional fare of the humble classes.[49]

Kegler, by contrast, did not prioritize the traditional regimens for moderating the six *res non naturales* but, rather, shifted the emphasis to the need to prevent or counteract the body's blockages. This was most likely a popular choice, since many in early Europe believed sickness to result from a clogging of the body's natural inward and outward exchange.[50] Most strikingly, Kegler begins his medical advice with purgative recipes, in contrast to Stromer's learned opening on the plague's origins.[51] Kegler also gives relatively few recommendations for food and drink, appearing near the end of his pamphlet after an abbreviated list of the six *res non naturales*. And, while his dietary recommendations resemble Stromer's in their aim to prevent external poisons from entering the body, they also mention the body's blockages. Kegler states that a person must always keep his/her body open during plague epidemics and not "stopped up," reflecting greater emphasis on this concern.[52]

When revising and expanding his plague pamphlet in 1529, Kegler added the promise to reveal secret "experiments" (*expermenten*), although these did not include the recipes for his own electuary and *aqua vitae*. Kegler's use of the word "experiment" reflects his long experience fighting plague, since the word is derived from the Latin "*experimentum*," or "proof from experience." But, despite claims that his pamphlet contains "many worthy experiments previously kept secret and never before brought to light," Kegler continued to guard his personal cures.[53] He explains that it is too difficult to communicate the exact techniques to make his own medicines since they involve complicated manipulations and alchemy. This passage comes after Kegler denies being able to describe how to make a special juniper wine:

> I certainly want to write about it, but no one can do so since one shows [by doing] with the hand. The same is true of my electuary, which is extracted from theriac and mithridate, the subtle spirit from the crude material – a process that belongs to alchemy.[54]

Kegler mentions that the audience could find the special juniper wine made with the powerful juniper berry oil at his own place, perhaps referring to his shop at Leipzig's city hall.[55] More importantly, this passage contains Kegler's only reference to an alchemical concept – that alchemical techniques can separate subtle healing essences from physical objects, which matches the alchemical thought of contemporary medical authors.[56] Regarding his own electuary, Kegler also adds an interesting detail: his superior remedy is made with unicorn horn.[57] It is not clear if Kegler is referring to the same electuary made from theriac and mithridate, yet this electuary of unicorn was the one that many physicians described later as "Doctor Caspar Kegler's Electuary."

By emphasizing his personal expertise and creative powers, Kegler fit among the artists and artisans of Renaissance Europe. In German-speaking lands in particular, artists began to sign their work with new symbols that emphasized the artist himself. Albrecht Dürer and Lucas Cranach the Elder were among the first to seize the commercial opportunities of the time by establishing workshops that reproduced their woodcuts and engravings for the market.[58] There was also growing attention to the expertise of specific healers in the sixteenth century. One of the earliest printed examples of a named plague cure appeared in a 1515 pamphlet by the Viennese medical professor Martin Stainpeiss.[59] Instead of discussing traditional medicines such as theriac and mithridate, he focused much of his text on his own herbal recipes, including "A Stainpeiss Prophylactic against the Pestilence."[60] Unlike Kegler, however, Stainpeiss revealed the recipe of this medicament.

Kegler's pamphlets of 1521 and 1529 built on the conventions of the earliest medical advertisement literature of German lands, which thrived in the fourteenth and fifteenth centuries as short manuscripts that promoted one specific medicine or traveling healer.[61] Another form was the single-leaf document that merchants displayed at fairs or sold with their products, many of which were "wonder drugs," ranging from natural substances to more complex products such as theriac or distilled brandy.[62] Kegler's use of secrecy and alchemy and his implication of novelty and ownership, however, departed from all conventions of previous commercial literary forms. The time was ripe for innovation, as advertisement literature proliferated in print, including lists of specific medicines at local apothecary shops. It was not unusual after 1520 for appointed city physicians to publicize the products at the local pharmacy during threatening times.[63] Collaboration between physician and apothecary in the sale of medicines appears in one 1528 pamphlet by Magnus Hundt of Magdeburg, concerning a special powder he ordered at the city's two pharmacies. There was no attempt at secrecy in this case, however, since Hundt gave the recipe in a lengthy Latin text and since the special powder was available at the low price of one groschen.[64]

It was not unusual for contemporary physicians to conceal special recipes in vernacular writing, although Kegler's secrecy was extreme, since many such authors expressed a willingness to share information upon request. For example, even though Johann Drachenfuss withheld the recipe for his precious antidote in his circa 1531 pamphlet, this physician of Gunzenhausen stated that he would reveal the recipe to a fellow scholar who inquired about it. In this case, Drachenfuss sought to draw authority and credibility from his cure's pedigree and efficacy; he had learned it from his teacher at Bologna, Doctor Benedictus Fauentinus Benedetto Vettori (1481–1561), who had used it in multiple epidemics.[65] Other physicians employed secrecy in a fashion more like Kegler, such as Adam Zwicker. This physician of Memmingen refused to reveal the recipe for the "golden electuary" in his 1537 pamphlet, but advised his audience to purchase it from the local apothecary, whom he trusted to make it properly. Unlike Kegler, however, Zwicker did not claim

Boeckele ?!

the cure as his own, nor did the cure achieve a commercial legacy in later decades.[66] Thus, not all secret medicines became brand-name medicines that bore the names of German physicians in markets across the empire.

Finally, the support of the Leipzig city council and Duke Georg I of Albertine Saxony is worth mentioning as one factor in Kegler's rise. Effective prophylactics and cures for plague promised great political and economic advantages, and Kegler's overlords in Leipzig and Saxony were certainly interested.[67] Kegler dedicated his 1529 pamphlet to the mayor and city council of Leipzig, but mentioned that it was the duke of Saxony who urged him to write. The role of the duke in 1529 contrasts with one of the earliest plague pamphlets printed in Leipzig, which mentions only the urging of the Leipzig city council.[68] Moreover, according to Kegler, the duke requested that he reveal some secrets for the good of the people.[69] Considering the continued secrecy of Kegler's signature cures, however, it seems that even Duke Georg could not persuade Kegler to reveal his special recipes. There is also no evidence that Kegler's cures or texts enjoyed commercial protections from political authorities before 1607.

A prescription for novel times: alchemy, plague, and the Reformation

Commercial motives and print were major factors in the creation of novel, secret medicines in the early sixteenth century, yet there is much more to the story. Alchemy, continuous cycles of epidemics, and the turbulence of the Reformation era hold clues as to why Kegler developed new medicines and why they drew interest. Kegler developed and publicized his cures during a time harried by seemingly new sicknesses and laden with eschatological expectation. As an author who wrote for a broad audience, Kegler responded to these fears as he presented novel cures for the seemingly novel problems that early modern Germans were facing.[70]

Kegler's introduction of 1521 emphasizes the novelty of contemporary events and urges the audience to repent amidst concern that the current plague was much stronger and intense than any known before. Kegler explains that the almighty God was acting like a fatherly punisher, moved by the sins of humanity to spread justice by introducing new dangers for the body and soul.[71] Kegler wrote this introduction at a time when fears of pestilence and the French Disease coincided with the initial events of the German Reformation and when physicians such as Alexander Seitz and Johann Copp predicted a flood of biblical proportions or other such upheavals, as seen above.[72] Thus, fears of new and unusual events were rampant in Kegler's era.

Kegler's revisions of 1529 reinforce the view that he offered novel cures for novel times and offer a glimpse of the decade's heightened fears. As the new English Sweating Sickness swept through central Europe in 1529, invading Ottoman forces lay siege to Vienna and the rift within western

Christendom continued to grow. Taking an anti-Protestant position much like Duke Georg I, Kegler denounced the growing divisions within the Church as the product of the Devil and humanity's divisiveness. Kegler saw himself fighting new evils in the world, interpreting the new epidemic as a divine punishment for the "new gestures, new curses, new clothes, and the new unchristian faith." Moreover, the text resounds with apocalyptic tones in its anxiety about the quickening pace of catastrophe in 1529. In Kegler's view, the English Sweating Sickness was not to be feared as much as the divine punishments that could follow, including a greater pestilence in the coming summer, ending with famine and war as occurred recently in Italy, perhaps referring to the sack of Rome in 1527. Kegler saw the state of souls as dire, and urged moral reform according to the example of the biblical Ninevites.[73] In an effort to boost the pamphlet's popular appeal, the Leipzig printer Valentin Schumann fitted the text with a title page illustration of St. Veronica holding the *sudarium* of Christ – an image that had a devoted following in the late Middle Ages as a channel of bodily and spiritual healing (Figure 3.4).[74]

Plague epidemics had been inspiring new medical approaches since the fourteenth century. Late medieval physicians struggled to understand the plague's origin and treatment in specific terms since they had little ancient precedent to follow. Plague seemed to be a novel phenomenon unknown to Greek and Roman physicians, and therefore it challenged the theoretical basis of medieval academic medicine. Moving away from ancient humoral theory, late medieval physicians categorized the fourteenth-century plagues within Avicenna's discourse on pestilential fever, adding their own discussion of poison, contagion, and swellings to the thought of this eleventh-century Persian physician. Physicians turned to poison to explain the sickness since the epidemic affected all regardless of age, status, and humoral composition and seemed to spread from person to person through occult means.[75] The new emphasis on poison in late medieval medicine resulted in greater emphasis on the antidotes of antiquity. Some fifteenth-century physicians also began to search for new medicines within alchemy, astrology, and magic.[76]

Alchemy merits deeper exploration as the source of Kegler's novel cures and one factor in their appeal. Kegler drew on both learned alchemy and artisanal practices to develop his own medicines, which was unusual for physicians and medical professors at the time, since alchemy was not taught at universities.[77] Much like Johann Vochs, Kegler's learned source for alchemical cures was the Pavian medical professor Antonio Guaineri (? – ca. 1446), who pioneered alchemy's integration into physicians' medical practice.[78] Guaineri's *Practica* appears as the alchemical reference work in Kegler's 1529 pamphlet, specifically for details on how to produce *aqua vitae*.[79]

At least a few physicians in Leipzig were even hostile to alchemy and its practitioners, including Heinrich Stromer, who denounced contemporary alchemists as mere "spice-sellers" in a 1526 letter to the humanist Willibald Pirckheimer.[80] The Leipzig physician Johann Reusch similarly did not recommend taking *aqua vitae*, amounting to an apparent rejection of Kegler's ideas. Reusch also denounced the "great deceptive lie" that one medicine can serve in all pestilences, as was a common strategy in selling powerful medicines.[81]

Despite contemporary challenges, the techniques described in Kegler's recipes show that this physician was deeply involved in the alchemical laboratory. Kegler's pursuit of alchemy is confirmed, if indirectly, by the inventory of the family estate that civic officials conducted in 1547, following the death of Kegler's synonymous son.[82] Since Caspar Kegler the younger was also a Leipzig physician employed at the St. Georg hospital and outlived his father by only nine years, there is a great likelihood of continuity in the professional possessions of father and son.[83] Of great interest is the detailed content list of the Kegler laboratory and library, which totaled over 200 prints and manuscripts in German and Latin. Numerous alchemical books reveal that Kegler drew on a rich medieval tradition. Alongside four books described as "alchemical" appear works by the Italian physician Antonio Guaineri and the Strasbourg surgeon Hieronymus Brunschwig, as well as older medieval texts by Arnald of Villanova, Petrus Hispanus, and (pseudo-) Albertus Magnus.[84] The description of instruments reveals equipment for distilling and assaying: "[F]ifteen long glasses that contain little water for alchemy, …a copper still with a helmet-lid in which one brews [distills] water, …a copper oven."[85] Furthermore, the inventory specifies many vessels of all shapes and sizes, some holding waters of various colors as well as the essential ingredients for family recipes: aqua vitae, unicorn, and juniper oil.[86]

Alchemy provided Kegler with products that presumably had a dramatic effect on the body and carried the mystique of occult powers, since alchemists believed that they accessed the immaterial and eternal powers of the natural world. By promoting his *aqua vitae* as the perfect medicine to counter quick and horrible sicknesses such as plague, Kegler was likely responding to consumers' hopes for a quick and penetrating remedy.[87] Distilled medicines may have also appealed to a broad audience in German cities because they were familiar. In German lands especially, distilling was rooted in domestic and artisanal practices, despite new interest from physicians.[88] Interest in distilled medicines also thrived among German noblewomen, such as Anna of Saxony (1532–85), who established a medical production facility, staffed by an apothecary, a distiller, a gardener, and the wives of physicians.[89] Not surprisingly, Kegler's cures attracted interest within Anna's circle of lay healers. A recipe for a plague electuary attributed to Kegler appears in a handwritten book of recipes that Katharina Wernerin gave to Anna of Saxony in 1563. This recipe calls for unicorn horn, but, since the recipe for Kegler's personal cure remained secret in his publications, it is impossible to confirm it as the true recipe for "Doctor Caspar Kegler's Electuary."[90]

The diverse set of authors of plague literature in the first decades of the sixteenth century helped to bring the experience of craftsmen and alchemists to bear on the knowledge of academic medicine.[91] Kegler's 1529 pamphlet in particular provides some of the most remarkable technical details and explicit instructions among contemporary plague pamphlets. Among the new recipes that Kegler revealed in 1529 was a special water of celandine (*Schelwurtz*), which depicts Kegler's unusual level of technical detail:

> First wash and cut the celandine and place the parts in a pot with as much wine or wine vinegar as will fit. Next take a different glass vessel that is specially fashioned so that it can be turned over on the first edge of the pot, so that its bottom stands at top. Make a gum from beaten egg whites and flour and seal it well. Set it near a fire's coals so that it dries well at all places. Then place the pot in a circular fire so that the coals do not touch it but are at a distance of a half ell. Let it boil without interruption for six hours. When these six hours have passed, take it from the fire, let it grow cold and break the seal. Place the plant with the root in a clean cloth and wring it out little by little until complete. Hold the liquid in glasses prepared so that no smell is allowed to enter. Keep this until it is needed.[92]

Provided that one had the equipment, professional and lay healers would have been able to follow these complete directions. Kegler added that he had used this inexpensive medicine to help over 300 people during four epidemics in Leipzig and recommended it for monks and country gentlemen who had to treat large groups.[93]

Kegler's most technical recipe reveals both alchemical learning and familiarity with the tools and methods of a goldsmith. Kegler recommends this "*aurum vitae*," or "gold of life," to induce vomiting in a patient as a purgative against poisons. The fourteenth-century Italian physician Gentile da Foligno was among the first to recommend potable gold for plague, but Kegler's recipe is much more extensive and adds a step of calcination.[94] The recipe opens with a mixture of mercury and gold and calls for methods that goldsmiths use to separate silver from gold. This mixture undergoes treatment with a "strong water," distillation, and calcination by fire. Most interestingly, Kegler warns against buying *aurum vitae* from salesmen, since they may use the writings of alchemists who omit the calcination or the gold, both of which are essential to temper mercury's harm.[95] Although Kegler's alchemical medicine is drawn from learned, if non-traditional, texts, his detailed discussion and references to goldsmiths reflect his knowledge of artisanal production. Furthermore, Kegler adds a personal note that he himself took the medicine on three occasions thirty years prior and that he had helped many young lads in Leipzig as well, thus dating his alchemical work to circa 1500.[96]

Kegler's knowledge of manipulating metals and chemicals was most likely encouraged by his surroundings in Saxony, one of the great mining areas of central Europe at the time. The minerals of the Ore Mountains attracted the interest of scholars, artisans, and princes and funded the political projects of the ruling houses of Saxony.[97] Georgius Agricola (1494–1555), hailed today as the father of mineralogy and mining science, is a prime example of what Saxon scholars could achieve in their attempts to relate ancient knowledge to their own observations of the world. His 1556 *De re metallica* was the most thorough description of minerals and mining techniques to date, and remained the authoritative text on these subjects for the next two centuries.[98] Most significant about Agricola's *De re metallica* is that it combined scholarly theories with the practice and experience of miners, and in this respect it is similar to Kegler's project. Agricola wrote based on direct observation of mining practices and products, much as Kegler claimed to write about his own personal experience from a lifetime of practicing medicine.[99] Although evidence is scarce, Agricola may have heard Kegler's lectures while he studied medicine at the University of Leipzig between 1522 and 1524 and boarded at Heinrich Stromer's house.[100]

Branding and marketing the Kegler family cures

Few details exist regarding how exactly Caspar Kegler the elder sold or distributed his medicines during his lifetime, not to mention how consumers reacted. Most evidence concerning the sale of Kegler's cures dates to the mid- and later sixteenth century and suggests that family members and merchants were responsible for turning Kegler's name into an early brand name within the marketplace. Whereas Kegler described his secret cures in distinctly possessive terms, these later figures cultivated the name "Doctor Caspar Kegler" in conjunction with his electuary of unicorn, promoting this brand well beyond Leipzig as a mark of authenticity and efficacy.

The earliest reference to the branded cure, "Doctor Caspar Kegler's Electuary," appears in a short advertisement tract of 1552 by the Leipzig surgeon Lorenz Misch. Kegler's electuary is one of two signature cures that dominate the text, along with "Doctor Mangolt's Electuary." Misch pitched such novel products to the high end of the market, since Kegler's cure is the most expensive, fetching twelve groschen per loth (ca. 15g) compared to eight groschen for Mangolt's cure.[101] Secrecy also continued to play an important role in the marketing of Kegler's cures, as Misch states in his title that Kegler's best recipes are not found in his book. Kegler's electuary was apparently worth promoting again in a similar fashion in 1565, even though Misch omitted Doctor Mangolt's cure.[102] It is unclear how or if Misch obtained the authentic, secret recipe.

Promoting and selling Kegler's cures outside Leipzig employed his sons Lukas and Melchior as well as his grandson Caspar. The family business took Lukas to Magdeburg, where circa 1545 he reissued his father's 1529 pamphlet, adding at the end of the original dedication:

> Thus you will find from me Lukas Kegler, citizen of Magdeburg, the described electuary, aqua vitae, and a little white powder for young children who can otherwise use no medicine, as my description on the poster [*anschlag Briff*] demonstrates.[103]

Not only does this reveal the Kegler family's growing commercial web, but also shows Lukas introducing a new powder and advertising in the local market with some sort of broadside, now lost. Lukas's move probably happened after 1539, since in that year Kegler's original text appeared in Magdeburg for the first time, promoting a different local distributor, Heinrich Eycksted.[104] It is again unclear how or if Eycksted obtained the Kegler family recipes.

Advertisement tracts show that "Caspar Kegler's Electuary" flourished in Magdeburg in the later decades of the sixteenth century. The appointed city physicians recommended it for plague protection in 1565, and it appears in two commercial pamphlets of 1582 and 1607 that list its price at the local pharmacy.[105] Magdeburg's merchants also marketed the remedy alongside the most prestigious and expensive products. In both texts Kegler's electuary appears with the "golden egg" at the culmination of a seven-day course designed to prepare the body for the plague's poisons. Both Kegler's electuary and the "the better golden egg" are the most expensive among the products, surpassing "the common golden egg," "the emperor's powder," "Doctor Copp's Liberantz Electuary," "the aqua vitae for pestilence," and the "Pestilence Pills of Doctor Augustus."[106]

Although he was a cleric at Breslau Cathedral, Melchior Kegler promoted the family medicines there, reissuing the 1529 text for the epidemic of 1566, adding his own dedication and some new recipes. When plague threatened, city officials prevailed upon him to see patients and prepare the Kegler family medicine with his own hands. Melchior allegedly used these family remedies during Breslau's plague of 1542 and thereby saved the lives of many poor people, treating them for free.[107] The need to fight impostor versions of the family medicine also drove Melchior to publish his work, as well as the fact that bookstores were sold out of the thousands of earlier copies. Most importantly, Melchior maintained the secrecy surrounding the recipes, claiming that only Caspar's children had the true recipes of the electuary, *aqua vitae*, and the *aurum vitae*, since their father had passed them on within the family before he died.[108]

Kegler's reputation grew steadily during the second half of the sixteenth century along with editions of his pamphlets. His work appeared in print in Wittenberg (1552), Eisleben (1565), Graz (1577), and Königsberg (1588), perhaps in support of local apothecaries and merchants.[109] Pamphlets from Halle (1575, 1581) reveal that city physicians placed "Doct. Caspar Kegler's Alexiteric" at the local pharmacy alongside other great antidotes, including theriac, mithridate, and "Emperor Maximilian's Electuary."[110] One of the last editions appeared on Wilhelm Lützenkirchen's press in Cologne in 1597 and demonstrates how far Kegler's pamphlets and medicines had traveled since 1521. This first edition on the lower Rhine spreads the news that Kegler's medicine is available in all places and pharmacies.[111] This text gained greater prominence later at the Frankfurt Book Fair.[112] Manuscript recipe books reveal further interest for Kegler's plague advice and recipes through the end of the sixteenth century.[113]

Attempts by Kegler's descendants to control the production and sale of Kegler's electuary reveal that they regarded this cure as the exclusive property of the family. The history of Kegler's electuary in Dresden best illustrates the product's success as well as the family's efforts to strengthen their proprietary claims. Behind much of this was Caspar Kegler the grandson, probably the "Doktor Kegler" appointed as Dresden's first city physician in 1594.[114] The 1584 Dresden edition indicates that Kegler's literature was in demand at the court of the elector of Saxony and that "Doctor Caspar Kegler's Electuary" was available in Dresden pharmacies.[115] In the final Dresden edition of Kegler's text, in 1607, the grandson's immediate task was to assail those who had printed the false recipe for the famous electuary of unicorn in Dresden, Cologne, and Leipzig, warning that such antics could do great harm to patients. Like a good businessman, Caspar the grandson also advertised his own wares and claimed exclusivity: "You shall also find more electuaries that are prepared according to the true and secret description at my own place in Dresden and also from Mr. Ernst Maßbachen of the Leipzig council, and from no one else."[116] Christian II, elector of Saxony, renewed his support for the ambitions of the Kegler family at this final publication in 1607. The elector hailed the life-saving powers of Kegler's electuary of unicorn and confirmed that only Kegler's male descendants had learned the true ingredients and hand preparation of the cure from their father, who instructed them to keep it as a "special, secret, and hidden treasure."[117] In an unusual move, the elector also granted the sole privilege to print Kegler's work to his grandson for a period of twelve years, and specified a fine of 300 gulden for infractions.[118]

Kegler's products and reputation remained of great interest long after 1607. During the Thirty Years' War, "Caspar Keglers Electuary" was a standard part of the Leipzig pharmacopoeia, appearing alongside theriac and mithridate as before.[119] Over the course of the sixteenth and seventeenth centuries, references to Doctor Kegler's electuary in other physicians' vernacular plague pamphlets remain steady up to 1680 in the central and eastern parts of Germany.[120] Since the recipe for Kegler's electuary does not appear in any of these later pamphlets, the secret remains to this day.

Conclusion

In his much-reprinted plague literature, Caspar Kegler the elder built on medieval ideas and practices related to secrecy, experience, and alchemy, and mobilized his innovations using the new medium of print. These innovations were mainly commercial in nature, since Kegler and his descendants were among the first to develop and market a new sort of brand-name medicine in the marketplaces of central Europe, if not in all of western Europe. Kegler also deserves credit for being among the first wave of German physicians to embrace alchemical medicines and their methods of production, and did so before Paracelsus. These findings reveal that commercial motives and growing interest in alchemy were changing the character of medicine from the early sixteenth century and well before the rise of Paracelsians and the consumer revolution of the later seventeenth and eighteenth centuries. Although Kegler did not reveal his greatest secrets, his accessible writing and novel cures drew great interest from professional healers and laypeople alike, including physicians, surgeons, apothecaries, and printers, as well as Saxon noblemen and noblewomen. One can also imagine that the urban middle classes of merchants and artisans were tempted to purchase Kegler's pamphlets and cures in times of need due to the broad appeal of distilled and alchemical products. Most importantly, one can detect in Kegler's writings a shift of emphasis away from ancient scholarly theory and towards a more practical medical profession oriented to consumer desires and the cultivation of personal experience in the field and laboratory.

Acknowledgments

An earlier version of this chapter was published as "The Plague Cures of Caspar Kegler: Print, Alchemy and Medical Marketing in Sixteenth-Century Germany," *Sixteenth Century Journal* 43, no. 2 (2012): 417–440.

Notes

1 Kegler was born in Thiersheim, Upper Franconia, circa 1461 and died on May 2, 1537, at the age of seventy-five. For his epitaph: Salomon Stepner, *Leipzigische Lorbeer-Blätter / das ist Alte und neue denckwürdige Uberschrifften / Grab- und Gedächtniß-Mahle...* (Leipzig: Lanckischen Buchladen, 1690), 195. For the date of death: Stadtarchiv Leipzig, Ratsbuch Vol. 7, fol. 16v [hereafter SAL]. An electuary was a paste-like confection often taken by spoon: Erika Hickel, *Die Arzneimittel in der Geschichte* (Nordhausen: Verlag Traugott Bautz, 2008), 543.

2 Neil McKendrick, John Brewer, and J. H. Plumb, *The Birth of a Consumer Society: The Commercialization of Eighteenth-Century England* (London: Europe Publications, 1982).

3 For this description in civic documents: SAL, Ratsbuch Bd. 8, 50v. A variant spelling of Kegler is "Kegeler." One Leipzig historian offers reliable but brief biographical information on Kegler: Carly Seyfarth, *Das Hospital zu St. Georg in Leipzig durch acht Jahrhunderte 1212–1940*, Vol. I (Leipzig: Georg Thieme Verlag, 1939), 76.

4 Erik Anton Heinrichs, "The Plague Cure: Physicians, Clerics and the Reform of Healing in Germany, 1473–1650," Ph.D. thesis, Harvard University, 2009, 274; Martin Luther, *Ob man fur dem sterben fliehen muge. Mart. Luther Wittemberg. M.D. XXVII* (Wittenberg: Hans Lufft, 1527). Luther's pamphlet was reprinted sixteen times up to 1607: *D. Martin Luthers Werke: Kritische Gesammtausgabe*, Vol. XXIII, *Predigten und Schriften 1527* (Weimar: H. Böhlau, 1901), 323–337.

5 Charles Webster has pointed out the problems of viewing Paracelsus as a "lone prophet": Charles Webster, "Paracelsus: Medicine as Popular Protest," in *Medicine and the Reformation*, Eds. Ole Peter Grell and Andrew Cunningham (London: Routledge, 1993): 57–77. For the tendency to view Paracelsus as the sole pioneer

of alchemy in German medicine: Heinz Zimmermann, *Arzneimittelwerbung in Deutschland vom Beginn des 16. bis Ende des 18. Jahrhunderts: Dargestellt vorzugsweise an Hand von Archivalien der Freien Reichs-, Handels- und Messestadt Frankfurt am Main* (Würzburg: Jal-Verlag, 1974), 182–184; Heinz Peickert, *Geheimmittel im deutschen Arzneiverkehr* (Leipzig: Alexander Edelmann, 1932), 13–34.

6 Christoph Friedrich and Wolf-Dieter Müller-Jahncke, *Rudolf Schmitz: Geschichte der Pharmazie*, vol. II, *Von der Frühen Neuzeit bis zur Gegenwart* (Eschborn: Govi Verlag, 2005), 230.

7 On apocalyptic expectation and Paracelsus's new medicine: Charles Webster, *Paracelsus: Medicine, Magic and Mission at the End of Time* (New Haven, CT: Yale University Press, 2008), 210–243. On the "common man": Joachim Telle, Ed., *Pharmazie und der gemeine Mann: Hausarznei und Apotheke in deutschen Schriften der frühen Neuzeit* (Wolfenbüttel: Waisenhaus-Buchdruckerei und Verlag, 1982).

8 Much like Kegler, Fioravanti gave his novel medicines unique and imaginative names, sometimes including his own name: William Eamon, *Science and the Secrets of Nature: Books of Secrets in Early Modern Culture* (Princeton, NJ: Princeton University Press, 1994), 235; David Gentilcore, *Medical Charlatanism in Early Modern Italy* (Oxford: Oxford University Press, 2006), 245; Roy Porter, *Health for Sale: Quackery in England 1660–1850* (Manchester: Manchester University Press, 1989); Andrew Wear, "Medical Practice in Late Seventeenth- and early Eighteenth-Century England: Continuity and Union," in *The Medical Revolution of the Seventeenth Century*, Eds. Roger French and Andrew Wear (Cambridge: Cambridge University Press, 1989): 294–320.

9 McKendrick, Brewer, and Plumb, *The Birth of a Consumer Society*, 1–6; Roy Porter, *English Society in the Eighteenth Century* (London: Penguin Books, 1982), 232–268. Most scholars place the German "common man" among the urban middle classes, including artisans and small-time merchants: Friedrich and Müller-Jahncke, *Rudolf Schmitz: Geschichte der Pharmazie*, Vol. II, 84–88. On the growth of practical vernacular literature, see: Miriam Chrisman, *Lay Culture, Learned Culture: Books and Social Change in Strasbourg, 1480–1599* (New Haven, CT: Yale University Press, 1982).

10 Kegler's name became a "brand name" when merchants attached it to one of his novel remedies within a marketplace. This brand name might have appeared with other products, such as "Doctor Caspar Kegler's aqua vitae." Essential to the definition of a brand name is a commercial context, since it is common to find medical recipes named after a person in late medieval and early modern recipe books. On the growth of brand names, trademarks and unique recipes: Zimmermann, *Arzneimittelwerbung in Deutschland*, 109–115, 183–184; Eamon, *Science and the Secrets of Nature*, 235; Gentilcore, *Medical Charlatanism*, 235–264.

11 Andrew Wear argues that the empirics who pushed novel pills did not introduce substantial changes to earlier medical traditions: Andrew Wear, *Knowledge and Practice in English Medicine, 1550–1680* (Cambridge: Cambridge University Press, 2000), 349.

12 Eamon, *Science and the Secrets of Nature*, 55–58.

13 Zimmermann, *Arzneimittelwerbung in Deutschland*, 33–35, 107–115.

14 Paula Findlen and Pamela H. Smith, "Commerce and the Representation of Nature in Art and Science," in *Merchants and Marvels: Commerce, Science,*

and Art in Early Modern Europe, Eds. Pamela H. Smith and Paula Findlen (New York: Routledge, 2002): 1–25.

15 Harold J. Cook, *Matters of Exchange: Commerce, Medicine, and Science in the Dutch Golden Age* (New Haven, CT: Yale University Press, 2007), esp. 56.

16 On patents and medicine: Zimmermann, *Arzneimittelwerbung in Deutschland*, 62–65. For the view that a medicine can be termed "proprietary" if its creator claimed sole rights with a secret formula rather than a patent: Michael H. Jepson, "From Secret Medicines to Prescription Medicines: A Brief History of Medicine Quality," in *Making Medicines*, Ed. Stuart Anderson (London: Pharmaceutical Press, 2005): 223–241.

17 Eamon, *Science and the Secrets of Nature*, esp. chaps. 3–6.

18 Alisha Rankin, *Panaceia's Daughters: Noblewomen as Healers in Early Modern Germany* (Chicago: University of Chicago Press, 2013); Tara Nummedal, *Alchemy and Authority in the Holy Roman Empire* (Chicago: University of Chicago Press, 2007); Deborah E. Harkness, *The Jewel House: Elizabethan London and the Scientific Revolution* (New Haven, CT: Yale University Press, 2007); Antonio Barrera, "Local Herbs, Global Medicines: Commerce, Knowledge, and Commodities in Spanish America," in Smith and Findlen, *Merchants and Marvels*: 163–181.

19 Karl Sudhoff, *Die Medizinische Fakultät zu Leipzig* (Leipzig: J. A. Barth, 1909), 3.

20 Seyfarth, *Hospital zu St. Georg*, 76.

21 Uwe Schirmer, "Die Leipziger Messen in der ersten Hälfte des 16. Jahrhunderts: Ihre Funktion als Silberhandels- und Finanzplatz der Kurfürsten von Sachsen," in *Leipzigs Messen 1497–1997*, Vol. I, Eds. Hartmut Zwahr, Thomas Topfstedt, and Günter Bentele (Cologne: Böhlau Verlag, 1999): 87–107, see 91.

22 Schirmer, "Die Leipziger Messen," 107; Gerhard Fischer, *Aus Zwei Jahrhunderten Leipziger Handelsgeschichte 1470–1650* (Leipzig: Felix Meiner, 1929), vii.

23 Fischer, *Aus Zwei Jahrhunderten Leipziger Handelsgeschichte*, 42–45.

24 Kegler and Stromer both hailed from small towns in nearby regions, Kegler from Upper Franconia (Oberfranken) and Stromer from the Upper Palatinate (Oberpfalz).

25 In Goethe's *Faust (Part One)*, Auerbach's Keller was the site of the "barrel ride" by Mephistopheles. It exists today in its original location in central Leipzig. Gustav Wustmann, *Der Wirt von Auerbachs Keller: Dr. Heinrich Stromer von Auerbach 1482–1542* (Leipzig: Hermann Seemann Nachfolger, 1902), 76–82.

26 Like Kegler, Melchior Lotter the printer also owned a "cammer under den bonen," presumably to sell books: Gustav Wustmann, Ed., *Quellen zur Geschichte Leipzigs*, Vol. I (Leipzig: Duncker & Humblot, 1889), 152 (Kegler) and 169 (Lotter). Kegler's widow, Anna, sold the storefront in 1542 to Johann Hutter, owner of Leipzig's Lion Pharmacy: SAL, Ratsbuch Vol. 8, 50v–51r.

27 Friedrich and Müller-Jahncke, *Rudolf Schmitz: Geschichte der Pharmazie*, Vol. II, 229–230.

28 Seyfarth, *Das Hospital zu St. Georg*, 75. Schiltel was appointed city physician in 1512. His father-in-law, Johann Hutter, was a city councilor and an apothecary.

29 On the "Turk Tax" survey of 1529, see: Wustmann, *Quellen*, Vol. I, 152, 165, 189.

30 Robert Jütte, *Ärzte, Heiler und Patienten: Medizinischer Alltag in der frühen Neuzeit* (Munich: Artemis & Winkler Verlag, 1991), 17–32.

31 Gianna Pomata, *Contracting a Cure: Patients, Healers, and the Law in Early Modern Bologna* (Baltimore: Johns Hopkins University Press, 1998), 120–139; Martin Gnann, "Populäres Heilen im kulturellen Umfeld der Vormoderne," Ph.D. thesis, Eberhard-Karls-Universität Tübingen, 1994, 54–60.

32 Seyfarth, *Das Hospital zu St. Georg*, 65. On early modern epidemics, see: Mary Lindemann, *Medicine and Society in Early Modern Europe* (Cambridge: Cambridge University Press, 2010), 39–42. Although retro-diagnosis of sixteenth-century epidemics is difficult, historical epidemiology suggests that forms of plague caused many, which is why I use this term rather than the general term "pestilence." Edward A. Eckert, *The Structure of Plagues and Pestilences in Early Modern Europe: Central Europe, 1560–1640* (Basel: Karger, 1996).

33 Caspar Kegler, *Eyn Nutzlichs vnd trostlichs Regiment wider dy Pestilentz vñ Gifftig Pestilentzisch Feber die Schweyssucht genannt / vnd sust mācherley gifftig vñ tödlich kranckheit / Durch Casparū Kegler / der ertzney Doctorn / zwsamen gebracht / vornewt vñ mit vil trostlichen experimentē gebessert / Die zuuor heymlich gehalten / vnd an den tag nyhe gegebē seyn. Anno 1.5.2.9. auß gegangen* (Leipzig: Valtenin Schumann, 1529), 1v. Kegler treated the English Sweating Sickness as a "Pestilentz" by revising and reissuing his original 1521 pamphlet for this new epidemic of 1529.

34 Ernst Müller, *Leipziger Neubürgerliste 1502–1556*, Vol. I, Ed. Annelore Franke (Leipzig: Stadtarchiv Leipzig, 1982), 11. Kegler is listed under "Begeler, Caspar".

35 Seyfarth, *Das Hospital zu St. Georg*, 76.

36 Universitätsarchiv Leipzig, Film 538, no. 80, fol. 128r (the notes of Wilhelm Ferdinand Vetter).

37 In addition to the Leipzig prints already cited: Caspar Kegler, *Eyn Nutzlichs vnd tröstlichs Regiment widder die Pestilentz vnd Gifftig Pestilentzisch Fever die Schweyssucht genant…* (Erfurt: Melchior Sachssen, 1530); Caspar Kegler, *Eyn Nutzlichs vñ tröstlichs Regiment wider die Pestilentz vnd gifftig Pestilētzisch Feber die Schweyssucht genant…* (Regensburg: Paulum Khol, 1530); Caspar Kegler, *Een seer costelic ende profitelije regiment / ey- principael bewijs hā crupdē / gebrande waterern / worterlen / eñ puluer. ec. Tot bewaringhe des ver schrickeliken ghebreck der pestilentiē…* (Constans: Johann Haselberck, ca. 1530).

38 Falk Eisermann, "Leipziger Einblattdrucke des 15. Jahrhunderts," in *Bücher, Drucker, Bibliotheken in Mitteldeutschland*, Ed. Enno Bünz (Leipzig: Leipziger Universitätsverlag, 2006): 373–400.

39 Thomas Döring, "Der Buchdruck in Leipzig zu Lebzeiten Luthers," in *Luther und Leipzig: Beiträge und Katalog zur Ausstellung*, Eds. Ekkehard Henschke and Klaus Sohl (Leipzig: Universitätsbibliothek Leipzig, 1996): 25–50, 27–29.

40 Helmut Claus, *Das Leipziger Druckschaffen der Jahre 1518–1539: Kurztitelverzeichnis* (Gotha: Forschungsbibliothek Gotha, 1987), 124–149.

41 Lisa Jardine, *Worldly Goods* (New York: Norton, 1998), 128.

42 Karl H. Dannenfeldt, "The Introduction of a New Sixteenth-Century Drug: 'Terra Silesiaca,'" *Medical History* 28 (1984): 174–188. For broader discussion of the "local" trend in science: Alix Cooper, *Inventing the Indigenous: Local Knowledge and Natural History in Early Modern Europe* (Cambridge: Cambridge University Press, 2007).

43 Caspar Kegler, *Einn Regiment durch Doctorem Casparum Kegler gemacht Darinnen sich / vor der Erschrecklichē kranckheyt / der pestilentz / preseruiren /*

bewaren vnd enthalten / Desgleichen Etzliche trostliche / vnnd vnder andern Außgeleßene / Medelen / hilff vnnd ertzeneyen / So etwer mit gedachter krancheyt / begriffen / Inficirt / ader vorgifft wurde / Wie man dem selben Dor mit tzu hilff komenn / errettenn vnnd vormittelst gotlicher hilff / widerumb / tzue voriger gesuntheyt verhelffen mag (Leipzig: Valentinum Schuman, 1521), sigs. A2r–3r.

44 Ibid., sig. A6r. All translations are the author's unless otherwise noted.

45 Ibid., sig. A7v. This is the first of Kegler's references to self-medicating, which is rare in plague pamphlets.

46 Heinrich Stromer von Auerbach, *Henrici Stromers Aurbachii, Medicine Doctoris, saluberrime adversus pestilentiam observations, recens editae:– Aeque pauperibus prosunt locupletibus aeque. Aeque neglecte pueris, senibus nocebunt* (Leipzig: Valentino Schuman, 1516); Heinrich Stromer von Auerbach, *Regiment Henrichen Stromers von Aurbach d ertzenney Doctors inhaltēdt wie sich wid die pestilentz tzubewarē / auch den ihenen die damit begriffen hilff tzureichen* (Leipzig: Melchior Lotther, 1516).

47 Kegler refers specifically to only two medical texts: Antonio Guaineri's *Practica* (as explored below) and a common herbal regarding the power of a certain remedy. Kegler, *Eyn Nutzlichs vnd trostlichs Regiment*, 1529, fols. 34v, 13r, 19r, 25v.

48 Jütte, *Ärzte, Heiler und Patienten*, 139.

49 Heinrich Stromer, *Regiment Henrichen Stromers von Aurbach*, sig. B2v.

50 Pomata, *Contracting a Cure*, 129–139. On similar beliefs in eighteenth-century Germany, see: Barbara Duden, *Geschichte Unter der Haut: Ein Eisenacher Arzt und seine Patientinnen um 1730* (Stuttgart: Klett-Cotta, 1987).

51 Kegler, *Einn Regiment durch Doctorem Casparum Kegler gemacht*, sig. A3r.

52 Ibid., sigs. B4r–v.

53 "[V]il trostlichen experimentē gebessert / Die zuuor heymlich gehalten / vnd an den tag nyhe gegebē seyn": Kegler, *Eyn Nutzlichs vnd trostlichs Regiment*, 1529, title.

54 Ibid., fol. 20r.

55 "Dis findeth man pey mir": ibid.

56 Hieronymous Brunschwig, *Liber de arte distillandi. de simplicibus. Das buch der rechten kunst zu distilieren die eintzigen ding von Hieronymo bunschygk…* (Strassburg: Johannes Grüeninger, 1500), sig. C1r.

57 Kegler, *Eyn Nutzlichs vnd trostlichs Regiment*, 1529, fols. 13v–14r.

58 Joseph Koerner, *The Moment of Self-Portraiture in German Renaissance Art* (Chicago: University of Chicago Press, 1996), 203–207.

59 Vivian Nutton, "Medicine at the German Universities, 1348–1500: A Preliminary Sketch," in *Medicine from the Black Death to the French Disease*, Eds. Roger French, Jon Arrizabalaga, Andrew Cunningham, and Luis García-Ballester (Aldershot, UK: Ashgate, 1998): 85–109, at 97.

60 Martin Stainpeiss, *Ain hailsame ertzney: mit ierem zwesatz: zu behuetten wider den lauff der Pestelentz…* (Vienna, 1515), sigs. A6v, B3r.

61 Gundolf Keil, "Das 'Costelic Laxatijf' Meister Peters von Dorth," *Sudhoffs Archiv* 50 (1966): 113–135; Karl Sudhoff, "Vier Niederlassungsankündigungen von Ärzten aus dem 15. Jahrhundert," *Archiv für Geschichte der Medizin* 6 (1913): 309–312.

62 Francis B. Brevart, "Between Medicine, Magic and Religion: Wonder Drugs in German Medico-Pharmaceutical Treatises of the Thirteenth to the Sixteenth

Centuries," *Speculum* 83 (2008): 1–57; Thomas Holste, *Der Theriakkrämer: Ein Beitrag zur Frühgeschichte der Arzneimittelwerbung* (Pattensen: Horst Wellm Verlag, 1977), 53.

63 Balthasar Lothwiger, *Eyn kurtz nutzbar Regiment und Rath vor die schweren vñ erschrecklichen kranckheit der Pestilētz...* (Leipzig: Wolffgang Stöckel, 1516); and Wolfgang Peysser, *Ordnung der fursichtigen Ersamenn Weisen herrn Burgermaister / vnd Rat / der loblischen stat Inngolstat...* (Ingolstat, 1521).

64 Magnus Hundt, *Durch den hochgelerten Magistrum Magnuse hundt weyth beruffen Artztten / eyn Erbarn Rathe der Altenstadt Magdeburgck / seynen Erbherren uñ sust guthenfreunden doselbst wyder dy schwere plage der pestilentz zwgestelth...* (1528), sig. A4v.

65 Drachenfuss advertises an effective antidote learned from "Doctor Benedictus Fauentinus," calling it a "great wonder." Johann Drachenfuss, *Ein köstbarliche / bwerte vnd gewisse Artzney / wie ein gesundter in sterbens leufftē / auch einer der schon mit der grausamen kranckheyt der Pestilentz ergriffen worden / von solchem schnellen vnnd tödtlichen gift / sein leben erretten soll* (ca. 1531), sig. A2v.

66 Adam Zwicker, *Ein kurtze wolgegründte vnderrichtung vnd eklerung von Doctor Adam Zwicker zů Memmingen / wie man sich der erschröcklichen kranckheit der Pestilentz präseruieren / vnnd bewaren soll...* (1537).

67 On the importance of political agendas in encouraging alchemical and occult studies: Bruce T. Moran, *The Alchemical World of the German Court: Occult Philosophy and Chemical Medicine in the Circle of Moritz of Hessen (1572–1632)* (Stuttgart: Franz Steiner Verlag, 1991).

68 Simon Pistoris, *Ein kurtz schon unnd gar trostlich regiment widder die sweren vñ erchreckliche̅ kranckheit der pestilentz...* (Leipzig: Martin Landsberg, 1506), B6r.

69 Kegler, *Eyn Nutzlichs vnd trostlichs Regiment*, 1529, fols. 3r–v.

70 Similarities to Paracelsus exist in this regard: Webster, *Paracelsus*, 210–243.

71 Kegler, *Einn Regiment durch Doctorem Casparum Kegler gemacht*, sig. A2r.

72 Heike Talkenberger, *Sintflut: Prophetie und Zeitgeschehen in Texten und Holzschnitten astrologischer Flugschriften 1488–1528* (Tübingen: Niemeyer, 1990), 154.

73 Kegler, *Eyn Nutzlichs vnd trostlichs Regiment*, 1529, fols. 5–5v. Jonah, 3:1–5 (NSRV): in this story, God sends the prophet Jonah to Nineveh to preach that God will destroy the city in forty days unless the Ninevites repent.

74 Robert W. Scribner, "Cosmic Order and Daily Life: Sacred and Secular in Pre-Industrial German Society," in *Religion and Society in Early Modern Europe 1500–1800*, Ed. Kaspar von Greyerz (London: George Allen & Unwin, 1984): 17–32, at 25.

75 Melissa P. Chase, "Fevers, Poisons, and Apostemes: Authority and Experience in Montpellier Plague Treatises," in *Science and Technology in Medieval Society*, Ed. Pamela O. Long (New York: New York Academy of Sciences, 1985): 153–171.

76 Danielle Jacquart, "Theory, Everyday Practice, and Three Fifteenth-Century Physicians," *Osiris* 2nd series 6 (1990): 140–160. On late medieval alchemy and plague: Chiara Crisciani and Michela Pereira, "Black Death and Golden Remedies: Some Remarks on Alchemy and the Plague," in *The Regulation of Evil: Social and Cultural Attitudes to Epidemics in the Late Middle Ages*, Eds. Agostino Paravicini Bagliani and Francesco Santi (Sismel, Belgium: Edizioni del Galluzzo, 1998): 7–39.

77 Bruce Moran states "the art of distillation in the sixteenth century had, by and large, not yet come into the hands of university-educated philosophers and physicians": Bruce T. Moran, *Distilling Knowledge: Alchemy, Chemistry, and the Scientific Revolution* (Cambridge, MA: Harvard University Press, 2005), 55.

78 Jacquart, "Theory, Everyday Practice," 153–154; Karl Sudhoff, "Pestschriften aus den ersten 150 Jahren nach der Epidemie des 'schwarzen Todes' 1348," *Archiv für Geschichte der Medizin* 16 (1925): 117–118; Lynn Thorndike, *A History of Magic and Experimental Science*, Vol. IV, *Fourteenth and Fifteenth Centuries* (New York: Columbia University Press, 1934), 230–231.

79 Kegler, *Eyn Nutzlichs vnd trostlichs Regiment*, 1529, 19r.

80 "Gewürzkrämer / aromatarii": Wustmann, *Wirt von Auerbachs Keller*, 61.

81 Reusch recommended the traditional plague medicines, preferring "true theriac," which he advertises was available from Michael Hoffmann, an apothecary in Leipzig: Johann Reusch, *Regiment Doctor Johan Reüschen Wie sich zur zeit der Pestilentz zu halten sey / Die einwoner der Stadt Leiptzigk / vornemlich belangendt* (Leyptzigk: Nickel Schmidt, 1539), sigs. A3v–4r, B1v–2r, B5v.

82 SAL, Richterstube Inventarien und Hilfsbuch, 1547–1549, fols. 2r–7r. For the contract dissolving the estate in 1548, see: Ratsbuch, Vol. 9, fols. 147v–148v.

83 On Caspar Kegler the younger: Seyfarth, *Hospital zu St. Georg*, 76–77.

84 The inventory officials described four books specifically as "alchemical," two in Latin and two in German, but provided few details: SAL, Richterstube Inventarien und Hilfsbuch, 1547–1549, fol. 5v. On medieval alchemists: Crisciani and Pereira, "Black Death and Golden Remedies," 7–39.

85 "Fünffzehen lange gleßer dorin wenigk wasser zur Alchemey," "[E]in kupffern blaße mit einem helm dorin man wasser brauet," "[E]in kupffern offen": SAL, Richterstube Inventarien und Hilfsbuch, 1547–1549, fols. 6v–7r.

86 Ibid., fols. 5v–6r.

87 Kegler, *Einn Regiment durch Doctorem Casparum Kegler gemacht*, sig. B1r. On the popularity of novel alchemical medicines: William Eamon, "Alchemy in Popular Culture: Leonardo Fioravanti and the Search for the Philosopher's Stone," *Early Science and Medicine* 5 (2000): 196–213, esp. 203.

88 Moran, *Distilling Knowledge*, 55; Robert James Forbes, *Short History of the Art of Distillation* (Leiden: Brill, 1970), 102–103.

89 Anna of Saxony was the wife of the Elector Augustus of Saxony (r. 1553–1586): Rankin, *Panaceia's Daughters*, 128–167.

90 Sächsische Landes- und Universitätsbibliothek Dresden, B201, fols. 3r–v.

91 For discussion of this process outside of plague literature: Eamon, *Science and the Secrets of Nature*, 93–133; Moran, *Distilling Knowledge*, 59; Forbes, *Short History*, 100.

92 Kegler, *Eyn Nutzlichs vnd trostlichs Regiment*, 1529, fol. 20v. An ell corresponds roughly to a yard.

93 Ibid., fols. 20v–21v.

94 For Gentile's recipe: Crisciani and Pereira, "Black Death and Golden Remedies," 12.

95 Kegler, *Eyn Nutzlichs vnd trostlichs Regiment*, 1529, fols. 24v–25v.

96 Ibid., fol. 25v.

97 Hans Prescher and Otfried Wagenbreth, *Georgius Agricola: Seine Zeit und ihre Spuren* (Leipzig: Deutscher Verlag für Grundstoffindustrie, 1994), 14–20.

98 Ibid., 112–197. See also: Friedrich Naumann, Ed., *Georgius Agricola 500 Jahre* (Basel: Birkhäuser Verlag, 1994).

99 Moran, *Distilling Knowledge*, 44–45.

100 Prescher and Wagenbreth, *Georgius Agricola*, 30–38.

101 Lorenz Misch, *Für die Pestilentz Zweyer köstlichen Latwergen rechter Brauch. Eine des hoch vnd weithberümpten Herrn Doctor Mangolts seligen / weilandt der Stadt Costnitz Physici. Die Ander des Hochgelarthen Herrn D. Caspar Keglers / des eltern / seligen / die so er fur seinen besten schatz stets gehalten / vnd in den büchlein sonst nicht gefunden wirt / mit welchen von beiden Doctoribus zur zeit der Pestilentz an vielen glücklichen practicirt…* (Leipzig: Valentin Bapst, 1552); the title page lists the cost as well as his address on Fleischergasse in Leipzig. In Leipzig, the loth standard was 1/16th mark or 14.6133g: Ronald E. Zupko, *Revolution in Measurement: Western European Weights and Measures since the Age of Science* (Philadelphia: American Philosophical Society, 1990), 349–351.

102 Lorenz Misch, *Eine Tröstliche / bewerte Kunst / in sterbens nöten / wieder die Pestilentz / die alte güldene Pillen genant / Verordtnet / durch den künstreichen / Meister Lorentz Misch / inn der Churfürstlichen Stadt Leipzig / Wundt vnd Schneidtartzt / jetzo in der Peterstras / Wonhafftig daselbst zu finden* (1565).

103 Caspar Kegler, *Eynn nützlichs Vnnd tröstlichs Regiment wider die Gifftigk Pestilentzisch Feber die Schweyssucht genant / Vnnd sunst mancherley gifftig vnd tödtlich kranckheyt…* (ca. 1545), fol. 4r.

104 Caspar Kegler, *Ein Regiment durch Doctorem Casparum Kegeler gemacht / Darynnen man sich / vor der Erschrecklichen kranckheit der Pestilentz / Preseruiren / bewaren vnd erhalten…* (Magdeburg: Hans Walther, 1539), fol. B8r.

105 Heimeran Bulderkar and Lucas Gercke, *Kurzer Nützlicher vnd Nötiger Bericht / wie man sich jtziger zeit der Pestilentz verhalten…* (Magdeburg: Joachim Walden, 1565); *Kurtzer Nützlicher vnd nötiger Bericht / Wie man sich zur zeit der Pestilenz vorhalten / vnd die Ertzeney / so Anno 76. auff des Rahts der Altenstadt Magdeburgk Apoteck vor ordnet / vnd jtzo dieses 82. Jahres daselbst auch zubekommen / gebrauchen sol* (Magdeburg: Wolffgang Kirchner, 1582); *Kurtzer Nützlicher vnd Nötiger Bericht / Wie man die Medicamenta praeservativa curative Pestis, so Anno 97. auff des Raths Apoteken der Alten Stadt Magdeburgk verordnet / vnnd jtzo dieses 1607. Jahrs aus Befehl eines Erbarn Raths von jhren ver-ordneten Medicins revidirt vnd verbessert / gebrauchen sol* (Magdeburg: Ambrosius Kirchner/Salomon Kichtzenhan, 1607).

106 *Kurtzer Nützlicher vnd Nötiger Bericht*, 1607, fols. D2r–3r.

107 Caspar Kegler, *Ein heilsam / nutzbar vnd hülffreichs Regiment Wieder die Pestilentz vnd das gifftige Pestilentz Fieber (die Schweissucht genant) vnd sonsten mancherley gifftige vnd todtliche Krankheiten…* (Dresden: Christian Bergen, 1607), fols. A2v–A3r; Caspar Kegler, *Ein Nützliches vnd Tröstlichs Regiment wider die Pestilentz / vnd gifftig Pestilentzisch Feber / die Schweissucht genant / Vnd sonst mancherley gifftige vnd todtliche Kranckheit…* (Leipzig: Johan Rhambaw, 1566), fols. A3v–4r.

108 Kegler, *Ein Nützliches vnd Tröstlichs Regiment*, 1566, fols. D1v–2r. See also: Kegler, *Ein heilsam / nutzbar vnd hülffreichs Regiment*, 1607, fols. 13r–14r.

109 *Verzeichnis der im deutschen sprachbereich erschienenen Drucke des XVI. Jahrhunderts- VD 16*, Part I, Vol. X (Stuttgart: Anton Hiersemann, 1987), 370–371; Caspar Kegeler, *Ein nützliches vnd tröstliches Regiment / wider die*

Pestilentz / vnd gifftig pestilentzisch Fieber / die Schweissucht genant / Vnd sonst mancherley gifftige vnd tödliche Kranckheit (Eisleben: Andreas Petri, 1565); Caspar Kegler, *Ein Nützliches vnd tröstlichs Regiment wider die Pestilentz / vnd gifftig Pestilentzische Fieber / die Schweissucht genant / Vnd sonst mancherley gifftige vnd todtliche Kranckheit...* (Königsberg in Preussen: Georg Osterberger, 1588).

110 An "alexiteric" is a medicine that counteracts poison. Balthasar Brunner, *Kurtzer vnd einfeltiger Bericht / Wie man sich / in jetzo verfallender Sterbenßzeit / praeseruiren vnd verhalten sol. Gestellet vor die Gemeine zu Halle* (Leipzig: Jacob Berwaldts Erben, 1581), sig. C2r; *Kurzer und Einfeltiger Bericht: Wie sich in diesen jetzigen sterbensleufften der gemeine Man zuuerhalten habe. Auff beger eines Erbarn Wolweisen Raths zu Halle / von den Medicis daselbst / gemeiner Stadt zunutz gestellet* (Eisleben: Andream Petri, 1575).

111 Caspar Kegler, *Nützlicher vnd wahrer Bericht wider die Pestilentz / vnnd wie man sich in zeit dero erschrecklichen regierung preseruiern / bewahren vnnd erhalten...* (Cölln: Wilhelm Lützenkirchen, 1597), sigs. B5r–v.

112 *Die Messkataloge des sechzehnten Jahrhunderts*, Vol. V (Hildesheim: Georg Olms Verlag, 1972), fall 1597, vernacular medicine category.

113 Universitätsbibliothek Heidelberg, Cod. Pal. germ 204 (fols. 190v–202r), 239 (17v–38r), 242 (105r–106r), 256 (470v–471v), 278 (87v), 285 (5r–6r).

114 Volker Klimpel, *Dresdner Ärzte: Historisch-Biographisches Lexikon* (Dresden: Hellerau Verlag, 1998), 165.

115 Kegler, *Ein Regiment / Durch Doctorem Casparum Kegeler gemacht*, 1584, sigs. A2r–v, C1r. This edition adds a list of medicines that are available to rich (for a fee) and poor (for free) from the barber Zacharias Blath on Wilßdorffer Gasse. The printer Gimel Bergen also appended an official public health announcement.

116 Kegler, *Ein heilsam / nutzbar vnd hülffreichs Regiment*, 1607, sig. A6v.

117 Ibid., sig. A2v.

118 Ibid., sig. A3r.

119 SAL, Tit. XLIV B Nr. 3 (F), fol. 46v, and Tit. XLIV B Nr. 4 (F), fol. 1r. This first document probably dates from the 1640s. The second document is dated April 16, 1644.

120 The latest pamphlet to cite Kegler: *E. E. Hochweisen Raths der Stadt Leipzig Verneuerte und verbesserte Ordnung / Wie es bey besorgenden ansteckenden Seuchen / da GOtt dergleichen über diese Stadt verhängen sollte / ...* (Leipzig: Christoph Günther, 1680), 52.

5 The flourishing of German medicine, 1530–1580

Humanism, empiricism, and Protestantism

In the decades after Caspar Kegler and Martin Luther became prominent plague authors, a new generation continued this reform of healing in plague texts. Like Luther, some physicians and clerics promoted Protestant reforms, sometimes even incorporating Luther's positions into their own writing. Like Kegler, some authors attempted to connect more directly to a broad audience, especially by promoting cures discovered or confirmed through personal experience. And, following the example of Johann Vochs and the great German botanists, some physicians showed renewed interest in a patriotic German medicine as well as in the particulars of local environments. While these various agendas had previously been separate, this chapter demonstrates how these innovative trends blended and reinforced each other in some of the more original and popular plague treatises composed after 1530. This unification of the innovative trends from Renaissance thought, Protestantism, and vernacular print is significant since it encouraged non-traditional ideas about plague and plague responses, and, overall, gave these texts their own distinct character. It is therefore during these decades around the mid-sixteenth century that one sees the full flourishing of a distinctly German reform of healing in print that had been decades in the making.

The continuing reform of plague advice in German lands is important for demonstrating the impact of authors such as Johann Vochs, but also for revealing the growth of a new network of physicians that began to connect academic medicine more directly with the local environmental and cultural contexts of German lands. Physicians became more interested in discussing specific causes of plague within the local environment, rather than relying solely on the traditional but general sayings about miasmas and poisoned air. Other changes in the social and political context encouraged this trend as well, as town physicians and magistrates after 1530 became more interested in creating public health guidelines for epidemics. The impulse for this change came to some extent from abroad, as physicians and magistrates throughout western Europe sought to imitate the public health efforts of Venice and other Italian cities.[1] But, regardless of where this trend originated, it encouraged German physicians to reflect on local causes of the plague as well as local responses, and drove a discussion about contagion, or how the plague spread from person to person, from town to town. Such changes also affected the rhetorical tone within some plague treatises produced after circa 1530, as physicians felt a new impulse to develop and publicize rules for behavior during plagues. This trend brought physicians to construct knowledge about plague at a finer, more local level, thereby diverging from previous academic approaches to the subject that were content with universal explanations and cures. Observation, experience, and specific causes were ascendant, thereby diminishing the role of ancient theory and scholarly authority.

This chapter explores a number of German physicians who penned some of the most reprinted or most original plague texts in the decades after 1530, yet who are nonetheless obscure today. These include Johann Reusch, Tarquinius Schnellenberg, Jodocus Willich, and Ernst Reuchlin. Johann Dryander appears here as well, as an influential editor of plague texts. Since some of these authors are obscure, this chapter investigates both their lives and their writings, in an effort to show how plague advice changed amid the medical, religious, and social concerns of the time.

Johann Reusch and the revival of Johann Vochs

The story of Vochs's continuing impact begins with the well-known humanist Johann Dryander, a professor of medicine and mathematics at Marburg. Dryander contributed much to the direction of German plague writing as an editor and commentator rather than an author. Not only did he republish Johann Vochs's plague text in 1537 but he also republished a Lutheran collection of plague texts in 1554, as explored further below. Dryander was clearly impressed with Vochs's positions since he took time to reissue the text relatively soon after taking his academic post at the University of Marburg. Dryander added little commentary to Vochs's work other than introductory remarks in support of Vochs's mission to protect Germania from the greed of medical swindlers. One other added preface offers a warning against the "egg of the philosophers" (*Ovum philosophorum*), an ostensibly alchemical cure that Dryander denounces as flawed in design and substance.[2] Like Vochs, Dryander did not reject alchemy *in toto* but targeted the deceit of greedy impostors, who threatened the health and wealth of Germania.

Vochs's ideas had a lasting impact on Johann Reusch (1490s? –1543), the Leipzig physician and one-time rector of the University of Leipzig. Reusch's plague treatises, published in 1527 and 1539, reveal an important continuation of Vochs's ideas and rhetoric, as well as many other important changes under way within plague advice after the tumultuous 1520s. Reusch was drawn to Vochs's text since they both shared the reforming spirit and patriotism of German humanism. Reusch's writings are marked by a local pride in Leipzig, perhaps due to the professional and economic success that Reusch found there, much like Kegler, after arriving in the city as a student in 1512.[3] In 1520 Reusch wrote to defend Leipzig's reputation against negative stories about its people and environment, as spun by rivals at the University of Wittenberg. In a position that he would repeat later when writing about plague, Reusch denied that Leipzig's environment produced dangerous swamp gasses that poison the air but, rather, praised the city's people, rivers, and forests.[4] Reusch was also interested in the reform of religion, and yet in 1520 he identified more with Erasmus than with Luther, as a letter to the Nuremberg humanist Willibald Pirckheimer makes clear.[5] This allegiance may have shifted by 1522, however, as Duke Georg of Saxony moved to eradicate Luther's Reformation from his lands, including Leipzig. At this time historian Gustav Wustmann describes Reusch as an early enthusiast of Luther's, guided by the views of the Leipzig medical professor Heinrich Stromer.[6] Two years later, in April 1524, Reusch was elected rector of the University of Leipzig, shortly after the death of Petrus Mosellanus, the local leader of reform-minded humanists.[7] As rector, Reusch had to defend himself from the bishop's criticism that he was not doing enough to root out Luther's heresy at the university. Perhaps because of the difficult religious politics of the time, Reusch soon began to study medicine, and he gained his baccalaureus in 1526.

After turning his attention to medicine, Reusch had much success, especially in growing his influence outside the university. Near the end of 1527 Reusch bore the cost of publishing a short Latin plague treatise dedicated to prominent members of the Leipzig city council. This text seems to have impressed the council so much that they granted him the privilege of citizenship at no cost the following year. Composed in Latin, the text demonstrates the knowledge that Reusch had obtained only recently in his medical studies. It is remarkable for traits that would grow more prominent in his later vernacular text, such as specific commentary on Germans and German lands, the occasional use of an ego perspective, as well as an interest in *secretum*, or proven cures that remained somewhat mysterious. For example, after listing the standard academic positions on the plague's origins, Reusch turns his attention to what he believed were the common causes among Germans (*Germanos*): disorderly use of food and drink, immoderate sex and exercise, and damp places and silver mines that release pestiferous exhalations, much like Pliny's example of the Italian Lake Amsancto. Reusch gives other contributing factors, such as the wretched state of Christian mores, public order, and cleanliness in German cities.[8] In a likely reference to Kegler, Reusch also praises an electuary "of my preceptor" made of unicorn horn that has the "most efficacious" power of *aqua vitae*.[9] A further similarity to Kegler's 1521 pamphlet is that Reusch sometimes uses an ego perspective to add details from his own experience, such as this statement: "I however have used not unfruitfully in this year the most secret, most experienced (*expertissimo*) powder with the written electuary."[10] Here Reusch refers to an herbal recipe that he believed could replace theriac among the poor, which sounds very similar to Vochs's goals and methods.

If it is not completely certain whether Reusch was drawing on Vochs's text as he wrote in 1527, his 1539 vernacular pamphlet removes all doubt.

Here Reusch echoes full sentences and even paragraphs of Vochs's text. These include passages on the special characteristics of German bodies as well as the dangers of imported theriac and foreign salesmen. Reusch even names Vochs as he praises his "German theriac" (*deüdtschen Teriacks*) made of native ingredients. Perhaps taking a cue from Kegler, Reusch advertises this powerful medicine as available from the Leipzig apothecary Michael Hoffman at an honest price.[11] Reusch mentions the German theriac multiple times as he substitutes it for the traditional theriac in the text.[12] Like Vochs, Reusch also believed that there was not one single cause of the plagues but, rather, that each plague had its own origin. This similarly led Reusch to deny that one powder can cure all plagues, so much so that one should "throw out the window all powders of bolus armenicus, terra sigillata and camphor rather than putting them into the body."[13] Furthermore, the following quotation about purging practices illuminates how this "German" approach to medicine encouraged the use of experience within medical thought, if not also practice:

> Because relieving the body of excess humidities is done differently among us Germans than among the Italians and Spaniards, do not employ the softening or purging from the same books as them, but rather do so out of good reasoning and certain experience.[14]

This quotation reveals that Vochs's message remained alive within the next generation of physicians, specifically his warning not to accept ancient or Mediterranean medical traditions uncritically and without the guidance of experience.

Reusch's embrace of Vochs's medical views in 1539 extended even to Vochs's non-traditional focus on water, rather than air, as important to the cause and spread of the epidemic. In his section on the plague's origins, Reusch comments specifically on environmental conditions at the regional and local levels. These passages show Reusch relying on personal observation to guide his medical views as he compares local realities to general ancient teachings. Much like his defense of Leipzig from its Wittenberg detractors in 1520, Reusch in 1539 flatly denies that Leipzig's air is poisoned and also dismisses the harmful effects of planets and comets on the atmosphere. Reusch's justifications for rejecting poisoned air include these statements:

> [B]irds such as hawks and sparrows, which avoid poisoned air, have remained with us up to now. One has also not noticed that unusual types of worms have crept up from their holes to the earth. Also this past summer and fall has had so much warm and clear sunshine that has completely cleaned and purified the air.[15]

Such observations led Reusch to suspect water as a cause of the plague in 1539. In an unusual move for the time, Reusch focuses on water as the main infectious agent behind the spread of the sickness:

> But according to my opinion, this sickness creeps around from one to another, since the earth has been penetrated and flooded for two or three consecutive years with great waters, which has poisoned the nature and qualities of the water.[16]

It is no surprise, however, that this unusual position is likely drawn from Vochs, who some thirty years earlier had rejected poisoned air and focused on water as the cause of the pestilence: "I say that the flooding of waters in this year and the past three years has poisoned and corrupted the nature and essence of the water."[17] Like Vochs, Reusch continues by saying that the putrefied water has fouled seeds in the fields and fruits on the trees, but here he adds the news that local farmers ("*Haussveter auff dem Land*") recently failed to preserve radishes and kraut with salt, "which has never happened before according to memory."[18] This leads Reusch to fear a general dying in German lands as many people must drink, cook, or bake with "stagnant, swampy, slimy and stinking water." Although Reusch draws heavily on Vochs in this passage, he adds his own personal observations and reports about harmful water elsewhere in the region. Reusch does not specifically say that the water around Leipzig is poisoned, but urges caution since it is nearly surrounded by "many swampy lakes," and since the dying started at watery places and seaports such as Lübeck and Danzig. In building his case on the connection between bad water and bad health, Reusch appeals to the authority of Galen, although he seems to ignore Galen's teachings that connect bad air and epidemics.[19] In this way, Reusch builds a particular view of the plague's origin by selectively applying teachings from Galen and Vochs to the local situation, as well as by drawing on personal observations and regional news.

The emphasis on water by both Vochs and Reusch is interesting, because it contradicts one predominant assumption of Galenic medicine: that the atmosphere of air was the most important avenue of transmitting a general sickness. Indeed, Latin Galenism considered the "air-environment" to be the most important of the six non-naturals for human health.[20] Certainly, water was important among the Galenic physicians, but in many cases only secondarily, due to its effect on the air. Water does appear among the causes of plague in earlier plague treatises, such as in the 1348 text by the Catalan physician Jacme d'Agramont. Agramont accepted that putrefied waters can cause a universal pestilence if vapors from the water rise and corrupt the air in its substance.[21] But, regardless of where the putrefaction originates, whether swamps, battlefields, or the influence of planets, Agramont and other early plague authors focused most of their attention on the air or general atmosphere when discussing the plague's origins and how it spread from region to region.[22] It is therefore unusual for Vochs and Reusch to deny that the local air is poisoned while focusing on water instead. Reusch may have received further encouragement to explore this idea since Martin Luther also rejected that the local air around Wittenberg was poisoned when discussing the plague of 1527, as discussed further below.

This position against poisoned air is also surprising since contemporary Italian thinkers who wrote on the connection between plague and flooding were hesitant to break with traditional ideas by excising the role of air. The Italian humanist Niccolo Leoniceno, for example, cited cases of flooding as behind the French Disease, and specifically the flooding and stagnant water that resulted from the great rains of 1495–96 in Italian lands. But Vochs and Reusch go beyond Leoniceno in their focus on water as the chief agent of infection, since even Leoniceno held the more traditional view that the water works through the air to spread the sickness. In Leoniceno's words, the French Disease resulted from "certain intemperances of the air" brought about by the stagnant water.[23] Overall, the unusual position staked out by Vochs and Reusch shows how widely German physicians could depart from the views of their colleagues elsewhere, and raises the possibility that this divergence is tied to their particular transalpine perspective. If one starts from the assumption that plague in German lands does not conform to the traditional views of the Mediterranean-based authorities, it inspires physicians to rethink the fundamental issues of plague's causes and cures.

Reusch's attention to poisoned water led to what may have been a therapeutic innovation. Due to Leipzig's swampy and potentially dangerous local environment, Reusch recommends that people strain their water through a clean cloth, boil it, and strain it once more before cooking or preserving food with it. Reusch understands this process to clean all of the slime or mire (*schleym*) from the water, preparing it for human consumption. Obviously, Reusch did not intend to kill waterborne microorganisms by boiling. As he viewed it, rather, this process made the food and water more digestible, since hard-to-digest nourishment creates foul humidities that can poison the body from within.[24] Although it likely had little impact on preventing bubonic plague, Reusch's suggestion would have proved helpful in protecting the body from waterborne illnesses, not to mention helpful in preparing a clean brine solution for the successful fermentation of sauerkraut.

Historians have written little on the early history of advice to boil water for human consumption. It appears occasionally in early modern plague treatises, and may stem from basic kitchen practices and popular notions of hygiene. Marsilius Ficino's 1481 plague treatise recommends that people boil their drinking water, although this advice did not strike historian Walter Pagel as unusual or significant.[25] Historian Samuel Cohn uncovered a little-known plague doctor Massuci, who recommended that his audience boil and filter their drinking water if it was drawn from rain or well water. Cohn finds that it was rare before 1575, however, for Italian plague doctors to warn about the dangers of certain types of drinking water, as well as to emphasize the importance of finding clean water sources. Yet attention to water became more prevalent in Italian plague tracts during the epidemic of 1575–76, when intense debates broke out between physicians on the role of contaminated water. One respected astrologer, Annibal Raimondo, resembles Vochs when he argued that Venice's air was not poisoned, but that the plague resulted from contaminated drinking water. Cohn also explains the growing attention to the quality of water in the Italian plague treatises as tied to the growth of awareness of public health issues during the sixteenth century.[26]

Despite Reusch's focus on water as a primary cause of the epidemic, his 1539 pamphlet considers other forms of contagion to help explain how the sickness spread between people. Reusch's exploration of contagion is tied directly with greater attention to public health issues in Leipzig, and especially to the creation of rules by civic authorities for regulating the population during epidemics. Reusch's discussion of contagion shows that he believed it to take place either directly, through contact with a person's breath, or indirectly, through contact with an infected person's clothes and bed sheets. "Because this sickness creeps easily from one person to the other," Reusch announces the city council's order that the heads of the household (*Hausvater*) should take their sick to the St. Georg Hospital outside the Ranstädter city gate. Reusch also bans the people who attend to the sick from circulating in the city, and bans people moving around the city to distribute the sacraments to the sick. Reusch reasons that, because the air inside such houses is infected by the sick person's breath, the sickness spreads when the healthy person takes it in with the breath and through the sweat pores. To prevent indirect contagion, Reusch says that the clothes and the bed sheets of the sick and dead must not be sold or given away, but that they be cleaned outside the city in flowing water. In 1539 there even seemed to be attempts to enforce such rules in Leipzig, as Reusch mentions "laws and earnest punishments, as is common for many honest regimes [*policien*]."[27]

Such public health statements reflect a rhetorical change in German plague treatises, as they moved away from providing general instructions for preventing and curing plague and began to publicize new rules that sought to regulate civic behavior. Magistrates and territorial rulers were only beginning to get involved in public health issues related to epidemics during the early sixteenth century. To some extent they were spurred to action by the arrival of the frightening French Disease in 1495.[28] Reusch's role in publicizing Leipzig's new "laws" for plague times was a first for a physician in the city and came after a long, slow growth of interest among local magistrates for creating civic policies for epidemics. One of the earliest plague pamphlets printed in Leipzig mentions that the city council urged the author, Simon Pistoris, to compose his text for the good of the city in 1506. But soon the city council sought more than just engaging the pens of local physicians, and sought institutions to counter the spread of the sickness. In 1520 Leipzig created its first plague hospital on the grounds of the St. Georg Hospital outside the city walls, where the city could isolate the sick during epidemics.[29] More serious attempts to regulate behavior to prevent plague came in 1536, when the city's territorial lord, Duke Georg of Saxony, issued rules on the practices of burying the dead.[30] Perhaps because Leipzig's city council had many local physicians to whom it could turn to compose plague treatises, the civic magistrates themselves did not publish comprehensive plague rules until 1607.[31] In contrast, authorities in Vienna published their first plague regulations in print in 1541, and in Nuremberg in 1562.[32] Overall, Reusch's 1539 vernacular pamphlet was at the leading edge of more intensive efforts by German rulers to regulate their populations during epidemics.

Reusch's attempts to change the medical behavior of the *Hausvater*, or male head of household, also reveal an important shift within German vernacular literature after 1530. After the first tumultuous decade of the Reformation, and given magistrates' growing interest in public health, religious and medical authors began more often to address their messages to the *Hausvater*, either directly or indirectly. The *Hausvater* were not just any men, but were property owners in town and country who oversaw the members of a large pre-modern household, which could include immediate and extended families, servants, and day laborers. By impressing their agendas upon the *Hausvater*, religious and medical authors sought to reform the behavior of even the lowest orders of society. The term *Hausvater* certainly pre-dates the 1530s within German plague treatises, but only later did it take on new importance amid the growing efforts to reform society.[33]

Protestant attempts to promote social stability in particular drove the proliferation of the term *Hausvater* after circa 1530. In this period Protestant reformers began to respond to a perceived crisis within families by publishing sermons intended to reorient the household and family along more "Christian" lines. This effort included spelling out the powers and responsibilities of husbands, wives, mothers, fathers, children, and servants, drawing on biblical principles. Protestant efforts reinforced the patriarchal family structure, since reformers reaffirmed the *Hausvater* as the leader of the extended household.[34] Luther himself played a role in popularizing the term *Hausvater*, since he included it in his German translation of the Bible and his Small Catechism of 1529, which were among the most-read books of the sixteenth century.[35]

Within plague treatises, appeals to the "common man" never disappeared but were often replaced with appeals to the *Hausvater* over the course of the sixteenth century. Since the term "common man" was connected to the protests of the 1520s or even the social catastrophe of the 1525 German Peasants' War, authors and printers turned to the male head of the household as a more reliable partner in reform. In German lands both Protestant and Catholic, physicians believed that the *Hausvater* served as an important link in a chain of medical treatment, whose help was becoming more important as physicians and magistrates confronted plague's contagious and infectious nature. Authors imagined that the *Hausvater* would act as a medical intermediary, the physician's representative, treating the sick and poor among one's own in order to stem the contagion. One wonders, however, how the medicine of the physician and *Hausvater* interacted with the folk household medicine, which was traditionally the province of women.

Reusch's use of the term *Hausvater* connects him to contemporary social and medical reform. Leipzig in fact was just beginning an official Protestant Reformation as Reusch wrote his vernacular plague treatise in September 1539. In the spring of 1539 Duke Georg of Saxony died, leaving his Protestant brother Heinrich to inherit the position. As the territorial lord of Leipzig, Duke Heinrich IV ushered in the city's Protestant Reformation. Given his long interest in religious reform, Reusch seems to have welcomed this change.[36] Overall, Reusch's plague texts reveal the blending of various reform efforts, from public health, German patriotism, and an emergent reform of religion and society. They also demonstrate how such reform efforts could spawn innovative ideas about plague and new approaches to its treatment.

Tarquinius Schnellenberg and the German medicine of the botanists

The effort to create a more German medicine grew significantly in the decades after Johann Vochs's text reappeared in print in 1537. By the mid-sixteenth century this disparate movement had expanded to include a broad array of authors from both medicine and botany. The story of the physician Tarquinius Schnellenberg (? –1561) reveals a champion of German medicine who drew new inspiration from the recent works of the great German botanists Otto Brunfels, Hieronymus Bock, and Leonhard Fuchs, while the thought of Vochs and the Protestant Reformation play key background roles. Schnellenberg's plague texts of 1540 and 1546 demonstrate how this German reform movement grew beyond its roots as new authors explored its wide creative potential.

The importance of Schnellenberg's plague texts is immediately apparent from their lengthy publication history. His 1546 book in particular, *Experimenta from 20 Plague Roots and Herbs, How They May Be Used for Poison and Plague*, counts among the most reprinted plague texts of the era, totaling at least twenty-seven editions between 1546 and 1700. This publication success rivals that of Caspar Kegler's works, and even surpasses it after 1600 as various printers and editors renewed it, incredibly, up to 1700.[37] But, despite the success of Schnellenberg's works in vernacular print, historians have largely forgotten him, much like Kegler.

Schnellenberg's success as an author came from his original vision of a plague medicine based thoroughly on German plants known through *experimenta*, which showcased knowledge derived from his own long experience. Schnellenberg's *experimenta* were much like Kegler's: recipes that had been proved to be effective through experience, but were nonetheless mysterious since no one could explain their efficacy through reason, logic, or learned authority. For Schnellenberg and Kegler, *experimenta* allowed them to highlight a new and more personal sort of knowledge based on experience, and provided an attractive alternative to the more traditional plague advice of the time. As seen in Chapter 4, this approach won tremendous success within the burgeoning world of vernacular print.

Schnellenberg's success in publishing is also remarkable given that he did not achieve great fame or status during his career, which otherwise left relatively few traces in the historical record. He identified the city of Dortmund as his homeland, although the date and exact place of his birth are unknown. The first evidence of Schnellenberg's medical practice comes in 1519/20, when he treated plague victims in Saxony, according to his own account.[38] Other records show him active in Erfurt and Schwarzburg by 1536/37, and serving as the physician to the city councils of Nordhausen by 1538 and Dortmund by at least 1546. In 1540 the poet Cyprian Stapert (Vomelius) described him as having recently obtained his doctor of medicine degree in Cologne. At some point after 1546 Schnellenberg left Dortmund, and later he died in Travemünde near Lübeck, in 1561.[39] In addition to his famous *experimenta* book of 1546, Schnellenberg published a more traditional plague treatise in 1540, as well as various almanacs and other astrological texts during his career.

Schnellenberg's first publication, his 1540 plague treatise, introduces an emphasis on proven cures that would later define his *experimenta* book. In his 1540 text and other works, Schnellenberg seems to promote the notion that experience should be at least an equal partner with texts and philosophy in building medical knowledge, if not a greater partner. Even when Schnellenberg draws recipes from other plague texts, he is careful to note their proven abilities, or even tells stories of how they were used successfully in the past. For example, Schnellenberg cites the Leipzig physician Simon Pistoris for one pill that purportedly protects people from plague for up to fourteen days, and notes that experienced doctors in Cologne used and valued it.[40] Schnellenberg does not advance a patriotic German medicine in his 1540 text, however, although he does seem to be aware of his vernacular audience, as he describes a pill that has been proven "within the borders of Germany."[41]

While his plague treatise seems to have had little influence on its time, Schnellenberg found success with his 1546 *experimenta* book for plague, in which he promotes German medical simples and proven cures with the zeal of a reformer. This text also has a more distinct German tone, as it focuses on twenty plants of the "German Nation" (*Deudscher Nation*) that the common man could use to fight plague and poison.[42] Indicative of his effort to reach a broad audience, Schnellenberg designed the text for ease of use. To ease reference, Schnellenberg lists the twenty plants in alphabetical order. To ease plant identification, he includes small woodcut images of each plant as well as a lengthy written description, including where to find such plants among the German regions. Schnellenberg also omitted some of the defining elements of the plague treatise genre: the scholastic discussion of causes and signs of the pestilence, the division between prevention and curative medicine, and advice based on the six *res non naturales*. Schnellenberg's *experimenta* book therefore falls outside the scholastic plague treatise genre, as established in the fourteenth century, and instead resembles a printed herbal of the later Renaissance, just like the sort that the great German botanists were publishing during the 1530s and 1540s. Since Schnellenberg cites Otto Brunfels, Hieronymus Bock, and Leonhart Fuchs at various times in his text, it is no mystery that their works provided key inspiration. Focusing a German herbal on plague and proven cures was Schnellenberg's signature innovation, however. This was certainly a shrewd idea, since he was blending two separate genres – the herbal and plague treatise – both of which had recently begun to thrive in the world of vernacular print.

Schnellenberg's *experimenta* book praises personal experience and German simples to an unusually high degree, apparent from the opening dedication to the syndic Michael Meienberg of Nordhausen. Here Schnellenberg introduces his *experimenta* as recipes and treatments known through experience: "[C]ompiled from long practice, named *Experimenta* or *Empirica*."[43] Later he describes his esteem for native botanical medicines as he states that he has used the "green woods" alone to practice medicine when apothecary shops were not available.[44] Schnellenberg was no rustic empiric, however, as his text relies on learned textual authority as well. In a poem to the reader, Schnellenberg praises Galen as a "prince and lord" and emphasizes Galen's own esteem for medical simples. Yet this poem also raises the possibility that experience is more important than learned authority, as Schnellenberg saves the highest praise for experience: "[E]xperience is the mistress above all / the sophist can say what he wants."[45] This love of experience is a natural consequence of his focus on native plants, since only he could claim to know the real German specimens based on experience, unlike Galen, Avicenna, and others.

Considering his broad reach within popular print in the sixteenth and seventeenth centuries, Schnellenberg became one of the era's great champions of German medicine, likely surpassing the influence of Vochs in due time. Schnellenberg's argument for German simples resembles that of Vochs, since he argues that German plants are better suited to the nature of German bodies: "[W]e have so many good and precious simples in the German Nation that are more trusted and closer to our nature than the overseas imports."[46] There is no explicit evidence that Schnellenberg was aware of Vochs's work, although it seems likely, especially given his studies in Cologne. Furthermore, many contemporary authors do not make such specific connections between the nature of the German body and native plants, including even Paracelsus in his *Herbarium*. Schnellenberg's text also demonstrates how far the German herbal had developed by the 1540s, since it provides images and descriptions of the plants in question, which were notably absent in Paracelsus's *Herbarium*.[47]

The influence of the German botanists Brunfels, Bock, and Fuchs deserves further comment. Schnellenberg's *experimenta* book is similar to contemporary herbals in both structure and content, including even discussion of the thorny issues of plant identification. All Renaissance botanists faced difficulty in relating ancient scholarship to the plants that appeared before them, since the plant names and descriptions from the past presented many uncertainties. Botanical scholarship therefore involved researching the history of names used in earlier texts in an effort to find an accurate name for the plant in question. Relating German plants to ancient Mediterranean-based texts ran up against the challenges of botanical diversity within Europe, however, since German lands often had their own distinct varieties of plants that were also found near the Mediterranean, if they appeared in both regions at all. On such issues of plant diversity and whether the ancients were aware of the German plants, Schnellenberg often sided with Hieronymus Bock. Both believed that ancient scholars such as Dioscorides were not ignorant about the plant in question but often lacked specific knowledge of German varieties. In most cases, Schnellenberg respected the work of his Greek and Roman predecessors, but was not shy to highlight the limits of their knowledge, especially in light of German particulars. For example, Schnellenberg notes that Dioscorides does not mention the flowers of the betonia plant and comments: "[M]aybe he has never seen them…because what we see, that we attest to, as the jurists say."[48] Here it is interesting to see Schnellenberg borrowing the method of jurists to support his experience-based medical views, as he sought to supplement or correct ancient knowledge.

Schnellenberg's discussion of the problems of botanical scholarship reveals further details of his view that personal experience must come before knowledge from texts. When discussing the medical simple brown betonia, he states that he and the "diligent" Bock have needlessly paid attention to the ramblings of scholars who have never seen the plant "with their bodily eyes" (*mit leiblichen augen*) but who have relied on writings alone. In a sweeping statement of his own philosophy of medical knowledge, Schnellenberg argues for experiencing the plants first, in order to know their nature and the lands and circumstances in which they grow, and only then to compare them to the books. Schnellenberg believed that an experience-first approach would solve the many contradictions among physicians' texts on the topic of medicinal simples:

> One wants to bring betonia from Spain because it was supposed to have been found there first, as Pliny writes in Book 25, Chapter 8. Another wants to fetch betonia from Britain, since the same can be found there in abundance. I, however, next to others who are experienced and knowledgeable about German lands [*deudschen Landen*], want to say and witness that I have seen and used the real betonia, both white and brown, seen most notably and for the first time in the Harz Mountains, in a spot called Elnelingerode. There the white flowers were visibly growing next to the brown. Thus [the knowledge] appears to me much more settled from him who has visually discovered the medical simple, applied it in

> practice, and has actually dealt with it, and thereupon compares it to the text. The same must be viewed as that much more believable and sure than he who deals alone with mere texts.[49]

To emphasize the universality of his outlook, Schnellenberg adds the following: "[S]uch experience should take place beforehand for all things."[50] Striking here is that Schnellenberg emphasizes the body's visual sense and personal real-world experience in his view of how to construct a more certain medical knowledge. Here Schnellenberg appears to be an early proponent of an active science of the body that historian Pamela Smith sees as emerging more broadly among scholars by the early seventeenth century.[51] On these issues Schnellenberg shares much with Bock, who placed the most emphasis on personal experience among his peers Brunfels, Fuchs, and others. Bock's herbal of 1539 relies on his own descriptions of the plants that he found in German lands, surpassing the particular knowledge found in his peers' herbals, which were derived more thoroughly from ancient sources.[52]

Schnellenberg's life and work also demonstrate that the reform of medicine and botany remained connected to the reform of religion in sixteenth-century German lands.[53] Schnellenberg seems to have embraced Protestant views, along with his contemporaries Brunfels, Fuchs, and Bock – the latter serving as a Lutheran minister for a time. Parallels between the reform of botany, medicine, and religion are strong in Brunfels's *Reformation der Apotecken* (1536), which was famous for modeling a pharmaceutical reformation on the basic principles and rhetoric of the Protestant Reformation.[54] And, much like Brunfels, Vochs, and Luther, Schnellenberg saw himself fighting foreign ideas and sophistication with simple, solid truths that were at home among Germans. Certainly, Schnellenberg's *experimenta* book appealed to such cultural sentiments as he sought to replace foreign compound medicines of dubious ingredients with German simples plucked from local fields and forests. In this spirit Schnellenberg added a "Protestatio" to the end of his text in which he summarizes his arguments for German medicines, including that they are most helpful to the "poor, common man" since they are closer to his "complexion in Germania than the overseas imports" (*transmarina*).[55]

Other details from Schnellenberg's life and writings show that he was sympathetic to the Lutheran Reformation. During his time in the imperial city of Nordhausen, around 1539, he was friends with some of the key figures in the local Reformation, including the syndic Michael Meienburg and the theologian Johann Spangenberg.[56] Schnellenberg even begins his 1540 plague treatise with a Latin poem dedicated to Johannes Gigas, a prominent Lutheran reformer. Schnellenberg's 1540 plague treatise also seems to echo Martin Luther's plague sermon when it emphasizes that people must help each other, rather than flee, during plague times.[57] A more explicit Protestant voice appears in Schnellenberg's 1546 *experimenta* book, although he tries to stay focused on plants rather than religious controversies:

> The old women in the times of popery [*Papisterey*] have indeed used this [herb elecampane: *Alant Wurzel*] as a main ingredient in their incense, not without cause. I know something to write on this topic, but will not go into it at this time. I will write alone about natural effects and experience in order to not strengthen anyone's anger.[58]

Here Schnellenberg senses that Protestant polemics would not aid the function and reception of his text, and omits them. In this way, even though the Reformation was an important part of the context for Schnellenberg's work and approach to medicine, he did not aim to contribute directly to the reform of religion. Protestant sympathies do seem to be a part of his identity, however, focused as it was on connecting contemporary medicine more directly to German realities.

The Lutheran reform of healing in plague literature after 1540

As seen with Reusch and Schnellenberg, the emerging Protestant Reformation was a part of the cultural context of medical reform, even as these two physicians were more interested in working out the details of a German medicine or local understanding of the epidemics. For the physicians explored in this section, however, the Reformation played a more direct role in shaping their ideas and plague advice more generally. The writings of Jodocus Willich, Johann Dryander, and Ernst Reuchlin are more explicit in their promotion of the Lutheran Reformation, and sometimes even enlist the aid of Martin Luther's ideas and social authority to support their attempts to remake plague advice. New concerns about contagion and public health measures appear in the writings of Willich and Dryander as well, prompting a particularly Lutheran discussion about civic health controls. Attention to a specifically German medicine continued after 1550 as well, as the innovative trends of the time blended and reinforced each other by the mid-sixteenth century.

Some of the most reprinted and discernably "Lutheran" plague pamphlets of the mid-sixteenth century came from Jodocus Willich (1501–1552), a medical professor at the University of Frankfurt on the Oder. Willich's work appeared in print at least eleven times between circa 1545 and 1582 in three different pamphlets, first in Frankfurt on the Oder (ca. 1545, 1549, 1550, 1564, and 1565), and posthumously in Leipzig (1553), Marburg (1554), Bremen (1565), and Dresden (1582). When he wrote his texts, Willich was a rising star at the new university at Frankfurt on the Oder and a personal physician to the margrave of Brandenburg, Joachim II. As a moderate supporter of evangelical reform, Willich received greater room to explore his theological interests after Margrave Joachim II converted to Protestantism in 1539. By 1540 Willich was drawing condemnation from the local Catholic bishop for preaching his own exegesis of the Bible. During this period Willich also translated sections of the Bible as well as the writings of Hippocrates and Galen.[59]

Willich's concern with the Reformation is clear at the start of his first plague treatise, appearing circa 1545. His opening prayer states that God is justified for sending war, plagues, and famine to punish humans, and singles out a particular group as most deserving: "[E]specially those who defy your Word / and who arrange false divine services against your commands and order." Such religious statements make up a significant part of this pamphlet's introduction, or, rather, the first five of the pamphlet's forty-five pages of text.[60]

An exceptionally strong Lutheran tone marks the opening spiritual advice in a later plague pamphlet by Willich, one of two short plague pamphlets he published in 1549.[61] Willich's instructions for spiritual prevention follow the teachings of St. Paul, moving a sinner through three steps: recognizing that humans are unable to fulfill God's law; recognizing God's mercy and Jesus's sacrifice; and, finally, living a God-fearing life in faith. Such spiritual medicine is ostensibly Lutheran, since it mimics Luther's own conversion experience:

> First have regret and pain for your sins, which are revealed by the law and incite the wrath of God, from which all punishments come. St. Paul acknowledged that the function of the law was to produce knowledge of sin, so that a person must despair for one's sins, but does not go further as Judas had done.

The second step of Willich's spiritual medicine for plague involves a Lutheran view of salvation, coming not from trust in one's own worthiness but from certain hope in the mercy of God and trust that Jesus's redemptive act absolves all sins. The third step contains a characteristically Lutheran reference to the Devil, as Willich instructs people to lead a God-fearing life of faith and relent from devilish beings and works.[62] Willich included this Lutheran spiritual guidance in later pamphlets as well.[63]

Willich's plague literature is important not only for its Lutheran spiritual advice and its success in print but also for its detailed discussion of contagion, which attracted the attention of none other than the Marburg medical professor Johann Dryander. In 1553 Willich's examination of plague contagion appeared in print, in which he sought to describe contagion's nature and workings in order to promote public cleanliness and order.[64] Reflecting the growing interest in contagion among contemporary physicians and magistrates, Willich emphasizes that contagion is more important than poisoned air in spreading the sickness. Willich states that plague arises from poisoned air only rarely, but is more commonly a "hanging-on" or "carried plague" (*angehenckte seucht*).[65] At the time, the nature of plague poisons and how they moved around cities and territories were matters of continual mystery and debate.[66] For his part, Willich believed that plague poisons were tenacious and long-lasting, able to cling to clothes and walls for years, which made it all the more important to keep one's house and clothes clean. Poisoned air can lie inert in an object such as a pillow if the household is lazy and neglects to shake or wash it. When this pillow is used again years later, the poisons are activated by the movement and warmth of a person. From this case, Willich concludes that the poisons of plague are often spread because of the laziness of unclean people.[67] Willich also recommends that hospitals be established near running water and winds to carry away filth, and that people should not visit crowded places that lack controls of admittance, such as wine and beer cellars, meat markets, and washing banks.

Just as Dryander played an important role in reviving the ideas of Johann Vochs in 1537, Dryander became instrumental in promoting Willich's plague thought during the 1550s. Dryander reprinted Willich's text in 1554, including it with selections of Luther's 1527 plague sermon and his own introductory comments on the texts. In the writings of Willich and Luther, Dryander saw deep implications for the soul, medicine, and civic plague prevention, especially since both texts undermined the traditional teachings that one should flee the plague and that the air was poisoned. As seen in Chapter 3, Luther's plague sermon addresses the ethics of fleeing the plague and recommends that Christians remain in their communities in order to show their trust in God. Most importantly, Willich and Luther agree that a poisoned atmosphere was not as important as other causes of the plague. Reflecting on the causes of the 1527 plague in Wittenberg, Luther believed that it was caused entirely by local filth, not poisoned air.[68]

Besides using the texts by Willich and Luther to build a case against the role of poisoned air, Dryander also used them to support his argument that cities should isolate the sick during plagues. Magistrates had long sought to keep the sick separate from the healthy when devising early plague controls, but convincing arguments were in short supply in the face of popular opposition. The authority of Luther here helped Dryander promote public order by discouraging the act of flight as well as by encouraging people to remain at home and to cooperate with physicians and magistrates. Although Dryander praises Luther's stance on flight in the introduction of his text, Dryander's selections from Luther's 1527 sermon contain some of Luther's most forceful justifications of medicine. Here Luther justifies medicine as a gift of God and considers those who do not use medicine as not only sinning but also committing suicide (as seen above in Chapter 3). Dryander's selections also include Luther's statement concerning the execution of the evil people who spread plague intentionally. Luther viewed plague spreading as a grave sin akin to murder. To further promote Lutheran piety, Dryander also includes Luther's advice to pastors on how to advise their flocks and deal with dying people.[69]

Overall, Dryander combines the messages from both Willich and Luther along with his own ideas to present a particularly Lutheran justification for more rigorous civic health controls in the fight against contagion. Dryander was well informed about contagion, and claims to have been teaching about it for some time. Dryander even encourages German cities to follow the Italian examples by isolating the infected to prevent the contagion from spreading. Against religious arguments that condemn isolating the sick as unchristian and "Turkish," Dryander emphasizes that it is more dangerous to risk spreading contagion by failing to isolate the sick. Here he draws support from Luther's view that it is a grave sin to spread the plague.[70] Final support for Lutheran piety appears at the end of the pamphlet, as Dryander includes Willich's spiritual instructions of 1549 that guide the reader through a Lutheran repentance or conversion process.[71]

Finally, the work of one other little-known plague author, Ernst Reuchlin (ca. 1525– ?), reflects how closely the historical trends examined here became intertwined after 1560. Reuchlin's plague pamphlets of 1565 and 1577 reveal an important continuation of this Lutheran reform of healing, and show how this trend remained tied to the other innovative trends of the time: Vochs's German medicine and Schnellenberg's botanical experience. Most apparent in Reuchlin's work is how Martin Luther's legacy continued to shape Lutheran physicians' medical and moral positions well after his death. The clearest expression of Lutheran medical views comes in Reuchlin's 1565 plague text as he holds Luther up as a model of medical behavior during plague epidemics:

> Even the theologasters and matheologians know well that Doctor Luther, my dear and friendly brother-in-law [*Schwager*], held out against the plague in Wittenberg not once, but four times, along with his dear wife, children, and entire household. He did this not out of arrogance, curiosity, or temptation, as though one should not flee the plague, but he did this because of his office [*Ampt*]. He truly visited the sick without being timid, as he desired. He also used diligently the advice of learned and experienced doctors, and in particular the highly learned Doctors Caspar Lindemann, Augustin Schurff, Jacob Millich, and Melchior Fendt, my dear preceptors, as I saw and experienced myself. He required that his children and household take their prescribed medicines on all days. He also used smoking devices [*Reuchwerg*] and other remedies in his entire house, and did in no way scorn them. Thus no one in his house was afflicted or died, by means of divine help.[72]

In this passage, Luther himself plays the role of Reuchlin's ideal patient and *Hausvater* as he uses medicines and other means to protect his body and household during plague times. In its emphasis on a person's duties during an epidemic, Luther's life also becomes an illustration of Luther's position on whether one should flee the plague. Physicians' idealistic vision for medicating society is also apparent here, as Luther acts as the ideal *Hausvater*, overseeing the medication of the entire household. Here Reuchlin specifies that Luther consulted learned physicians and acted upon their advice, thus protecting the entire household, which would have included extended family, servants, and even the university students who boarded with the Luther family. Furthermore, Reuchlin's words tie the authority of physicians to the authority of Martin Luther, revealing much about the dynamics of social authority in Lutheran German lands in the mid-sixteenth century. Luther was becoming such a cultural hero that even his medical teachings were celebrated within Lutheran culture.

The most surprising part of Reuchlin's discussion of Martin Luther is that he appeals to his own experience with the reformer and his doctors, even calling Luther his "friendly, dear brother-in-law" (*Schwager*). Reuchlin was in fact Luther's nephew-in-law, since he had married Luther's niece Magdalena. Luther may not have characterized his relationship to Reuchlin as friendly or dear, however. Luther's first impression of Reuchlin was not warm, since he wrote to the Bishop of Pirna in 1545 to complain that Reuchlin was improperly scheming to marry his widowed niece. Luther's complaints about Reuchlin were considerable: that he was less than twenty years old at the time, had not sought the counsel or consent of Luther and his family, and that he had not provided information about his own family, much less news of his own father's consent. Luther feared that Reuchlin was attempting to marry the widow for her money, part of the Devil's scheme to humiliate him and his family in retaliation for the Reformation. Besides shedding light on Luther's fears in the year before his death, Luther's letter helpfully provides a rough birth date for Reuchlin (circa 1525?) and gives his hometown as "Geusing" (Geising) in Saxony.[73]

Luther was unsuccessful in blocking Reuchlin's marriage to his niece Magdalena. And, fortunately for Reuchlin, this episode does not seem to have had a negative effect on his career. According to Reuchlin's own account, he began to study medicine at the age of twenty-one at the University of Wittenberg, where he was classmates with Caspar Peucer and others who found fame as physicians and theologians.[74] By 1549 Reuchlin was working as a young *medicus* during a plague in Brandenburg.[75] Only later, in 1563, did Reuchlin receive degrees in medicine from the University of Wittenberg: the licentiate degree under the direction of Dr. Johann Hermann, as well as the doctor of medicine later that year.[76] Reuchlin seems to have been practicing medicine continuously since 1549 in the Margraviate of Brandenburg, as he states in 1565 that he had served the subjects of the margrave of Brandenburg for sixteen years.[77] His authority expanded in 1565, when he began to serve Margrave Joachim II as the appointed physician (*medicus*) for the seven cities of Brandenburg. In 1568 Reuchlin began medical practice in Lübeck, serving there as the appointed physician (*medicus ordinarius*). When he composed his second plague pamphlet in 1577 he had held this position for nine years. This pamphlet's imagined audience includes the people of Hamburg and Lüneburg as well, where Reuchlin seems to have had friends and patients.[78]

Besides holding up Luther as a moral example for plague times, Reuchlin continues other parts of the Lutheran reform of medicine in his 1565 and 1577 pamphlets. As far as his ideas echo and elaborate on Luther's own writings on plague, there should be no doubt about the appropriateness of the term "Lutheran reform of medicine." Much like Luther's 1527 plague sermon, Reuchlin attacks the fatalistic view that one should not take medicines to resist the plague. Echoing similar statements by Luther, Reuchlin argues that such a view is like a hungry person who rejects food.[79] His adoration of Luther's plague sermon goes so far that he provides a fanciful elaboration on Luther's unusual position that evil spirits cause the plague. In his 1527 plague text, Luther states that "all plague is brought among the people through the evil spirits, just like all other scourges. They poison the air or otherwise blow with an evil breath and thereby push the deadly poison into the flesh."[80] Even though such explanations were uncommon among Galenic physicians of the time, Reuchlin elaborates on it by appealing to the Devil's work and ideas from Greek mythology. Reuchlin views the evil spirits that poison air, water, grain, and hay as extensions of the Devil, and associates them with the nymphs of ancient Greece. Reuchlin associates the devil of well and stream with the Naiades, the devil of sea and lake with the Nereides, the devil of forest and bush with the Dryades, the desert devil with the Onosceli or donkey-footed beasts, and the air devil with the Aeroplictas. According to Reuchlin, such devils produce much suffering, pain, and anger on earth every day. Most interesting is how Reuchlin appeals to his own experience to support his ideas about these spirits. To illustrate the activities of the devil of forest or bush, Reuchlin mentions that he often saw in Brandenburg how this devil pulled up many thousands of trees and put them down in other places. To illustrate the work of the air devil, he refers to an historical example of a plague in Constantinople.[81] Such views fit with contemporary Lutheran interest in the Devil and the Devil's activities during the last age of the world, drawing on Luther's own eschatology. The connection to Greek mythology, however, represents an unusual attempt to connect classical lore to the contemporary Lutheran worldview.

Two final examples show Reuchlin participating in the Protestant reform of spiritual medicine in more traditional ways. Both his 1565 and 1577 pamphlets end with a statement that attacks the cult of the saints and the papacy:

> Our Lord Jesus Christ, the sole source of spiritual and bodily medicine (and not St. Anthony, St. Sebastian or St. Christopher as the foolish and even blasphemous papacy allows to be dreamed), wants to relieve and take away from our dear neighbors this punishment that we deserve a hundred times over, this rapid, horrible and frightening epidemic, through his groundless grace and mercy, and thereby protect and save us, Amen, Amen, Amen.[82]

Reuchlin encourages Protestant devotions instead, apparent when he encourages his readers to live a moderate lifestyle, to rejoice in the Lord and "to diligently hear and read God's Word, to hang this on the heart like an amulet or anti-poison compound, so that it is less able to be sickened by the poisoned air."[83] Here it is interesting to see God's Word enacting a physical effect on people, and even compared directly to physical things, including medicines, that offer worldly protection. This treatment therefore resembles a late medieval sacramental, although here the physical form that contains the divine power is imagined, rather than tangible. In these ways, Reuchlin continues the Protestant reform of spiritual medicine into the later sixteenth century. That these reform efforts continued, even among physicians, is perhaps a sign of how much difficulty Protestant reformers were having as they attempted to reform traditional beliefs within the broad population.

In addition to continuing Martin Luther's legacy, Reuchlin also accepted the other great reform effort of the time: the promotion of a more German or local medicine. In the preface to his 1565 pamphlet, Reuchlin states that he does not include "Calicut, Indian, or African medicines," but draws on medical resources that can be found in the prince's own lands and without payment, for the sake of the common man.[84] Most impressive, however, is the extent that Reuchlin incorporates local knowledge into his text for the help of his audience, in some instances revealing where to find certain herbs growing in the wild. When discussing the plants to perfume a house against harmful air, Reuchlin includes this:

> For this purpose one can use especially oak leaves, birch bark, juniper branches along with the berries, rosemary, "gele Müntze" which is called "Conyza Maior" and grows in abundance around Stendel, and scordion or garlic plant, which you can find in great abundance in front of St. Anna's gate in Brandenburg, and all around Stendel.[85]

Despite the local botanical advice in this instance, Reuchlin elsewhere recommends some products that can be purchased only from apothecary shops, and even advertises for certain ones. For high-quality theriac, and not the Venetian or Alexandrian theriac that the adulterators sell, Reuchlin advertises the "well-learned and experienced Herr Caspar Pfrundt, apothecary of Wittenberg," as well as Magister Maurice Steinmetz of Leipzig.[86] Such attacks on imported medicines, the concerns about false theriac from abroad, and attention to local botanical resources recall the legacies of both Vochs and Schnellenberg. Later Reuchlin seems to echo the thoughts of Vochs on the specific characteristics of German bodies as he states that he is attempting to cure Germans (*Deutsche*), and therefore does not include information about the diets and cures of "Manardus, Guaineri, Valescus, Bertruti, the French and Italians." Here he refers to influential foreign scholars of earlier times who had written on plague: Giovanni Manardi, Antonio Guaineri, Valescus de Taranta, and Niccolo Bertucci. Reuchlin also states that he avoids recipes that draw on expensive imported ingredients, such as lemon or orange juice, pearls, emeralds, sapphires, and other precious stones.[87] In this way Reuchlin advances the anti-foreign aspect of this German reform of medicine as well as its interest in native resources. Overall, Reuchlin's texts reveal how the legacies of Luther and the various authors who promoted a more German medicine came together and thrived in the decades after 1560.

Conclusion

The plague writing of Reusch, Schnellenberg, Willich, Dryander, and Reuchlin demonstrate how trends established earlier during the Renaissance and Reformation continued to encourage new directions in plague advice into the 1570s. The cause of German medical localism, faith in the ideas and independent spirit of Martin Luther, and new interest in public health and contagion became especially important to physicians who sought to challenge contemporary medical traditions. Underlying such trends was increasing confidence in German experience as distinct and more reliable as a foundation for knowledge and practice. As efforts grew to reform medicine and society and to develop civic plague policies, such new directions in medical thought became more important and pressing. It is clear that, by the mid-sixteenth century, the German reform of healing had blossomed fully within plague writing, as later authors brought innovative trends together, exploring their potential to encourage new traditions of knowledge and culture.

Notes

1 Venice's lazaretto was the world's first permanent plague hospital, founded in 1423. Jane L. Stevens Crawshaw, *Plague Hospitals: Public Health for the City in Early Modern Venice* (Farnham, UK: Ashgate, 2012), 3.

2 Johann Dryander, Ed., *Opusculum praeclarum de omni Pestilentia, sive sit ab aere corrupto, sive ab aquis putridis, aut a cavaderibus: & de diuturna peste morbi Gallici…* (Cologne?, 1537), sigs. Aa2r–Aa4v.

3 Various university records identify Johann Reusch as from the town of Eschenbach, although historians disagree whether this was Eschenbach in Middle Franconia or Obereschenbach in Lower Franconia. Otto Clemen, "Johannes Reusch von Eschenbach: Humanist, Theologe, Mediziner," *Neues Archiv für Sächsische Geschichte* 21 (1900): 111–145, 122; Carly Seyfarth, *Das Hospital zu St. Georg in Leipzig durch acht Jahrhunderte 1212–1940*, Vol. I (Leipzig: Georg Thieme Verlag, 1939), 75.

4 Clemen, "Johannes Reusch," 114.

5 Ibid., 128–129. Conradin Bonorand also describes Reusch as an Erasmian and cool to Luther's messages: Conradin Bonorand, *Vadians Humanistenkorrespondenz mit Schülern und Freunden aus seiner Wiener Zeit: Personenkommentar 1–4 zum Vadianischen Briefwerk* (St. Gallen: Verlagsgemeinschaft St. Gallen, 1988), 4, 161.

6 Gustav Wustmann, *Der Wirt von Auerbachs Keller: Dr. Heinrich Stromer von Auerbach 1482–1542* (Leipzig: Hermann Seemann Nachfolger, 1902), 54.

7 Clemen, "Johannes Reusch," 133.

8 Johann Reusch, *Praecavendae et curandae pestilitatis methodus Ioanne Reuschio auctore* (Leipzig: Nicolaus Fabri, 1527), sigs. A3r–v.
9 This appears in a list of much-tested preservative medicines: ibid., sig. B1v.
10 Ibid., sig. B2r.
11 Johann Reusch, *Regiment Doctor Johan Reüschen Wie sich zur zeit der Pestilentz zu halten sey / Die einwoner der Stadt Leiptzigk / vornemlich belangendt.* (Leyptzigk: Nickel Schmidt, 1539), sigs. B5r–v.
12 Ibid., sig. C1r.
13 Ibid., sig. A4r.
14 Ibid., sig. B2r.
15 Ibid., sig. A4v.
16 Ibid.
17 Johann Vochs, *De pestilentia Anni p[raese]ntis et ei[us] cura* (Magdeburg, 1507), sig. B3r.
18 Reusch, *Regiment Doctor Johan Reüschen*, sig. A4v.
19 Ibid., sigs. A5r–v.
20 Jon Arrizabalaga, "Facing the Black Death: Perceptions and Reactions of University Medical Practitioners," in *Practical Medicine from Salerno to the Black Death*, Eds. Luis García-Ballester, Roger French, Jon Arrizabalaga, and Andrew Cunningham (Cambridge: Cambridge University Press, 1994): 237–288, 248.
21 C.-E. A. Winslow and M. L. Duran-Reynals, Trans., "Texts and Documents: Regiment de Preservacio a Epidemia o Pestilencia e Mortaldats," *Bulletin of the History of Medicine* 23 (1949): 57–89, 67–68.
22 Melissa P. Chase, "Fevers, Poisons, and Apostemes: Authority and Experience in Montpellier Plague Treatises," in *Science and Technology in Medieval Society*, Ed. Pamela O. Long (New York: New York Academy of Sciences, 1985): 153–171, 154–156.
23 Jon Arrizabalaga, John Henderson, and Roger French, *The Great Pox: The French Disease in Renaissance Europe* (New Haven, CT: Yale University Press, 1997), 75.
24 Reusch, *Regiment Doctor Johan Reüschen*, sig. A5v.
25 Ficino in general focuses on poisoned air as the cause: Walter Pagel, *Paracelsus: An Introduction to Philosophical Medicine in the Era of the Renaissance* (Basel: Karger, 1982), 174–177.
26 Samuel K. Cohn, Jr., *Cultures of Plague: Medical Thinking at the End of the Renaissance* (Oxford: Oxford University Press, 2010), 186–192.
27 Reusch does not actually use the term "contagion": Reusch, *Regiment Doctor Johan Reüschen*, sigs. A8v–B1v.
28 Augsburg, for example, established a civic "pox house" in the wake of the 1495 arrival of the French Disease: Claudia Stein, *Negotiating the French Pox in Early Modern Germany* (Farnham, UK: Ashgate, 2009).
29 Carly Seyfarth, *725 Jahre Hospital zu St. Georg in Leipzig* (Leipzig: Hermann-Eichblatt-Verlag, 1939), 4.
30 Craig Koslofsky, *The Reformation of the Dead: Death and Ritual in Early Modern Germany, 1450–1700* (New York: St. Martin's Press, 2000), 40–77; Beate Berger, Bodo Gronemann, and Jakuf Pacer, *Vom Aderlass zum Gesundheitspass: Zeittafel zur Geschichte d. öfftentl. Gesundheitswesens in Leipzig* (Leipzig: Leipziger Univ-Verlag, 2000), 6.
31 *Ordnung Eines Erbarn Hochweisen Raths der Stadt Leipzig…* (Leipzig: Michael Lantzenberger, 1607).

32 *Infection Ordnung / der Stat Wienn* (Vienna: Hanns Syngrienner, 1551); *Ains Erbern Raths der Stadt Nürmberg / vernewete Gesetz und Ordnung / in gegenwertigen sterbsleufften diß M.D.LXII. Jars auffgericht* (1562).
33 Gundolf Keil, "Der Hausvater als Arzt," in *Haushalt und Familie in Mittelalter und frühe Neuzeit*, Ed. Trude Ehlert (Sigmaringen: Jan Thorbecke Verlag, 1991): 219–243.
34 Julius Hoffmann, *Die "Hausväterliteratur" und die "Predigten über den christlichen Hausstand"* (Weinheim: Verlag Julius Beltz, 1959). Many accept the importance of the Hausvater ideology in the social history of early modern Germany. See, for example: Joel F. Harrington, *Reordering Marriage and Society in Reformation Germany* (Cambridge: Cambridge University Press, 1995). On the basic structure of pre-modern households, see: Otto Brunner, "Das 'ganze Haus' und die alteuropäische 'Ökonomik,'" in *Neue Wege der Sozialgeschichte: Vorträge und Aufsätze* (Göttingen: Vandenhoeck & Ruprecht, 1956): 33–61.
35 Hoffmann, *Die "Hausväterliteratur,"* 60–80.
36 Clemen, "Johannes Reusch," 136–138.
37 Tarquinius Schnellenberg, *Experimenta von XX. Pestilentz Wurtzeln und Kreutern, wie sie für Gifft unnd Pestilentz gebraucht mögen warden...* (Frankfurt am Mayn: Weygand Han, 1546). Starting in 1588, Walther Hermann Ryff edited and reissued Schnellenberg's text, which continued its popularity throughout the seventeenth century. See VD16 R 3965 and subsequent entries under Ryff and Schnellenberg in the *Verzeichnis der im deutschen Sprachbereich erschienenen Drucke des XVI. Jahrhunderts* (Stuttgart: Anton Hiersemann, 1983–2000), R 3965.
38 Schnellenberg, *Experimenta von XX. Pestilentz Wurtzeln*, sigs. A8v–B1r.
39 Rüdiger Wulf, "Tarquinius Schnellenberg alias Ocyorus: Doktor der Freien Künste und Arznei, Stadtphysikus zu Dortmund," *Heimat Dortmund* 3 (2005): 11–17; Franz Tetzner, "Zur Lebensgeschichte Schnellenbergs," *Westfälisches Magazin* (1910): 2–5.
40 Tarquinius Schnellenberg, *Ein kurtz Schön vnd tröstlich Regiment wider die alte schwere erschreckliche kranckheit der Pestilentz...* (Erfurt: Melcher Sachssen inn der Archen Noe, 1540), sig. B4v. Here Schnellenberg describes a pill recipe from Pistoris that can protect a person for up to fourteen days. He says it was much used and valued by physicians in Cologne during a plague.
41 Ibid., sigs. B7r–v.
42 Schnellenberg, *Experimenta von XX. Pestilentz Wurtzeln*, sig. *5r.
43 Ibid., sigs. A2r–v; Alisha Rankin, *Panaceia's Daughters: Noblewomen as Healers in Early Modern Germany* (Chicago: Chicago University Press, 2013), 39.
44 Schnellenberg, *Experimenta von XX. Pestilentz Wurtzeln*, sigs. A7v–8r.
45 Ibid., sig. A3v.
46 Ibid., sig. A2v.
47 Bruce T. Moran, "The Herbarius of Paracelsus," *Pharmacy in History* 39 (1993): 104–105.
48 Schnellenberg, *Experimenta von XX. Pestilentz Wurtzeln*, sig. B4v.
49 Ibid., sig. B4r.
50 Ibid., sig. B3v.
51 Pamela H. Smith, *The Body of the Artisan: Art and Experience in the Scientific Revolution* (Chicago: University of Chicago Press, 2004).

52 Brian Ogilvie, *The Science of Describing: Natural History in Renaissance Europe* (Chicago: University of Chicago Press, 2006), 143–148.
53 On this connection in Wittenberg: Karl H. Dannenfeldt, "Wittenberg Botanists during the Sixteenth Century," in *The Social History of the Reformation*, Eds. Lawrence P. Buck and Jonathan W. Zophy (Columbus, OH: Ohio State University Press, 1972): 223–248.
54 William Eamon, *Science and the Secrets of Nature: Books of Secrets in Medieval and Early Modern Culture* (Princeton, NJ: Princeton University Press, 1994), 98.
55 Schnellenberg, *Experimenta von XX. Pestilentz Wurtzeln*, sig. I3v.
56 Tetzner, "Zur Lebensgeschichte," 4.
57 Schnellenberg, *Ein kurtz Schön vnd tröstlich Regiment*, sig. A4r.
58 Schnellenberg, *Experimenta von XX. Pestilentz Wurtzeln*, sig. B3r.
59 *Allgemeine Deutsche Biographie*, Vol. 43 (Leipzig, 1898): 278–282.
60 "[V]nd sonderlich denen / so dein Wort vorachten / vñ ein andern falschen Gottesdienst / wider deinen befelch vnd Ordnung anrichten." Jodocus Willich, *Vonn der Pestilentz ein nützlich Regiment / auff diese zeit gestellet. Darzu auch / wie man schwangern frawen vnd Kindlin / in der kranckheit rathen sol.* (Frankfurt/Oder, ca. 1545), sig. A2r.
61 The pamphlet on curation: Jodocus Willich, *Wie man denen helffen sol / welchem mit der pestiletzische gifft begriffen seind. Durch D. Jodocum Willichium von Kesell* (Frankfurt/Oder: Johann Eichorn, 1549).
62 Jodocus Willich, *Wie man sich in einer stadt für der Pestilentz behüten sol vnd möchte / ein kurtz vnd seer nützliche vnderrichtung. Durch Doctorem Jodocum Willichium von Kesell / dem armen volck vorgestalt* (Frankfurt/Oder: Johann Eichorn, 1549), sigs. A2r–v.
63 It appears in the 1550 reprint and Johann Dryander's edited pamphlet of 1554 (see below). Jodocus Willich, *Wie man sich in einer stadt für der Pestilentz behüten sol vnd möchte / ein kurtz vnd seer nützlich vnderrichtung. Durch Doctorem Jodocum Willichium von Kesell / dem armen volck vorgestalt* (Frankfurt/Oder: Johann Eichorn, 1550).
64 Jodocus Willich, *Wie man sich vorhalten vnnd bewaren sol in den Heuseren / in welchen jemandes an der Pestiletz gestorben ist / Auff das es nicht leichtlich einreissen vnd weiter schaden thun möge. Item ein Radtschlag / vor die schwangere weiber vnd die kleine Kinder* (Leipzig: Wolff Günter, 1553).
65 Johann Dryander, *Von dem ytzigen Sterben oder Pestilentz. D. Jo. Eychmans genant Dryander / Ordinarij zů Marpurg / bedenckens. Sampt D. Luthers / vnd D. Jodoci Wilichii zweyen Büchlin von dem Sterben* (Marburg: Andreas Colben, 1554), sig. B1r.
66 For a long history of physicians attempting to understand the nature of plague's poisons: Erik A. Heinrichs, "The Live Chicken Treatment for Buboes: Trying a Plague Cure in Medieval and Early Modern Europe," *Bulletin for the History of Medicine* 91 (2017): 210–232.
67 Dryander, *Von dem ytzigen Sterben oder Pestilentz*, sig. B2r.
68 *D. Martin Luthers Werke: Kritische Gesammtausgabe*, Vol. XXIII, *Predigten und Schriften 1527* (Weimar: Böhlau, 1901), 369.
69 Dryander, *Von dem ytzigen Sterben oder Pestilentz*, sigs. C1r–C6v.
70 Ibid., sig. A5v.
71 Ibid., sigs. C6v–8r.
72 Ernst Reuchlin, *Zwey kurtze Büchlein / Aus welchen iedermenniglich Arm vnd Reich lernen kan / wie er sich jtziger zeit in der Schrecklichen straffe der*

Pestilentz vorhalten sol. Dem durchleuchtigsten / Hochgebornen / Fürsten vnd Herrn / Herrn Joachim des Namens dem andern / Churfürsten zu Brandenburg / etc. Zu gehorsamer vnd vnderthenigster dienstbarkeit… (Madgeburg: Andreas Ghene, 1565), sigs. A4r–v.

73 *Dr. Martin Luthers Sämmtliche Schriften*, Ed. Johann Georg Walch, Vol. XXI, Pt. 2, *Dr. Luthers Briefe* (St. Louis, MO: Concordia Publishing, 1904), 3111–3113.

74 Ernst Reuchlin, *Zwo Haußtafeln und underricht vor die Reichen unnd Armen / zur Sommer und Winter zeit / wider die fürstehende / schreckliche und wegkfressende Pestilentz / die nicht allein (wie der Königkliche Prophet / Psal: 91 saget) im finstern schleichet / sondern auch im Mittage / als ein wütender Mörder eilends unzeliche Menschen tödet* (Lübeck: Asswerus Kröger, 1577), sig. A3r.

75 Ibid., sig. A2v.

76 *PRAESIDE IOHANNE HERMANNO ARTIS MEDICAE DOCTORE, AD SEQVENtes propositiones pro Licentia in arte Medica consequenda, respondebunt honesti ac docti Viri. Ad Priores XLI. (DE FLVXIONIBVS ALVI) MAGISTER CLEMENS CHELNERVS ISLEBIENSIS. Ad Posteriores et Practicas. (CVRATIO FLVXIONVM ALVI.) MAGISTER ERNESTVS REVCHLINVS GEVSINGIVS Die primo Octobris. Anno 1563* (Wittenberg: Jakob Lucius, 1563). Andreas Sonnemann, *Elegia ad clarissiumum & integerrimum virum, D. Doctorem Ernestum Reuchlinum Geusingensem ordinarium medicus veteris Marchiae…* (Wittenberg: Laurentus Schwenk, 1564).

77 Reuchlin, *Zwey kurtze Büchlein*, sig. B1r.

78 Reuchlin, *Zwo Haußtafeln und underricht*, sigs. A2v–A4v.

79 Reuchlin, *Zwey kurtze Büchlein*, sig. A3v.

80 *D. Martin Luthers Werke*, Vol. XXIII, 355.

81 Reuchlin, *Zwo Haußtafeln und underricht*, sigs. B4r–v.

82 Reuchlin, *Zwey kurtze Büchlein*, sig. L3v.

83 Ibid., sig. B2r.

84 Ibid., sig. A4v.

85 Ibid., sig. B2v.

86 Ibid., sig. D3v.

87 Ibid., sig. L3r.

Conclusion

One of the great cultural trends of the Northern Renaissance and Reformation was the new impulse among Germans to define themselves and their lands as different from the lands and people of southern Europe. As northern humanists began to discover the importance of place, and as a chasm opened in western Christianity between north and south, it fell to German physicians to explore the meaning of locality and German identity within medicine. These cultural trends inspired a particularly German reform of healing for body and soul, viewed here within plague treatises from the first century of print. During this time of great cultural change the quest for a better plague medicine for Germans shared much with the movement to form a Christianity that respected local cultural concerns. Perhaps the most significant similarity between the Protestant Reformation and the German reform of healing was a willingness to question authority and to develop new traditions. Both sought a new and more certain standard on which to base their knowledge and teachings. Both wanted their teachings to be accessible and relatable to Germans more broadly, as seen in the embrace of vernacular print. Protestant reformers found this ultimate foundation in the text of the Bible, just as German physicians and botanists placed new emphasis on their own experiences and observations of their own locality, so far removed from the ancient authorities. Standing behind both movements was a profound sense of difference between peoples and lands, part of a broader reassessment of culture and institutions. Historians should not underestimate how these emergent cultural trends spurred the reevaluation of medicine and religion in the sixteenth century.

Given the importance of plague to society in the sixteenth century, this book also argues that physicians and their plague treatises deserve to be central to historians' understanding of the Renaissance, Reformation, and early modern sciences. The practicing physicians of town and court embraced the new possibilities of the printed media, and used the plague treatise genre to explore new ideas and a broader audience. In each decade between 1473 and 1573 plague authors were not merely repeating stale scholastic positions within a moribund medical genre. In each decade innovative physicians responded to their cultural context in their search for new solutions to plague, writing plague treatises that participated in the reform movements of the time. New interest in religious reform and alchemy, as well as in German bodies, medicines, and public health, are among the many trends that make the plague treatises a dynamic genre. These trends encouraged physicians to adapt their scholarly learning to popular expectations and the world they saw in front of them. By asserting their authority over local causes and cures for plague, and by reaching further into local marketplaces, German physicians discovered a new world within their midst.

Perhaps most importantly, the German physicians explored here were also at the leading edge of change in the early modern sciences as they altered the traditional path to medical knowledge. By learning to prioritize their own experiences and observations in order to become better acquainted with local realities, they challenged long-held assumptions in medicine and weakened the hold of ancient authorities in the production of medical knowledge. These medical and cultural innovations of the early and mid-sixteenth century thereby encouraged the empirical values that played such an important role during the Scientific Revolution.

This survey of German plague treatises from the first century of print has brought little-known physicians to light and has revealed their sometimes surprising contributions to contemporary plague advice and culture. Chapter 1 demonstrated how late medieval plague authors began to explore the potential of vernacular print to shape attitudes about spiritual and natural health, sometimes anticipating trends that became central to the Reformation. Chapter 2 traced the origins of German medical localism in the 1507 plague text by the little-known Johann Vochs, marked as it was with the broader concerns about German medical, cultural, and economic autonomy amid the Renaissance. As depicted here, Vochs initiated a particular German reform of healing, which would inspire many later physicians who sought to reform the natural and spiritual response to plague. Chapter 3 explored the broadening of the German reform of healing during the Protestant Reformation, as many German physicians and clerics, including Martin Luther, used plague writings to contribute to the Reformation. These efforts included reforming spiritual medicine for plague, as well as shaping attitudes to natural medicine. Chapter 4 introduced the innovative and popular plague treatises of Caspar Kegler, who used vernacular print to pitch his novel alchemical plague cures, thus exploring the new commercial potential of the genre. Chapter 5 traced the continuing German reform of healing in the plague treatises of Johann Reusch, Tarquinius Schnellenberg, and others, who combined the innovative trends that had emerged in earlier plague texts, thus marking the full flourishing of this particularly German movement in vernacular print. In these later plague writings, the long-term impact of German medical localism becomes clear, as well as the legacy of the Reformation, and Martin Luther specifically. Considering plague treatises written up to the mid-sixteenth century, it is Luther himself who deserves to be known as the "Luther of physicians," rather than Paracelsus.

The rise of the Paracelsians after 1560

Given the great stature of Paracelsus within medical history as the most radical and influential of the early modern reformers, it is surprising that his writings on plague had little impact on German plague treatises until the 1560s, or well after his death. Moreover, the first printed plague pamphlet attributed to Paracelsus, published in Salzburg in 1554, is an unoriginal work that even borrows a significant part of its content from Caspar Kegler's 1529 text.[1] Twelve consecutive pages of this 1554 text borrow heavily from Kegler, even lifting verbatim Kegler's recipe for *aurum vitae*, *electuarium liberantis*, and others.[2] In this case it is stunning to see a text attributed to the (allegedly) most innovative early modern alchemist lift its alchemical content from a predecessor. There is little doubt that this 1554 pamphlet is the work of someone else, who used Paracelsus's name to sell the text locally, drawing on Paracelsus's notoriety in Salzburg, where he died in 1541. This text appeared in print two more times with few changes in Straubing in 1561 and 1563.[3]

Paracelsus's own plague texts are less derivative, of course. During his lifetime Paracelsus wrote three works on plague, beginning in the later 1520s, in addition to dealing with plague briefly in other writings. In an exploration of these texts, historian Walter Pagel has shown that Paracelsus developed his own understanding of plague and plague medicine by elaborating on Marsilio Ficino's chemical and Neoplatonic notions.[4] Regardless of its Italian precedents, Paracelsus's innovative thought would inspire a different tradition of medical reform, largely separate from the German reform of healing explored here in the works of Vochs, Luther, Schnellenberg, and others. One major reason for the delay in the reception of Paracelsus's thought is that he was slow to embrace printed publication, unlike the authors explored here. Paracelsus's own writings on plague did not appear in print until 1564, when Adam von Bodenstein issued his *Two Books on Plague*.[5]

By the 1560s Paracelsus's writing on plague had become widespread enough in manuscript or print to inspire a handful of authors to continue his non-Galenic approaches to plague medicine. New and innovative plague treatises by Georg Phaedro (1562), Johannes Vogt (1564), and Wilhelmus Triphyllodaenus (1567) show that a new direction in plague medicine was taking shape, thanks to the inspiration of Paracelsus. These authors refer commonly to chemical medicines, personal experience, and case histories and sometimes even refer adoringly to Paracelsus himself. The pamphlet by Vogt also makes clear that other champions of personal experience were having an impact as well by the 1560s, including Georg Handsch and Pietro Mattioli, both of whom served as physicians to the Habsburg rulers of the day. That Vogt refers to Handsch and Mattioli at times in addition to Paracelsus reveals that the field of innovative physicians was more crowded than the standard historical narratives about Paracelsus would allow.[6]

Paracelsus was not a lone hero of reform but one of a number of German physicians working to devise better methods of healing.

But, even as this new iatrochemistry or "Paracelsian" movement began to have an impact on printed plague treatises, it also continued the familiar rhetoric of this earlier German medical localism. Vogt and Triphyllodaenus repeat some of the same sayings about foreign and local medicine first voiced by Vochs and others much earlier. Vogt's lament about popular medical belief reveals both the continuity and change of medical reform in the 1560s:

> One only wants medicine that comes from over the sea out of Calicut. The things that grow in German lands [*Teütschen Landen*] – metals, roots and herbs, as well as decreed and experienced doctors – are held in little regard among the local peasants.[7]

Familiar here is the contrast between German products and imports from Calicut. New, however, is that Vogt adds metals to the list of natural medicines that grow from German soil, revealing the rise of such non-Galenic chemical medicines among physicians. Vogt's reference to "experienced doctors" growing from German soil like roots and herbs is also striking, as he assumes that "experience" is characteristic of the German terroir of medical thought. Such statements reveal how ingrained this emphasis on experience in medical practice had become among German physicians by the 1560s, thanks in no small part to the earlier figures studied in this book. In this way, the nascent Paracelsian movement owed an enormous debt to reformers such as Vochs, who prepared the cultural and intellectual ground for this new assault on traditional medicine. By the time that Paracelsus grew in popularity among German physicians, many of them were well aware of the problems with imported medicine and the advantages of local medicines known through experience. But, much like the religious reformers of the time, German medical reformers found that overcoming tradition and habit within the broader population was no easy task.

The beginning of a Paracelsian movement forms a fitting end to this book, since this topic is among the most thoroughly studied in German medical history. Paracelsus and his admirers took medicine in new directions, even as they drew on some older notions about experience, alchemy, and native medicines. References to chemical cures and hermetic ideas in plague treatises increased in the later sixteenth century, while references to earlier reformers, such as Vochs and Luther, declined. Disputes between Galenic and Paracelsian physicians drove many medical debates after 1560. Even Ernst Reuchlin, the last author explored in Chapter 5, called Paracelsus unlearned and cast doubt on the medical use of mercury and arsenic.[8] It is important to note, however, that neither this German reform of healing nor the coming Paracelsian movement was able to end the dominance of Galenic medicine during the sixteenth or seventeenth centuries. The plague treatise genre continued into the eighteenth century with many Galenic notions, even though approaches to medical knowledge had begun to shift since the early sixteenth century, thanks to the German reform of healing in print.

Notes

1 Karl Sudhoff noted the lack of a Paracelsian spirit in this work: Karl Sudhoff, *Bibliographia Paracelsica*, Reprint Edn. (Graz: Akademische Druck- und Verlagsanstalt, 1958), 52; Paracelsus, *Für Pestilentz ain seer nützlicher vnnd bewerter Tractat / der Christlichen gemayn zů nutz vnd wolfart / auß deß weitberüembten vnd hocherfarnen Doctoris Philippj Theophrastj Paracelsj Bůch gezogen. Welches Er / von diser Khranckhait beschriben. Dariñ vil vnnd manicherlay Latwergen / Püllel / Wasser / Confect vnd Pulver / Sampt annderñ Preseruatifen erfunnden warden Damit sich die Gesunden in disen geschwinden leüffen der regierenden Pestilentz bewaren mügen: Auch / wie den Khrannckhen / so mit disem Gebrechen behafft / soll geholffen werden rc. Diß alles / nach ordnung jnnhalt volgunds Registers / jñ sechs Thayl: Vormals in Truckh nye kommen: verfertigt* (Salzburg: Hans Bawman [von Rottenburg auf der Tauber], 1554).

2 Compare Paracelsus, *Für Pestilentz*, sigs. 32r–37v, with Caspar Kegler, *Eyn Nutzlichs vnd trostlichs Regiment wider dy Pestilentz vñ Gifftig Pestilentzisch Feber die Schweyssucht genannt / vnd sust mächerley gifftig vñ tödlich kranckheit / Durch Casparū Kegler / der ertzney Doctorn / zwsamen gebracht / vornewt vñ mit vil trostlichen experimentē gebessert / Die zuuor heymlich gehalten / vnd an den tag nyhe gegebē seyn. Anno 1.5.2.9. auß gegangen* (Leipzig: Valtenin Schumann, 1529), sigs. 6v–9r, 24v–25v.

3 Paracelsus, *Von der Pestilentz. Ein seer Nutzlichs / vnnd bewertes Büchlein der Christlichen gemein zu nutz vnd wolfart / auß des weitberümbten vnd hocherfarnen Doctoris Philippj Theophrastij Peracelsi Buch so er von diser kranckheit beschriben / gezogen den gesunden/ sich in den geschwinden leüffen der regirenden Pestilentz / zuuerwaren / auch den krancken so mit disem brechen behafft / zur hilff vnd retrung / sonderlich nutz vnd dienstlich* (Straubing: Hans Burger, 1561); Paracelsus, *Von der Pestilentz. Ein seer Nutzlichs / vnnd bewertes Büchlein der Christlichen gemein zu nutz vnd wolfart / auß des weitberümbten vnd hocherfarnen Doctoris Philippj Theophrastij Peracelsy Buch so er von diser kranckheit beschriben / gezogen den gesunden/ sich in den gschwinden leüffen der regirenden Pestilentz / zuuerwaren...* (Straubing: Hans Burger, 1563).

4 Walter Pagel, *Paracelsus: An Introduction to Philosophical Medicine in the Era of the Renaissance* (Basel: Karcher, 1982), 172–182.

5 Paracelsus, *Zwey Bücher Theophrasti Paracelsi des erfarnesten Artzets / von der Pestilentz vnd ihren zůfällen. Durch den Edlen vnd Hochgelerten Adamen von Bodenstein / in Druck verfertiget* (Strasburg: Paulo Messerschmidt, 1564). These two books were originally composed in Nordlingen in 1529 or 1530: Karl Sudhoff, ed., *Theophrast von Hohenheim gen. Paracelsus Sämtlich Werke*, Vol. VIII (Munich: Otto Wilhelm Barth, 1924), 371–396.

6 Georg Phaedro, *Ge. Phaedronis Rhodochaei Medici Halopyrgice siue Iatrochemica pestis epidemicae curatio. Oder Warhaffte Cur der erschröcklichen sucht der Pestilentz / an den Hochwürdigsten in Gott Fürsten vnd Herrn Johann Jacob Ertzbischoff zů Saltzburg rc.* (Ingolstat, 1562); Johannes Vogt, *Ein nutzliche anzeigung gebrauchter Artzneyen / von gelerten Doctoribus in der hohen Not der Pestilentz / wie die Exempla außweisen / auch yetzunder zů Straßburg in*

der hohen Not in Brauch geordnet: Bey jnen Diastimios vnd precipitatis cum Auro genannt / die beide fast einer Würckung / Ich aber habs mein Aurum vitae / auch Confectionem vitae ettlich vnd dreissig Jar in meinen Schrifften genannt vnd gebraucht: Die Ertzney würt gebraucht wider allerley verborgne ‖ vnbekannte / wie sie genannt mügen werden / Kranckheitten… (Ulm: Oßwald Gruppenbacher, 1564); Wilhelmus Triphyllodaenus, *Gifftiager, Das ist: Von vrsach / reynigung / bewahrung vnd Cur Pestilentzischer lufft / fürnemer Artzten rath vnd bedencken / mit angehencktem vnterschied der Schüler Paracelsi vnd Galeni / in der Cur gemelter Kranckheyt* (Franckfurt: Martin Lechler in verlegung Sigmund Feyrabends and Simon Hüters, 1567). On Handsch: Michael Stolberg, "Empiricism in Sixteenth-Century Medical Practice: The Notebooks of Georg Handsch," *Early Science and Medicine* 18 (2013): 487–516.

7 Vogt, *Ein nutzliche anzeigung*, sig. B2v.

8 Ernst Reuchlin, *Zwo Haußtafeln und underricht vor die Reichen unnd Armen / zur Sommer und Winter zeit / wider die fürstehende / schreckliche und wegkfressende Pestilentz / die nicht allein (wie der Königkliche Prophet / Psal: 91 saget) im finstern schleichet / sondern auch im Mittage / als ein wütender Mörder eilends unzeliche Menschen tödet* (Lübeck: Asswerus Kröger, 1577), sig. I4r.

Appendix 1: Publication history of Caspar Kegler's pamphlets

Original pamphlet: composed by Caspar Kegler in 1521

1. 1521 (Leipzig: Valent Schumann) Jf I 155 (TUB)
2. 1521? (?: ?) HA 2 Tm 7670: F716 (SB)
3. ca. 1530 (Constance: Johann Haselbergk) H00 / Misc.A 342 (EUB)
4. 1539 (Magdeburg: Hans Walther) Jl 8060 #3 (SB)
5. 1584 (Dresden: Gimel Bergen) A: 111 Med. (2) (HAB)
6. 1597 (Cologne: Wilhelm Lützenkirchen) Path 158 #3 (BSB)

Second edition: revisions and additions by Caspar Kegler in 1529

1. 1529 (Leipzig: Valent Schumann) Res/ Path 98 #3 (BSB)
2. 1530 (Erfurt: Melchior Sachssen) Res/M.med 494 (BSB)
3. 1530 (Regensburg: Paul Khol) 999 IM/97.1588 (SBR)
4. ca. 1545 (Magdeburg?) 50 MA 26211 (SB)
5. 1551 (Leipzig: Wolff Günter) Nw. 457 c (8) (GNM)
6. 1553 (Leipzig) Bibl. Sud. 2429 (BSB)
7. 1565 (Eisleben: Andreas Petri) 109.7 Med. (4) (HAB)
8. 1598 (Leipzig: Abraham Lamberg) H61/4 TREW.T 303 (EUB)

Third edition: additions to 1529 pamphlet by Melchior Kegler in 1566

1. 1566 (Leipzig: Johann Rhambaw) Mx 239 (1) (HAB)
2. 1588 (Königsberg: Georg Osterberger) H00/4 MED-I 400# 9 (EUB)

Fourth edition: additions to the 1566 pamphlet by Caspar Kegler the grandson

1. 1607 (Dresden: Christian Bergen) 4 Path 434 u (BSB)

Locations:

BSB = Bayerisches Staatsbibliothek
EUB = Erlangen Universitätsbibliothek

GNM = Germanisches National Bibliothek, Nuremberg
HAB = Herzog August Bibliothek, Wolfenbüttel
SB = Staatsbibliothek Berlin
SBR = Staatliche Bibliothek Regensburg
TUB = Tübingen Universitätsbibliothek

Unexamined exempla:

1531 (Nuremberg?) (location unknown, see Gruner, 1847).[1]
1544 (Nuremberg?) (location unknown, see Gruner, 1847)
1552 (Wittenberg, Veit Kreutzer) 121, Sp. 570 (British Museum)
1566 (Leipzig: Johann Rhambaw) Third edition, title variation.
1568 (Breslau: Crispin Scharffenberg) Third edition (National Library of Medicine)
1577 (Graz: Zacharias Bartsch) Third edition (location unknown)

Note

1 Christian Gottfried Gruner, *Scriptores de sudore anglico superstites* (Jena: Sumtibus Friderici Maukii, 1847), 187–188, fn 1.

Appendix 2: Vernacular plague texts 1473–1607 in chronological order

This appendix gives additional bibliographical details, when possible, by using the following format. Double vertical lines indicate a line break within the title, as given on the original title page. Parentheses signify print information that appears on the last page of the text, rather than on the front page. Brackets indicate information that is not explicit in the text but is known through bibliographical research or library catalog information. These additional details may help in the identification of further editions or printings of these texts.

Heinrich Steinhöwel
Undanckberkeit (alsz die altern wÿsen schriben) ist für andere laster zeschelten. So aber ich Hainricus Stainhöwel von wÿl doctor in den ercznÿen / so vil gütheit er gunst vnd nucz / ÿecy zweÿ vn zweinczig iar / von den fürsichtigen ersamen vnd wÿsen burgermiestern / rät vnd ganczer gemaind der stat Vlm / mÿnen lieben herren / enpfangen habe! Ulm: Johann Zainer, 1473

Anon.
[Augsburg, ca. 1473] Single-leaf broadside

Heinrich Steinhöwel
Undanckberkeit ‖ alß die alten wi- ‖ sen schriben) ist ‖ für andere laster ‖ zeschelten. So. ‖ aber ich heinricus ‖ Stainhöwel vō ‖ wil doctor in den ‖ ertznyen so vil / … [Strasburg], (1474)

Hans Andree?
Vil menschen weren d pestelentz frey… [Augsburg?, ca. 1476/78] Single-leaf broadside

Anon.
Eyn trackat von der dotlichen sucht der peste ‖ lentz mit grosem fliß vß vjlen bücheren de nā- ‖ haftigesten lerern in der ertznij gezogen vnd in ‖ das dütsche bracht. [ca. 1480]

Anon.
Eyn traktat von der dotlicken sucht der pestle ‖ ntz mit grosem fliß uß vielen bucheren der nā ‖haftigesten lerern in der ertzny gezogen und ‖ in das dutsche brocht [1482]

Heinrich Steinhöwel
In vnda-ckberkait alß die alten wysen schri- ‖ ben ist für andere laster zeschelten So a- ‖ ber ich Hainricus Stainhöwel vō wyl do ‖ ctor in den ertznyen... (Ulm: Cunrat Dinckmut), [ca. 1482]

Johannes Jacobi
[Z]V lob vnd zu ere der heiligen vñ ‖ vegeteiltē trinitet. vñ der seligen ‖ erentreichen iūckfrawen marien ‖ Zu gut vnd zu nucz einer ganczē gemein ‖ zu auffenthaltung der gesunden. vnd erko ‖ berūg od widerpringūg der siechē. wil ich ‖ auß den geschriftē der namhaftigē vñ fur- ‖ nēstē maysterñ in d erczney etwas schrey ‖ ben von dem gebrestē od pestelencz dy zu ‖ zeyten vberhand nympt... [ca. 1482/83]

Heinrich Steinhöwel
Undnachberkeyt (als die alten weysen schreiben) ist fur andere laster zerschelten. So aber ich heinricus stainhowel von wyl docter in den ertzneyen. so vil guthey er gunst und nutz. yetz zwey vnd zweintzig jar. von den fursichtigen ersamen vnnd zeysen burgermeystern. rath vnd gantzer gemein d stat Ulm meynen lieber herren enpfangen habe... Nuremberg, [ca. 1484]

Hans Folz
Item ein fast köstlicher spruch von der pestilencz und anfenglich von den zeichen die ein künfftige pestilencz beteuten. [Nuremberg, 1482]

Anon.
Das Leben des heiligen herrn sant Rochus. Nuremberg, 1484

Ulrich Ellenbog
Hie nach volget ein gut regimēt vnd ordnūg vnd ‖ bewert p-seruatiua vnd ler. wie man sich wider dē ‖ geprechen der pestilentz aufhalten vnd bewaren ‖ sol. Auch gute Curatiua vñ bewert ertzney. Wie ‖ man den menschen die mit solchem geprechen be ‖ griffen werden. helfen sol. Die durch hochgelert ‖ doctores vnd meystē der ertzney. auf das kurtzist ‖ aufgezogen. vnd hie mit durch disen truck zu ge- ‖ meynem nutz. fur reich vnd arm geoffenbart sein. [ca. 1485/90]

Anon.
Hie vohet sich an der schatz des lebens ‖ vor inne man findt eyne warafftige arcte ‖ ney wider die schwree vnde snelle sucht ‖ der pestilentzie. Bewert von vil doctoren ‖ in der arczeney. (Erfurt: 1493)

Ambrosius Jung
Ein außerrvelt loblich tractat ‖ vñ regiment in dem schwären zeit der pestilentz. auß ‖ gezogen. auß den bewärttn vñ weysisten alten gsch ‖ rifften der artzney. Durch Ambrosium jung der sil- ‖ freyen künst vñ der artzney doctor. D zeit der wirdigē ‖ herrn vom thům zů Augspurg geschworner doctor. (Augsburg: Hans Schönsperger, 1494)

Ulrich Ellenbog
Ain wunderbäre instruction vnd ‖ vnderwysung wider die pestilentz ‖ herfliessend von kayserlichem hoff ‖ vnd aller bewärtesten doctoribus ‖ jn cristenlicher vñ haydescher na- ‖ cion funden wärden müge. (Memmingen: Albrecht Kunne, 1494)

Anon.
Wie sich der mensch halten sol wider die Pestilentz. Und auch wie er sich regiren sol wenn sy ist. Und den rat soll man dick überlegen. Augsburg: Hanns Schauren. [ca. 1495] Single-leaf broadside

Philippus Culmacher
Regimen zu deutsch Magistri philippi Culmachers von Eger wider die grausamen erschrecklichenn Totlichen pestelentz. von vil grossen meistern gesamelt außgezogen: do durch sich ein mensch tzu pestelentz tzeit: nicht allein enthalden. Sunder auch wol gefreyen kan: gegeben allen menschen zu sunderm nutz vnd grosserwoltat. Leipzig, [ca. 1495]

Hieronymus Brunschwig
Liber pestilentialis de venenis epidimie. Das bůch der vergift der pestilentz das da genant ist der gemein sterbent der Trüsen Blatten. Strassburg: Hans Grüninger, 1500

Heinrich Laufenberg
Ein tractat contra pestem. Preseruatiue vnd regiment. Wie du dich halten solt in der zeyt so die pestilentz regnieret daß gar nützlich ist den menschen zu wissen. Strasburg: [Grüneck von Bartholome?, 1500]

Conrad Schelling
Ein kurtz Regiment von dem hochgelerten meister ‖ Conradt Schelling von Heidelberg doctor der artze ‖ ny / vnd vnsers gnedigsten herrn Pfaltzgrauen kurfür ‖ sten rc. lib artzet / zů Eren vñ gefallen sein fürstlichen gnaden / Auch seiner gnaden vnderthanen zü nůtz / vß ‖ den fürnemsten Philosophen mit fliß gezogen vnd zů ‖ samen bracht. Wie man sich vor der Pestilentz enthal- ‖ ten / vnd ouch ob der mensch damit begriffen würd jm ‖ helfen sol. (Heidelberg, 1501)

Conrad Schelling
Ein kurtz regiment von dem hochgelerten meister Conardt Schelling von Heydelberg doctor der ertznei / vnd vnsers gnedigsten herrn Pfaltzgrauen kurfursten / leib artzet. Zu eren vnnd gefallen seinn fürstlichen gnaden Auch seiner gnaden vnderthanen zu nutz Uß den fürnemsten Ppylosophen [sic!] mit fleis gezogen vnd zesamen bracht Wieman sich vor der Pestilentz enthalten vnd auch ob der mensch da mit begriffen würd helfen sol / Speyer: Hartman Biber, 1502

Conrad Schelling
Eyn kurtz Regiment von ‖ dem Hochgelerten meister Conradt Schelling von ‖ Heidelberg doctor der Artzeny / vnd vnsers gnedigstē ‖ herñ Pfaltzgrauē kůrfürstē etc. lyb arzet / zu Eren vñ ‖ gefallen sein fůrstlichen gnaden Auch syner gnaden ‖ vñderthanen zu nutz / vß den fůrnemstē Philosophen ‖ mit fleyß getzogē vnd zusamen bracht Wie man sich ‖ vor der Pestilentz erhalten / vñ auch ob d mensch da ‖ mit begriffen wůrd jm helffen sol. (1502)

Anon.
Hie in disem büchlin vindest ‖ du Ein gut regimēt Für dye ‖ Pestilentz / Wer sich nach diser weyß als hie nach ge- ‖ schriben stad regiert / Dem getrew ich ym sol geraten ‖ werdē vñ büß wider die pestilētz Durch die gnad vnsers ‖ Herren Jhesū christi / on den nichts gůts beschehē mag. (Strasburg: Mathis Hüßfuff, 1502)

Heinrich Steinhöwel
Een korth schon vnde gar trostelick regimet... Braunschweig: [Dorn], 1506

Simon Pistoris
Ein kurtz schon vnnd gar trost ‖ lich regiment widder die sweren vñ erschrecklichē kranckheit ‖ der pestilentz. Durch den achtbaren hochgelartē herren Si ‖ mon Pistoris doctor yn der artzney eylendt begriffen / vnd ‖ dem Erbaren Rate zcu Leiptzick yn seynem wegzyehen zu ‖ geschryben vnd gelassen. (Leipzig: Martin Landsberg, 1506)

Ulrich von Kalw
Ein kurtz regiment vor die ‖ pestelentz / dem Erbarn Radt zcu Freyberg / durch den ‖ achtbaren höchgelarten Herren Udalricum von kalw ‖ Doctorem yn der Ertztey / zcu geschryben. (Leipzig: Martin Landsperg, 1507)

Anon.
Vur die pestilentz ‖ Vu schoner recept vnd lere wie man sich mit guedem ‖ regiment / wanne grois sterffden synt halden sal / sinder ‖ yr yn diesem boych allen mynschen sere nutzlich der ‖ pestilentz wederstrant tzo doyn in kurtz begriffen. (Köln: 1509)

Anon.
Eyn Geistlich Regiment fürzůkom-en vnd zůvertreiben den Onheilsamen vnnd Gifftigen gepresten der Pestilentz leib vñ Sel vñ den Ewigē tot. Noch dem volgt ein gemein Regimēt iñ zeit der Pestilentz sich zů gebrauchē. (Oppenheym, 1511)

Andres Reichlin
Pestilentz ‖ bůchlin / das da antzaigt Wie vñ ‖ wamit man sich vor der Pestilentz bewa- ‖ ren soll Vñ ob ain mensch damit vergifft ‖ wurd / wie vñ mit was artzney er jm helf- ‖ fen mag. Gemacht von dem Hochgeler- ‖ ten Maister Andres von Vberlingen der ‖ artzney berümpten Doctor rc. ‖ Item ain ander regiment / durch mai- ‖ ster Andres Reichlin / auch Doctor der ‖ artzney / gar maisterlich gesetzt. (Augsburg, 1512)

Martin Stainpeiss
Ain hailsame ertzney: mit ierem zwe- ‖ satz: zu behuetten wider den lauff der ‖ Pestelentz: aus bewertten geschriften ‖ der Ertzt: angezaigt durch Martinū ‖ Stainpeiss von Wienn: lerer der ertz- ‖ ney: zw haill vnnd nutzperkait allen ‖ menschen. (Vienna, 1515)

Anon.
Ein kurtze underri- ‖ chtūg heilbarer krefftiger ertzēney. ‖ mit welchen sich der mensch. ‖ wider die pestilentz bewa ‖ ren. auch die ienigen ‖ die do mit begrif- ‖ fen hulff zurey ‖ chen mag. (Leipzig: Melchior Lotther), [ca. 1515]

Balthasar Lothwiger
Eyn kurtz nutzbar Regiment und ‖ Rath vor die schweren vñ erschrecklichen kranckheit der Pe ‖ stilētz: Einem Erbarn Rathe tzu Halle vnd Jnwonern do ‖ selbist gunstlich tzugeeygent: durch den Achtbarn Hern Bal ‖ thasar Lothwiger Doctorem vffs kortzte begriffen. (Leipzig: Wolffgang Stöckel, 1516)

Heinrich Stromer von Aurbach
Regiment Henrichen Stromers von ‖ Aurbach d ertzenney Doctors inhal- ‖ tēdt wie sich wid die pestilentz tzubewarē / auch ‖ den ihenen die damit begriffen hilff tzureichen. (Leipzig: Lotther, 1516)

Simon Pistoris
Ein kurtz schon und ‖ gar trostliche regiment wider ‖ die schweren vnd erschrecklichen krancheyt der pestilentz. ‖ Durch den achtbaren hochgelartē herrē Simonē Pistoris ‖ Doctorem in der artzney eylendt begriffen vnd tzu den an ‖ dern mal vor andert dem Erbarē Rate tzu Leyptzck in sey ‖ nez weg zyehen tzugeschrieben vñ gelassen. (Leipzig: Martin Landesperg, 1517)

Heinrich Stromer von Aurbach
Regiment Henrichen Stromers von Aurbach der ertzeney Doctoris inhaltendt wie sie wyder die Pestilentz tzubewaren. Auch den ihenen dye damit begriffen hilff tzureichen. Leipsick: Melchior Lotther, [1517]

Heinrich Stromer von Auerbach
Regiment Hen- ‖ richen Stromers vō Aur ‖ bach der ertzney Doctors ‖ inhaltendt wie sich wider ‖ die Pestilentz zu bewaren ‖ auch den jhenē die damit ‖ begriffen hilff zu reichen / ‖ nach vleissiger vbersehūg ‖ gemehert vnd gebessert. Mainz: (Johann Schöffer, 1517)

Anon.
Ein Warhaftige Ertzney vñ Schatz des ‖ lebens wider die schwere vñ schnelle ‖ sucht der pestilentz. bweret von ‖ vil doctoren der ertzney. Leipzig: Wolfgang Stöckel, (1517).

Anon.
Ein warhaftige Ertzney und Schatz des ‖ lebens wider die schwere vñ schnelle ‖ sucht der pestilentz. bewert von ‖ vil doctoren der ertzney. Leipzig: Wolfgang Stöckel [ca. 1517]

Anon.
Ein warhaftige ertzney ‖ und Schatz des lebens wider die ‖ schwere uñ schnelle sucht der ‖ pestilenty. bewert uō uil ‖ doctoren der ertzney. Erfurt: Matthes Maler, [ca. 1517]

Johann Engel
Tractat von der Pe ‖ stilentz Joanni Engel / der Freyen künsten ‖ vnd artzney Doctor / aufs der leer der ‖ Doctorn der artzney vnd Astro- ‖ nomey gezogen. (Augsburg, 1518)

Sixtus Kolbenschlag
Ein nutzbarlichs ‖ Regiment von Doctor Six ‖ ten Kolbenschlag von Mergathem ‖ wider die pestilentz zů bewaren ‖ und Ihenen die do mit ‖ begriffen hilff ‖ zů reichen. (Nürenberg: Fryderichen Peypus, 1519)

Johann Lotzer von Horb
Ain Nützlich Regimen ‖ vnd vnderwysung / welcher massen den ‖ menschen mit dem gifft der Pestilentz bela- ‖ den / mit hailsamer Artzney zůhelffen sey. ‖ Durch den Hochberümbten Johannem ‖ Lotzer von Horb Doctorem des Hochwir ‖ digen fürsten vnd herrn herrñ Wilhelmß ‖ Bischoffen zů Straßburg / vnd Landt ‖ grauen zů Elsaß der zyt Lybartzet / ‖ zů hilff vnd trost dem menschen ‖ gemacht im Neunzehen- ‖ den Jar. (Hagenaw), 1519

Joachim Vadianus
Ein kurtz vnd trüwlich vnderricht / wider die sorgklich kranckeyt der Pestile-tz / nach aller notturfft vnd ordnung so in söllichem fal / betracht vngehalte- werden mag: neulich ußgangen / vn- zu nutz gemeyner Lantschafft der eydgnoschafft zusamen bracht / im xv. hundert vnd xix. Jar. Zusamen bracht uß dem Latin durch den hochgelerten Joachim Vadianu- / der syben freyen künsten vnd Ertzny Doctor. Basel: Adam Petri, [1519]

Anon.
Ein Neüw ge ‖ ordent Regimēt / wy- ‖ der den tödtlichen ge- ‖ bresten der Pestelentz. ‖ Auß viln bewertē schrifftē / gemei- ‖ nem volck zů uffhalt des lebens / iñ ‖ Reymen (vmb kürtz willē) zů ‖ sammen gesetzt / volgt hyer ‖ nach. Oppenheim, (1519)

Johann Stocker
Ein Kurtz ‖ Regiment für dē ‖ geprestē der pestilentz. So ‖ d hoch gelört herr Jo- ‖ hañ Stockar Doctor ‖ der ertzney / uñ Stat ‖ artzt zů Ulm / ge- ‖ schriben / vnd be- ‖ griffen vñ biß ‖ her in übūng vñ geprau ‖ ch ghabt hatt. (Nürmberg: Peypus, 1520)

Anon.
Ein kurtz ‖ Regiment auß vil ‖ treffenlichen zůsamen ge- ‖ prachten tractaten ver- ‖ stendiger artzt ge- ‖ zogen / wie sich ‖ zu zeitē der pe ‖ stilentz zu- ‖ halten ‖ sey. (Nuremberg: Friedrich Peypus, 1520)

Johann Magenbuch
Ain nützlichs vnd ‖ Bewärts gemains Regiment / vnd für ‖ kommen des vergyfften luffts / in der zeyt des ‖ Sterbens oder Regierūg der Pestilentz / ‖ Durch den Hochgeleerten Doctor ‖ Johann Magenbůch von ‖ Nürnberg / menigklich ‖ one schaden zů ‖ brauchen. (Nuremberg?), [ca. 1520]

Johann Stocker
Ain Regiment für die ‖ Pestilentz / Durch den hochgelertē ‖ Johañ Stockar / Doctor der ‖ Ertzney / vñ Stat Artzt zů ‖ Vlm beschriben vnd in ‖ seynē lebē gebraucht ‖ vnd geyebt. [Nuremberg, ca. 1520]

Anon.
Ein nutzlichs regiment fur die kranckheyt der pestilentz. [ca. 1520] Single-leaf broadside

Johann Copp
Ein nutzlich Regiment wie man ‖ sich halten sol das man gesunden leyb behalt / vñ ‖ sunderlich vor die pestilentz / zu gut allen Chri ‖ sten vnnd nemlich denn eynwondern der ‖ löblichē statt Erffordt / durch Joan ‖ nē Copp

vō Lantspurg Docto- ‖ rem mit höchstem fleyß ‖ gemacht. (Erfurt: Matthes Maler, 1521)

Ambrosius Jung
Ain nutzliche trostliche ‖ vnd kurtze vnderrichtung / wie man sich ‖ in disen schwären leüffen der pestilentz ‖ halten sol / durch Doctor Ambro- ‖ sium Jungen / statartzt zu Aug ‖ spurg / dem gemainen mañ zů ‖ hilff vnd gůttem / der nit ‖ andern beystand hat / ‖ verordnet. 1521

Ambrosius Jung
Ain nutzliche trostliche ‖ vnnd kurtze vnderrichtung / wie man ‖ sich in disen schwaren leüffen der pe ‖ stilentz haltenn sol / durch Doctor ‖ Ambrosium Jungen / statartzt ‖ zů Augspurg / dem gemainen ‖ man zů hilff vnd güttē / der ‖ nit andern beystand hat / ‖ verordnet. 1521

Caspar Kegler (Casparum Kegeler)
Einn Regi- ‖ ment durch Doctorem ‖ Casparum Kegler gemacht Darinnen ‖ sich / vor der Erschrecklichē kranckheyt / ‖ der pestilentz / preseruiren / bewaren vnd ‖ enthalten / Desgleichen Etzliche trostli- ‖ che / vnnd vnder andern Auß geleßene / ‖ Medelen / hilff vnnd ertzeneyen / So et- ‖ wer mit gedachter krancheyt / begriffen / ‖ Inficirt / ader vorgifft wurde / Wie man ‖ dem selben Dor mit tzu hilff komenn / er- ‖ rettenn vnnd vormittelst gotlicher hilff / ‖ widerumb / tzue voriger gesuntheyt ver- ‖helffen mag. (Leipzig: Valentinum Schuman, 1521)

Johannes Klainmüller
Ain hymlischen unn Natürlichen anzaygung diser sterblichenleüff mit ainem nutzlichen und trostlichen regiment wie sich des Mensch hallten soll / mit aderlassen Ertzneyen / unn gutter regierung / zü Eren ainer gantzen gemain der kayserlichen Stat Augspurg geordnet durch Doctore Johannes Klainmüller od Walhopter. Augsburg: “Hansen Schönsperger auff dem Weinmarckt”, 1521

Johann Lotzer
Ain nützlich Regimen und unnderweysung / wellicher massen den menschen mit dem gifft der pestilentz beladen / mit heylsamer ertzney zühellffen sey / durch den Hochberüembten Johannem Lotzer von Horb Doctorem des hochwirdigen Fürsten un herren herrnn Wilhelmß bischoffen zü Straßburg / unn lant graven zü Elsaß der zeit leybartzet / zühillff und trost dem menschen gemacht in dem XXI jar. 1521

Johann Lotzer von Horb
Ain nutzlichs re ‖ gimen vnnd vnnderweysung / ‖ wellicher massen den menschen ‖ mit dem gifft der pestilentz bela- ‖ den / mit heilsamer ertznej zůhelf ‖ fen sey / durch den hochberüem- ‖ ten johannem Lotzer von Horb

‖ doctorem des hochwirdigen ‖ Fürsten vnd herren herrñ ‖ Wilhelmß Bischofen zů ‖ Straßpurg / vñ landt ‖ grauen zů Elsaß der ‖ zeyt leybartzet / zů ‖ hillff vnd trost ‖ dem menschē ‖ gemacht. 1521

Wolfgang Peysser
Ordnung der fursichtigen Ersamenn Weisen herrn Burgermaister / vnd Rat / der loblischen stat Inngolstat / wie sich die mennschen der swern zeit / vnd krannckhait der Pestilentz halten sollen so durch die hochgelerten herrn doctores der Artznei der facultet / auf ir begern beschlossen vnd durch jren bevelch gemacht / durch den hochgelerte- Wolfgangen Peysser doctor vnd Ordinari benanter vniuersitet / Anno:c. XXI. Ingolstat, 1521
Other edition of Peysser: VD16 P 2084.

Nikolaus Pol
Vndericht Nicoly pol ‖ d erzney docters i halt ‖ wie sich d gemain man ‖ im lauff des sterbens zu Insprugg des ‖ 1521 jars / bewarn sol / Auch so es ‖ ayns an käm / wie es in ‖ der erstē eyl im selbs ‖ helffen müg auffs ‖ kurtz begiffen. (Schwatz: Joseph Piernsieder), 1521

Ulrich Rülein von Calw
Ein vnderweysūg ‖ wie mann sich tzu ‖ der tzeit der pesti= ‖ lentz halten sol. Al= ‖ len einwoneren der ‖ stat Freybergk tzu ‖ gut yn einn kurtze ‖ summe gebracht. (Leipzig: Valent Schumann, 1521)

Johannes Salius (Hans Saltzman)
Ein nutzliche ordnu-g vnd regime-t wider die Pestilentz durch Doctor Hansen Saltzman vo- Steir / des Durchleichtigisten Fuersten vnnd herren herrn Ferdinanden Ertzhertzogen von Osterreych. c. Leybartzt. dem gemainenn man zw nutz furchtperlich gemacht. Vienna: Johannes Singriener, 1521

Alexander Seitz
Ain schöner Tra- ‖ ctat von dem Saturnischē gschoß ‖ der Pestilentz mit ettlichen klü ‖ gen fragstucken / dariñ der vn ‖ gelert man sich irret / zü gfer ‖ lichem abbruch seins leb ‖ ens / ee zeit / alles durch ‖ den hochgelerten phi ‖ losophum Alexan ‖ der Seitzen von ‖ Marckbach ‖ Doctor zü ‖ München, auß ‖ menschlicher lieb ‖ trewlich beschriben / vnd verantwurt. 1521

Georg Tannstetter
Regiment für den lauff ‖ der Pestilentz durch Georgē ‖ Tañstetter von Rain der ‖ siben freyen künst vnnd ‖ Ertzney doctor:kurtz- ‖ lich beschriben. ‖ Anno. 1521

Anon.
Ain Pater noster zů be- ‖ ten Vnd zü Betrachten vnns Der ‖ Allmechtig got zů sendet Die pestilentz Krieg / wider wert- ‖ igkait / vnser gwissen zů

rainigen. Got vnser sünd bekla ‖ gen / vnd in bitten sein zorē vō vns wendē / Dañ auß ‖ erñstlich bitten / der berewten hertzñ / verhoffen ‖ wir / got der allmechtig wurde lassen von ‖ seinem zorē / vñ vns barm-hertzigkait ‖ beweysen / wie wol er vns strafft Zů hail vnßer seel / vnd auß vnßer ‖ sünd / Aber er der in allem vil barm-hertzig ist / Růffen wir an ‖ got vnsern erlößer vmb genad vñ barmhertzigkait. (1521)

Anon.
Ein kostlich regiment vor die grau- ‖ sam vnd erschrecklich plage der pesti ‖ lentz mitsampt der aderlassunge auß ‖ den buchern Auicenne Galieni und ‖ Iporactis genōmen: nicht mehr ynn ‖ solcher form gesehen. (Leipzig: Wolffgang Stöckel, 1521)

Anon.
Ain Pater noster zu beten / Und zu Betrachten so vnns Der Allmechtig got zu sendet Die pestilentz Krieg / wider wertigkait / vnser gewissen zu rainigen… [Augsburg], (1521)

Anon.
Das leben vn legedt des heiligen hern sand Rochus: der ain besund grosser nothelffer ist: fur die graussam plag der Pestilentz. (Vienna, 1521)

Caspar Kegler (Gasparum Kegeler)
Ein regiment durch Docto ‖ rem Casparum Kegeler gemacht / Dar- ‖ yñen sich / vor der erschrecklichen kranck- ‖ heit der Pestilentz / Preseruiren bewarē ‖ vñ enthaldten / Der gleichen Ettliche trostliche vñ ‖ vnnther anndern / außgelesen Medelen Hilff ‖ vnnd Ertzeneien / So etwer mit gedachter ‖ kranckheit / begriffen Inficirt / oder ‖ vorgifft wurde / Wie man denn ‖ selben darmit zuhilff komen ‖ erretten vnd vormittelst ‖ Gotlicher hulff / wi- ‖ derumb / zu vori ‖ ger gesūtheit ‖ verhelffē ‖ mag. [1521?]

Anon.
Ain regime-t wider Die pesitlentz vast güt Vnd nutzlich zu dyser zeyt. [ca. 1525]

Anon.
Ein geystliche erzeney fur die grausam erschrecklich pestilentz / Gemacht durch ein liebhaber der heyli ‖ gen geschrifft / fast nutzbar vñ trostlich yetlichē cristen menschen zu brauchen. [Nuremberg: E. Schoen, ca. 1525]

Martin Luther
Ob man ‖ fur dem ster ‖ ben fliehen ‖ muge. ‖ Mart. Luther ‖ Wittemberg. ‖ M.D. XXVII. Wittenberg: Hans Lufft, 1527

Martin Luther
Ob man ‖ fur dē ster ‖ ben fliehen ‖ muge. ‖ Mart. Luther ‖ M.D.XXVII. 1527

Magnus Hundt
Durch den hochgeler- ‖ ten Magistrum Mag- ‖ nuse hundt weyth beruffen Artztten / ‖ eyn Erbarn Rathe der Altenstadt ‖ Magdeburgck / seynen Erbherren ‖ uñ sust guthenfreunden doselbst wy- ‖ der dy schwere plage der pestilentz ‖zwgestelth / vnd nuhn? So Godt ‖ wyll? zw vyler enthaltung / des ‖ 14 tags Septembris. Anno ‖ 1528. in gemtyn auß- ‖ gangenn. 1528.

Heinrich Stromer von Aurbach
Heilbarer krefftiger Ertzney / mitt welchen sich der mensch wider die pestilentz bewaren / auch den ihenigen die do mit begriffen hulff reichen mag. Leipzig: Melchior Lotther, 1529

Wenceslaus Bayer von Elbogen (Cubito)
Richtiger rathschalg vnd bericht der ytzt regierenden Pestilentz / so man den Engelischen schweyß nennet / Durch Doctor Wenceßlaum Bayer von Elbogen / Cubito genandt / außgegangen. Leipzig: Nickel Schmidt, 1529

Anton Brelochs
Eyn kurtzer gegründ- ‖ ter vnderricht / vnnd erklerung einer ‖ geschwinden / vnd überscharpffen seüchten / yetzo von ‖ vielen / der Englisch schwayß / aber von den Alten ‖ das Pestilentzisch fieber genant / mit nützlicher vnd vast tröstlicher anzeygung / weß sich der ‖ mensch vorhin… (Nuremberg: Jobst Gutknecht, 1529)

Magnus Hundt
Eyn Kurtzes vnd sehr ‖ Nutzbarlichs Regiment wi- ‖ der dye schwynde vnd erschreckliche kranckheit ‖ der Pestilentz auß bewerten vn- geubten Ertzten ‖ tzu samen getragen / sampt einem kurtzen bericht ‖ der schweyßkranckheyt. ‖ Meher eyn nutzlichs Regiment wide die welt- ‖ leuftigen vn- vnsauberkranckheit der Frantzosen. ‖ Dortzu eyn bericht der gebranthen wasser zu ‖ gebrauchen druch Magistru- magnu- Hundt von ‖ Magdeburgk de Fursten- Collegiums tzu Leip- ‖ zigk Collegaten außgegangen. Inn. 29. Jar. Leipzig: Valentin Schuman, 1529

Anthonius Klump
Eyn kurtz Regiment und Consi- ‖ lium für die erschrockenlichen schnellen kranck- ‖ heyt / der Englisch schweiß genant / so der hochge ‖ lert Anthonius Klump / der Artzney Doctor / ‖ säßhafft in des Heyligen Reychs Stat Uberlin- ‖ gen / seynen herrn Burgermeyster vnd Räten ‖ daselbs gemacht und uberantwort hat. ‖ Anno. 1529. (Freyburg (Breisgau): Johann Juliacensen), 1529

Philip Novenianus
Eyn schone verordnung vo- den / der Pestilentz / vrsachen / Zceychen / Erczneyen / mit sampt eynem nützlichen Regiment / Einem Erbarn- Rathe der Churfürstlichen Stadt Halle / von dem Achtbarn- vnd Hochgelarten Herrn Philippo Noueniano Hasfurtensi der Etzney Doctorn zugeschrieben. Leipzig: Valentin Schumann, 1529

Caspar Kegler
Eyn Nutzlichs ‖ vnd trostlichs Regiment wider dy ‖ Pestilentz vnd Gifftig Pestilentzisch ‖ Feber die Schweyssucht genannt / vñ ‖ sust mächerley gifftig vñ tödlich kran ‖ ckheit / Durch Casparū Kegler / der ertzney ‖ Doctorn / zwsamen gebracht / vornewt vñ mit ‖ vil trostlichen experimentē gebessert / Die zu-‖ uor heymlich gehalten / vnd an den tag nyhe gegebē seyn. Anno 1.5.2.9. auß gegangen. (Leipzig: Valten Schumann), 1529

Caspar Kegler
Eyn Nutzli- ‖ chs vnd tröstlichs Re ‖ giment widder die Pestilentz vnd ‖ Gifftig Pestilentzisch Fever die Schweys ‖ sucht genant / vnd sunst mancherley gifftig ‖ vnd tödtlich kranckheit / Durch Casparum ‖ Kegler / der ertzney Doctorn / zu samen ge ‖ bracht / vornewt vnd mit viel trostlichen ‖ experimenten gebessert / Die zuuor ‖ heimlich gehalten / vñ an den tag ‖ nyhe gegeben sein. Anno ‖ 1529. auß ‖ gegangen. (Erfurt: Melchior Sachssen, 1530)

Caspar Kegler
Eyn Nutzlichs vñ ‖ tröstlichs Regiment wider die Pestilentz vnd ‖ gifftig Pestilētzisch Feber die Schweyssucht ‖ genant / vnd sünst mancherley vnnd gifftig ‖ tödtlich kranckheyt / Durch Casparum ‖ Kegler / der ertzney Doctorn / zu samē ‖ gebracht / vernewt vñ mit vil tröst ‖ lichen experimenten gebessert / ‖ Die zuuor heymlich gehaltē / ‖ vnd an den tage nye gege- ‖ ben sein. Anno. 1.5.3.0. ‖ auß gegangen. (Regensburg: Paulum Khol), 1530

Wenceslaus Bayer vom Elbogen
Eyn Nutzlicher ‖ kurczer vnterricht / wie ‖ man sich ynn der tzeyt der Pestilentz hal- ‖ ten / auch wass man vor ertzney brauchen ‖ soll / getzogen aus den büchlein so hieuor ‖ Er Wenceslaus Bayer vom Elbo- ‖ gen der Ertzney Doctor / von ‖ der Pestilentz Lateinisch ‖ hatt außgehen ‖ lassenn. Leipzig: Nickel Schmidt, 1530

Hans Folz
In disem büechel und Tractetl: ist beschriben ain seer güt nützlich und cöstlich Regiment und Ertzney / wider die Pestilentz / und andere Pestilentzische Fieber / als Preün und dergleich / so diser zeit und jar / fast umbgend und regierend / wie sich an yeder mensch / zu der zeit / lauf und regierung derselben… [1530]

Sebald Nebel
Ein kurtz ge- ‖ mein vnderricht / wie ‖ man sich zur zeit der Pestilentz hal- ‖ den sol / mit einem kleinen anhang der zufelle / ‖ so sich ynn sterbs leufften / nach vñ vor pfle- ‖ gen zu ereugen. An den Erbarn Radt vñ ‖ gantze gemein Churfürstlicher Stad Aldenburgk / druch Magistrum ‖ Sebaldum Nebelium Bür- ‖ ger daselbst / Zu samen ‖ gebracht. (Erfurt: Melcher Sachssen), 1530

Moses Staffelsteiner
Regiment wid- ‖ der die Pestilentz aussgan ‖ gen durch Moyses Staf- ‖ felsteiner Juden medicus ‖ wōhafftig zu Weymar aus denn alten Judischen bü ‖ chern ynns deutsch ge ‖ zogen Menni- ‖ glich zu nutz. (Marburg), 1530

Conrad Wickner
Das man sich vor ‖ dem zukünfftigen ster- ‖ ben oder Petsilentz ‖ nicht entsetzen ‖ soll. ‖ Conradt Wickner. ‖ Anno. 1530. Nuremberg: Friderich Peypus, 1530

Conrad Wickner
Gewise und warhaff- ‖ tige Practica auß der heyligen ge- ‖ schrifft / was eygentlich zůkünfftig sey / vñ ‖ was man warten / oder sich zu vertrösten ‖ hab / vnd das man sich dise zeyt vor ‖ der Pestilentz nicht entse- ‖ tzen dürffe. (Nuremberg: Friedrich Peypus), 1530

Sebald Nebel
Ein Kurtz ge- ‖ mein vnderricht / wie ‖man sich zur zeit der Pestilentz hal- ‖ den sol / mit einem kleinen anhang der zufelle / ‖ so sich ynn sterbs leufften / nach vñ vorpfle- ‖ gen zu ereugen. An den Erbarn Radt vñ ‖ gantze gemain Churfürstlicher Stad ‖ Aldenburgk / durch Magistrum ‖ Sebaldum Nebelium Bür- ‖ger daselbst / Zu samen ‖ gebracht. 1530

Hans Folz
Ain kostlicher vnd ‖ fast gründtlicher Spruch / wie ‖ man sich zů der zeyt der ‖ Pestilentz mit allen ‖ dingen hal- ‖ ten soll. [ca. 1530]

Caspar Kegler
Een seer costelic ende ‖ profitelije regiment / ey- principael bewijs hā crupdē / ‖ gebrande watern / worterlen / eñ puluer. ec. Tot bewaringhe des ver ‖ schrickeliken ghebreck der *pestilentiē* / Hoemen eles maken / eñ in- ‖ der noot ghebrunckē sal / het ñ van Electuariē / Pillelen / Plaste ‖ ren goeden rueck / oft anderē aromated.ec. Hoe ende in wat ‖ manierenhem die mēsche daghelies onderhonden sal met ‖ ader later / purgeringe / coppē / spyse ende dranck te nut ‖ ten / *Item wat edel gliestcvnte* om bloot aen dē lich ‖ aem te dragljen / *Doc diergelincken / wat worte* ‖ *len ende curnden* goet om te riecken zihn / ‖ voor die boose verghiftigen suchte te ver ‖ drinē / door *Meester Kaspar Kege-* ‖ *ler* van Lijbs doctoor der Mede ‖ cinen / cortelyck

begrepē / en- ‖ de int licht ghebrocht. a4, b2 (last verso blank), 11 pages. Constans: Johann Haselberck, ca. 1530

Johannes Sommerfelt
Ein Regiment ‖ vnd Ertzney widder die ‖ schwinde vnnd erschreckliche ‖ plaga der Pestilentz / wie sich ein ‖ mensch vermittelst Göttlicher ‖ hülffe / dauor bewaren / vnd auch ‖ derselben zu hülff kommen magk / ‖ auffs kürtzste anzuzeigen begriff ‖ en / aus der schrift vnd erfarung ‖ gezogen / sehr nützlich zuwissen. [ca. 1530]

Johann Stockar
Ain Regiment für die Pestilentz / Durch den hochgelerte- Johan- Stockar / Doctor der Ertzney / vn- Stat Artzt zu0 Vlm beschriben vnd in seyne- lebe- gebraucht vnd geyebt. [ca. 1530]

Theobald Fettich
Ordenung vnd Ee ‖ giment / sich vor der überscharpff- ‖ en vñ gifftigen kranckheit der Pestilentz zuenthalten / Vnd ‖ denen so damit begriffenn / mit Gottes hülff / wider ‖ zehelffen. Sampt den zůfellen. ‖ Mit angehenckter natürlichen vrsach des Englischenn ‖ Schweyßs. Alles Inhalt nachgehnds Registers… Frankfurt: Christian Egenolph, 1531

Theobald Fettich
Ordenung vnd Ee- ‖ giment / sich vor der überscharpffen ‖ vnd gifftigen kranckheit der Pestilentz zůent- ‖ halten / Vnd denen so damit begriffen / mit Gottes ‖ hülff / wider zehelffen. Sampt den zůfellen. ‖ Mitt angehenckter natürlichen vrsach des Englischenn ‖ Schweys… (Strasburg, 1531)

Sebald Heyden
Wie man sich in allerlay nötten / des Türcken / Pestilentz / Theürung / r.c. trösten / den glauben stercken / vnd Christliche gedult erlangen soll / Auß siben sprüchen heyliger schrifft kürtzlich angezeigt / Durch Sebaldum Heyden. Nuremberg: Friderich Peypus, 1531

Hieronymus Hüniger
Spiegel zů der ‖ zyt der Pestilentz. ‖ Misit verbum suum, & sanavit eos. Psal.106. Basel: Thoman Wolff, 1531
Luis (Abulensis) von Lobera (Ludouice de Avila y de Lorbera)
Ein nutzlich Regiment der gesundt ‖ heyt / Genant das Vanquete / oder Gastmal der Edlen diener ‖ von der Complexion / Eigenschafft / Schad / vnd nutz allerley ‖ Speyß / Trancks / vñ von allem / darmit sich der mensch in ge- ‖ sundtheyt enthelt / Mit sampt einem kurtzen Regiment / ‖ Wye man sich in der Pestilentz / Pestilentzischen fieber ‖ vnnd Schweyß halten soll. (Augsburg: Heynrich Steyner, 1531)

Anon.
Regimẽt ‖ weß man ‖ sich ytzund / vnd fort an ‖ zůr zeyt der Pestilentz / mit ‖ essen / trincken vnd pa- ‖ den halten sol. ‖ Auch findestu hierjnne manch- ‖ erley bewerter Artzeney zů ‖ den Zösen Zenen. ‖ Von des geprantẽ weins tugendẽ / ‖ Zwen vnd zwaintzig Artickel. ‖ M. D. XXXI. (Wolffgang Resch Formschneyder), 1531

Johann Drachenfuss
Ein köstbarliche / bwerte ‖ vnd gewisse Artzney / wie ‖ ein gesundter in sterbens leufftẽ / auch ‖ einer der schon mit der grausamen kranckheyt der ‖ Pestilentz ergriffen worden / von solchem ‖ schnellen vnnd tödtlichen gifft / sein ‖ leben erretten soll. [1531?]

Johann Magenbuch
Ain nützlichs und ‖ Bewärts gemains Regiment / vnd für ‖ kommen des vergyfften luffts / in der zeyt des ‖ Sterbens oder Regierũg der Pestilentz / ‖ Durch den hochgeleerten Doctor ‖ Johann Magenbůch von ‖ Nürnberg / menigklich ‖ one schaden zů ‖ brauchen. 1532

Adam Zwicker
Ein kurtze wolgegründte vnderrichtung vnd erkelerung von Doctor Adam Zwicker zu Memmingen / wie man sich vor der erschröcklichen kranckheit der Pestilentz präseruieren / vnnd bewaren soll / vnd wenn eins darmit angriffen würde / wie es sich halten soll / mit bewerten köstlichen stücken brauchen Gott dem herren zu lob vndehr / zü nutz gemeiner löblichen statt Memmingen. [1532]

Anon.
Ein kostlich Regi- ‖ ment vor die grau ‖ same vnd erschrockenliche ‖ plag der Pestilentz / sampt ‖ der Aderlassung / aus den ‖ Büchern Auicenne / Gale- ‖ ni / vñ Ipocratis genomen ‖ Allen menschẽ nützlich vñ tröstlich zuhaben. (Dresden: Wolfgang Stöckel), 1532

Anon.
Ein kurtz Regiment ‖ wie sich zu zeiten der Pestilentz ‖ zu halten sey. Nuremberg: Johann Petreium, 1533

Michael Fencken
Ain gut nützlich ‖ Regiment / wie man sich hal ‖ ten soll / vor / in / vnd nach der ‖ zeyt d erschröcklichẽ kranck ‖ hayt der Pestilentz / durch ‖ Michaelem Fencken / der ‖ Artzney Doctoren / di- ‖ ser zeyt Ordinarien ‖ der löblichen Vni ‖ uersitet zů In ‖ goldstat. (Augsburg: Alexander Weyssenhorn), 1533

Sebastian Petzher
Ordnung vnd Eegimēt ‖ wider die erschrocklichē kranckhait ‖ der Pestilentz / weß sich ein mensch damit bela ‖ den halltenn… (Regensburg: Hans Kohl, 1533)

Sebastian Petzher
Ordnung vnd Regime-t wider die erschrockliche- kranckhait der Pestilentz / weß sich ein mensch damit beladen halltenn auch wie man sich mit gotts hilffe vor der bewaren solle / durch Sebastianum Petzher vo- weyssenburg / der Freyen kunst vn Artznei Doctor / Stat artzet zu Straubing Aufs kurtzt zusamen pracht. Im 1533 Jar. Regensburg: Hans Khol, 1533

Marcus Deas Veringer
Ein Kurtz nützlichs Regi- ‖ ment / Wie sich ein egklicher vor der Pe- ‖ stilentz bewaren / vnd der selben entpfliehen / auch ‖ mit hilff des Allmechtigen Gottes / seines ‖ leibs gesundthait / erhalten soll / Dar- ‖ tzů den krancken mit diser sucht ‖ der Pestilentz beladen / ‖ fast dienstlich. (Augsburg: Heynrich Stainer, 1533)

Andreas Osiander
Wie vnd wohin ein ‖ Christ die grausamē ‖ plag der pestilentz ‖ fliehen soll. ‖ Ein predig / aus dem 91. Psalm. Nuremberg: (Johann Petreium), 1533

Heinrich Stromer von Aurbach
Regimēt Hē- ‖ richen Stromers vō ‖ Aurbach der ertzney Doc ‖ toris inhaltendt wie sich wi- ‖ der die Pestilentz zubewa ‖ ren / auch den yhenen die ‖ damit begriffen hilff ‖ zu reichen. Nuremberg, 1533

Andreas Osiander
WIe vnnd ‖ wohin / ain Christ die ‖ grausamen plag der ‖ Pestilentz flie- ‖ hen soll. [1533?]

Johan Agricola
Ain grüntlicher fleis- ‖ siger außzug / auß allen bewerten Kriechischen vñ ‖ Lateinischen lerern / dermassen bißher hoch nye beschehen / Von ‖ vrsachen / zaichen / fürsehung / vnd haylung der grewlichen ‖ Pestilentz / sampt allē zůfellen die sich in diser Kranck- ‖ hait begeben mögen / Alles auß gůtem grund / on ‖ all Sophistisch oder Arabisch / in der Artzney ‖ vngegründt / zůsetz vñ erdichtes geschwetz. ‖ Durch Doct. Johan. Agricola- / der Artzney ‖ vnd Kriechischen sprach leser zů Ingolstat. (Augsburg: Philipp Vlhart), [1533?]

Sebastian Petzher
Ayn Khurtzer Nützlicher ‖ begriff vnnd anzaygung den Armen jn vnnd ‖ vor dem Walde / der zeyt des Ster ‖ bens oder Regierung der ‖ Pestilentz

/ mit gerin- ‖ gen leichten vnd treglichen ko- ‖ sten zube- ‖ langen. (Regensburg: Hanns Kohl), ca. 1533

Johannes Milchtaler
Ain kurtz vnd notwendig vnderricht vnd Regiment / wie sich zu zeyten der Petilentz / vorhin vn- so ainer mit / oder ohn außwendige zaychen des leybs antast wurde / auffs fürderlichst halten vnnd artzneyen solle / Durch Doctor Johansen Milchtaler / Leybartzet zu Schwatz. [Augsburg?: Heinrich Steiner?], 1534

Georg Hobsinger and Leonhart Prechtl
Ein Khurtze Ordnung ‖ wie sich jngegen würtigen Sterblichen Leüff- ‖ en zu halten / durch Georgen Hobsing- ‖ er vnd Leonhartn Prechtl bede der ‖ Ertzney Doctores / von ainem ‖ Ersamen Chamerer vnd ‖ Rhatt / diser stat Re- ‖ gēspurg / darumb ‖ ersucht in Eyll zu sa- ‖ men getragē. ‖ [Regensburg?], 1535

Ambrosius Jung
Ain nutzliche trost- ‖ liche vnd kurtze vnderrichtung / wie man ‖ sich in disen schwären leüffen der Pestilentz haltē ‖ soll / durch Ambrosium Jungen / der Artzney ‖ Doctor zů Augsburg / dem gemainen ‖ mann zů hilff vnd gůtem / der ‖ nit andern beystand ‖ hat / verord- ‖ net. MDXXXV. Augsburg: Philipp Vlhart, 1535

Ambrosius Jung
Ein nutzliche trostliche ‖ vnd kurtze vnderrichtung / wie man ‖ sich in disen schwaren leüffen der Pestilentz hal- ‖ ten soll / dem gemeinen mann zů hilff ‖ vnnd gůtem / der nit andern bey- ‖ stand hat / verordnet. (Strasburg: Wendel Rihel), 1535

Adolph Occo, et al.
Was die Pestilentz an jr selbs ‖ sey / mit jren vrsachen vnd Ertzneyen / Den Er- ‖ same n vnd Weysen Burgermaister vnd Rathe / auch gantzer ‖ gemain der statt Augspurg / durch die bestelten Doctores da- ‖ selbst / zů nutz vnd gůt gemacht vnd beschriben. ‖ Mit kurtzer widerlegung etlicher grober einfallen- ‖ der jrsal / so sich bey vns wider der alten schrifft vnd ‖ gegründte vrsachen zůtragen. Augsburg: Philipp Ulhart, 1535

Anon.
Ein schön Regiment ‖ widder die erschreck ‖ liche kranckheit der ‖ Pestelentz / dem ge- ‖ meinen einfeltigen man zu ‖nutz vnd frumen / zusa ‖ men gebracht / Auch ‖ gantz nutzlich den / ‖ so damit begri ‖ ffen sind. (Wittenberg: Nickel Schirlentz), 1535

Anon.
Ein Kurtz Regiment wie man sich zuer ‖ zeit der Pestilentz halten soll. [Regensburg?, 1535?]

Hans Hörburger
Ain gůt vnnd vast nutzliches Regiment / ‖ wie man sich / in der Pestilentz / halten soll. 1536 Single-leaf broadside

Anon.
Der ain vñ neintz- ‖ ichst Pslam tröstlich in der ‖ Gemain zu der Zeyt ‖ der Pestilentz zu ‖ singen. 1537

Adam Zwicker
Ein kurtze wolgegründ- ‖ te vnderrichtung vnd erklerung von Do- ‖ ctor Adam Zwicker zů Memmingen / wie man sich ‖ vor der erschröcklichen kranckheit der Pestilentz prä- ‖ seruieren / vnnd bewaren soll / vnd wenn eins dar- ‖ mit angriffen würde / wie es sich halten soll / ‖ mit bewerten köstlichen stücken brauchen ‖ Gott dem herren zů lob vnd ehr / zü ‖ nutz gemeiner löblichen statt ‖ Memmingen (1537)

Johan Rympffer
Ein kurtz Regiment wi- ‖ der die grausame plag der Pestilentz / wie ‖ sich der mensch vor solcher plag teglichs vber bewa- ‖ ren sol. Und so ein mensch damit begriffen wirt / wie ‖ jm vnter xij. stunden / ehe dan ers beschlaffen ‖ hat / mit Gottes hilff durch vormittlung ‖ der Ertzney / one zweifel geholffen ‖ mag worden. (Nuremberg: Johan Petreio, 1538)

Ulrich Wolffhart
Ain kurtzer bericht von Doctor Ulrich Wolff- ‖ hart zů Memmingen / wie man sich vor der erschrockenlichen ‖ kranckhait des geprechens der Pestilentz Preseruiern vnnd be- ‖ waren mög / Auch wañ ains darmit angriffen / wie es sich hal- ‖ ten / vñ die bewärten kostlichen stuck / darzů dienstlich / so er auf ‖ das best in seiner Appentegk / so die alt geneñt wirt / hat lassen ‖ zůrichten / gebrauchen / Got zů lob vñ ehr / gmainer stat Mem ‖ mingen / auch menigklich zů nutz vnd wolfart. [Augsburg?: ca. 1538]

Ambrosius Jung
Ain nutzliche trostliche ‖ vnd kurtze vnnderrichtung / wie man sich in di- ‖ sen schweren leüffen der Pestilentz halten solle / ‖ durch Ambrosium Junngen / der Artzney ‖ Doctor zů Augsburg / dem gemainen ‖ mann zů hilff vnd gůtem / der nit ‖ anndern beystand hat / ‖ verordnet. M.D.XXXIX. (Augsburg: Silvanum Ottmar), 1539

Caspar Kegler
Ein Regiment ‖ durch Doctorem Casparum ‖ Kegeler gemacht / Darynn- ‖ nen man sich / vor der Erschrecklichen ‖ kranckheit der Pestilentz /

Preseruiren / ‖ bewaren vnd erhalten / Des gleichen / ‖ Etzliche tröstliche / vnd vnter andern ‖ Aus gelesene Medelen / hülff vñ Ertze- ‖ neyen / So etwer mit gedachter kranck ‖ heit begreiffen / Inficirt / oder vergifft ‖ würde / Wie man dem selbigen dar- ‖ mit zu hülffe kommen / erretten / ‖ Vnd vormittelst Göttlicher hilff / ‖ Widderumb / zur vorigen ge- ‖ sundheit verhelffen mag. ‖ Das auch mit sonderlichem vleis ‖ Corrigirt / vnd zu fromen eines jederen ‖ Christen menschen / jnn Druck ge- ‖ bracht. (Magdeburg: Hans Walther), 1539

Sebald Nebel
Ein kurtz ge- ‖ mein vnderricht / wie ‖ man sich zur zeit der Pestilentz hal- ‖ den sol / mit einem kleinen anhang der zufelle / ‖ so sich ynn sterbs leufften / nach vñ vor pfle- ‖ gen zu ereugen. An den Erbarn Radt vñ ‖ gantze gemein Churfürstlicher Stad ‖ Aldenburgk / durch Magistrum ‖ Sebaldum Nebelium Bür- ‖ ger daselbst / Zu samen ‖ gebracht. 1539

Johann Reusch
Regiment Do- ‖ ctor Johan Reüschen ‖ Wie sich zur zeit der Pestilentz ‖ zu halten sey / Die einwo- ‖ ner der Stadt Leip- ‖ tzigk / vornemlich ‖ belangendt. (Leyptzigk: Nickel Schmidt, 1539)

Heinrich Stromer von Aurbach
Eyn kurtze vnterrichtung getzogen auß den Regimenten Doctoris Heinrichen Stromers / heilbarer krefftiger Ertzney / mit welchen sich der mensch wider die Pestilentz bewaren / auch den ihenigen die da mit begriffen hülffe reichen magk. Leipzig: Nickel Schmidt, 1539

Alban zum Thor
Wie man sich ‖ vor der grausamen / erschrock- ‖ lichen kranckheit der Pestilentz ent ‖ halten / vnnd denen so domit bela- ‖ den / wid (mit Gott) helffen mög / ‖ rechte vnderwysung vñ regiment / ‖ durch Albanum zům Thor / der fry ‖ hen künsten vnd Artzny Doctor / ‖ des durchlüchtigen hochgebornen ‖ F. vnd H. hern Ernsten / Margro- ‖ fen zů Baden / etc. lybartzet / vffs ‖ kürtzst vß den ältsten vnd berümpt ‖ sten Ertzten / mit sonderm ‖ flyß zůsamen ge- ‖ lesen. (Basel: Balthasser Ruchen, 1539)

Johannes Siegmund Goerlitzer
Ein kurtzer Vnter- ‖ richt vnd Regiment, wie ‖ man sich zurzeit der Pestilentz bewaren ‖ vnd halten sol, auf das man nicht leicht- ‖ lich Inficirt / vnd vergifftet werde / Vnd wo ‖ jemand mit dieser erschrecklichen Plage ‖ vbereilet / und behafftet wird / wie ‖ man jm widerumb durch Gottes ‖ Hülffe helffen / vnd jn er- ‖ retten sol. (Wittenberg: Joseph Klug), 1540

Sixtus Kolbenschlag
Ein Tröstliche frustbare Ordnung vn- Unterricht / Wider die schröcklichen schnellen Kranckhait der vergifften Lufft vnd Pestilentz. Einer Erbarn Gemain

zu Würtzburg zu sonderm trost zugeschrieben / Durch den hochgelerten vnd weitberümbten der freyen kunst vn- Artzney Doctor Sixtum Kolbenschlag von Mergathaym. Darneben etliche zufell / jnn diser Kranckhait / mit mancherley Artzneyen angezeygt. Nuremberg: Leonhart Milchtaler, 1540

Anon.
1.5.4.0. Wie man sich zů zeiten ‖ der Pestilentz fürse- ‖ hen vnd erhall- ‖ ten mög. (Vienna: Hanns Syngrüener, 1540)

Tarquinius Schnellenberg
Ein kurtz Schön vnd tröstlich Regiment wider die alte schwere erschreckliche kranckheit der Pestilentz... Erfurt: Melcher Sachssen inn der Archen Noe, 1540
Matthias Boeham (with help from Johann Vogts II, and Wolfgang Talhauser)
Ain nutzliche / vnnd für den gemainen Mann / genůgsam ‖ gegründte vnderricht / wie sich diser ‖ zeyt der Pestilentz halben ‖ zuhalten sey. (Augsburg: Philipp Ulhart), [1540?]

Jacob Ebel
Ein gar kurtz vnd not- ‖ wendiges Regiment für den jetzschwe- ‖ benden Presten der Pestilentz / mit vielen Prae- ‖ seruatiuen vnd Curen / von dem Ehrwirdigen vnd ‖ Hochgelerten Herren / Herrn Jacoben Ebeln ‖ der Ertzney Doctorn / Scholastern vnd ‖ Canonicken zu Bunn rc. ‖ Artzt / Beschrie- ‖ ben. ‖ Mit andern vielen bewerten Re- ‖ cepten aus langer erfarung / ge- ‖ recht gefunden / mit fleiss ‖ herzu gesatzt. St. Victory bey Mainz: Francis Behem, 1541

Johan Castner
Wie man sich in Pesti- ‖ letzischen sterbsleuffen vor der vergiff- ‖ tung bewaren möge / vnd dargegen den ‖ vergifften mit artzney wider helffen / ein ‖ klare vnterrichtung / sampt andern natür ‖ lichen nottürfften / menschliche ge- ‖ sundtheyt zuerhalten / (Nuremberg: Johan Peterio, 1542)

Georg Sturtz
Ein tröstlich ‖ vnd vhast nützlich Regiment vor ‖ die Pestilentz / mit vielen schönen ‖ Regeln / Preseruatiuen / vnd Re- ‖ cepten / Einem Erbarn Rathe / ‖ der newen Bergkstadt / S. ‖ Marienbergk / Durch den Achtbarn vnd hochge- ‖ larten Herrn. ‖ Georgium Sturtzen der Artz- ‖ ney Doctor gestellet. ‖ Anno. M. D. XLII. (Erfurt: Merten von Dolgen an der breitten Strass), 1542

Andreas Aurifaber (Goltschmid)
Ein gut Eegiment [sic!] fur ‖ die gifftige Kranckheit der Pestilentz / ‖ etwan durch Magistrum Andream Goltschmid ‖verordenet / vñ nun widerumb

von etlicher ‖ notwendigen ursachen wegen ge- ‖ bessert vnd inn Druck ver- ‖ fertiget. Leipzig: (Nickel Wolrab), 1543

Andreas Osiander
Wie / vnd wo him / ein ‖ Christ / die grausamē ‖ plag der pestilentz ‖ fliehen sol. ‖ Ein predig / aus dem 91. Psalm. ‖ Vormals im 1533. jar außgegangen / vnd jetzo von ‖ newem wider vbersehen vnd gepessert. Nuremberg: Johan Petreius, 1543

Anon.
Ein kurtz Regiment / ‖ wie sich zu zeiten der Pestilentz ‖ zu halten sey. ‖ Durch die Gelerten vnd erfarnen der ‖ Ertzney Doctores / gemert vnd ‖ gebessert. anno 1543. Nuremberg: Johan Petreius, 1543

Veit Dietrich
Der XCI. Pslam. ‖ Wie ein Christ in sterbß- ‖ leufften sich trösten soll. ‖ Zu Nürnberg gepredigt / durch ‖ Vitum Dietrich ‖ M. D. XLIIII. (Nuremberg: Johann vom Berg und Ulrich Newbaw), 1544

Achilles P. Gasser
Ainfeltiger vñ gegrün- ‖ ter bericht / wie menigklich sich in Pestilen- ‖ tzischem vbergang / mit artznyen / vnd anderer lybs ‖ not / halten / bewaren / vnd genören soll / durch ‖ Achillem P. Gassarum L. natürlicher ‖ künsten vnd baider artznyen Do- ‖ ctorn zu Veldkirch ‖ gemacht. (Nuremberg: Johann Petreius, 1544)

Urbanus Rhegius
Ein schön ‖ vnterrichtung vnd ‖ trost / wie sich alle Chri ‖ sten in der grausamen ‖ plage der Pestilentz hal- ‖ ten sollen / sampt etzlichen Trostbrieffen allen Chri- ‖ sten nütze vnd von nöten / gestellet. (Hannover: Henningk Rüdem, 1544)

Dionysius Sibenbürger
Ein Nützlichs / Vnnd ‖ Tröstlichs Regiment / Wider das Gyff- ‖ tig Fieber der Pestilentz / wie unnd wo ‖ hyn / ein yeder die grausamen Plag fliehen / und Christ- ‖ lich vonn diser Welt abzuschayden / Menigklich zů nůtz ‖ vnd gut / Durch Dionisium Sibenbürger / ‖ Freyer Natürlicher Kůnst und bayder ‖ Ertzney Doctorn ‖ beschryben. Nüremberg: Christoff Gutknecht, (1544)

Ulrich Summer
Regiment vnd ordnung ‖ wie man sich in den geferlichen zey- ‖ ten / der Pestilentz halten soll / vnd der kranck ‖ heyt widerstreben müg / Menigklich zü nutz vnd ‖ gůt / durch Vdalricum Summer der Artz- ‖ ney Doctorn beschriben. ‖ 1544

Johannes Theophilium
Zwů Gotselige / Gna- ‖ denreiche vnd Christliche Bekantnussen ‖ vnser heyligen Christlichen Glaubens / Darmit ein ye- ‖ der Christ / so selig begert zu werden / zu yeder zeyt seines ‖ lebens gewapnet vnd gerüst sein sol / Vorab in disen ‖ fehrlichen leüfften vnnd vnfall der grausamen ‖ Pestilentz / So vber alle ander Artzney ‖ gantz nützlich / dienstlich vnd tröstlich ‖ sein / zu disem Newen Jare. Durch ‖ Joannem Theophilium sum- ‖ marie verfast / Damit ‖ sich ein yeder mensch ‖ in aller seiner ‖ not / ‖ habe zu trösten vnnd zu ‖ stercken / biß ins ewig ‖ leben. Nuremberg: Christoff Gutknecht, 1544

Caspar Kegler
Eynn nützlichs ‖ Vnnd tröstlichs Regiment ‖ wider die Gifftigk Pestilentzisch ‖ Feber die Schweyssucht genant / ‖ Vnnd sunst mancherley gifftig ‖ vnd tödtlich kranckheyt / durch ‖ Casparum Kegler / der Ertz- ‖ ney Doctorn / zusammen ge- ‖ bracht / vernewt vnd mit viel ‖ tröstlichen Experimenten ‖ gebessert / Die zuuor heim ‖ lich gehalten / vnnd an ‖ den tag nyhe gege- ‖ ben seyn. ‖ Anno 1.5.2.9. auss gegangen. [ca. 1545]

Jodocus Willich
Vonn der ‖ Pestilentz ein nütz- ‖ lich Regiment / auff ‖ diese zeit gestellet. ‖ Darzu auch / wie ‖ man schwangern fra- ‖ wen vnd Kindlin / in ‖ der kranckheit ‖ rathen sol. Frankfurt/Oder, [ca. 1545]

Philipp Wulff
Wider die erschreckliche ‖ grausame geschwinde plage der Pestilen- ‖ tzie / ein scöner Proceß / mit viel bewerten Recep- ‖ ten vnd Preseruatiuen / für den Armen so wol als ‖ den Reichen gestellet / Wie sie sich selbst helffen sol- ‖ len / so sie die Doctoren oder die Apoteken durch jre vnmögenheit nicht bekomen mögen / Auß vie- ‖ ler Hochgelerter Dcotoren der Hebrai- ‖ schen vnd Caldeischen / auch ande- ‖ rer sprachen verstendigen ‖ zusammen colli- ‖ giert. ‖ Durch ‖ Philippum Wulff / Medicum zu ‖ Ossenbrück. Lemgo, 1546

Tarquinius Schnellenberg
Experimenta von XX. Pestilentz Wurtzeln und Kreutern, wie sie für Gifft unnd Pestilentz gebraucht mögen werden… (Frankfurt am Mayn: Weygand Han, 1546)

Johann Hener
Ein Radtschlag wie man ‖ sich mit hilff Gottes / vor dem grausa- ‖ men prästen der Pestilentz hüten vnd bewaren ‖ sölle. Vund so einer damit angegriffen / wie unnd mit was ‖ Ertzneyen jm zehelffen. Auß den berümptesten der heilsa- ‖ men kunst der Artzny Doctorn / sonderlich was für die Ar ‖ men vnd vmb ein ring gelt wol zůbekummen / Einem

Er- ‖ samen Radt vnd gemeiner burgerschafft der loblichen ‖ Reychstatt Lindow zů eeren vnnd wolfart zůsa- ‖ men getragen durch Johann Hener / der ‖ leyb vnd wunderartzney Doctorn Phy- ‖ sicum vnd burger daselbst. (Zürich: Christoffel Froschouer, 1548)

Johannes Draconites
Von des Todes ‖ Gifft vnd der Hellen Pestilentz: ‖ IESV CHRISTO. [Lübeck]: (Georg Richolff, 1549)

Jodocus Willich
Wie man ‖ denen helffen sol / ‖ welchem mit der pesti- ‖ letzische gifft begrif- ‖ fen seind. ‖ Durch D. Jodocum Willi- ‖ chium von Kesell. Frankfurt/Oder: Johann Eichorn, 1549

Jodocus Willich
Wie man sich in einer ‖ stadt für der Pestilentz behüten sol ‖ vnd möchte / ein kurtz vnd ‖ seer nützliche vnder- ‖ richtung. ‖ Durch ‖ Doctorem Jodocum Willichium ‖ von Kesell / dem armen volck ‖ vorgestalt. Frankfurt/ Oder: Johann Eichorn, 1549

Anthoni Nigri
Regiment Anto ‖ nij Nigri / der Artzneien ‖ Doctoris vnd Leibartzt / ‖ der Erbaren Stadt Braun ‖ schweig / Inhaltendt / ‖ wie sich wider die Pesti- ‖ letz zubewaren / auch ‖ den jenen die damit ‖ begriffen / hülff ‖ zu reichen. Hannover: Henningk Rüdem, (1550)

Hieronymus Oder
Radt vnd Artz- ‖ ney / zu verhütung vnd zu ‖ rettung wider die Pesti- ‖ lentz / mit Gottes hülffe nützlich / ‖ trewlich gestellet / Durch ‖ Hieronymum Oder vom Annen- ‖ berg / der löblichen Kunst ‖ der Artzney / Doctor. Wittenberg: Veit Creutzer, 1550

Haymeran Schweller
Ein Christli- ‖ che vnderricht wie man sich ‖ zů den zeiten / der trübsal vnnd ‖ plagen Gottes / vnd sunderlich ‖ zůr zeit der Pestilentz / haltē soll. ‖ Beschribē durch Haymeran / ‖ Schweller Pfarrer ‖ zü Tirol. Ingolstat: Alexander Weissenhorn, 1550

Jodocus Willich
Wie man denen helf- ‖ fen sol / weliche mit der pesti- ‖ lentzische gifft begrif- ‖ fen seind. Frankfurt/Oder: Johann Eichorn, 1550

Johan Behem
Ein Regiment ‖ widder die Pestilentz / Vnd ‖ sonderlich wie man sich mit dem ‖ aderlassen halten soll. ‖ Zu Martini Lutheri zeiten / ‖ durch den

hochberuümpte Me- ‖ dicum / M. Johan Behem zu Wit- ‖ temberg gestellet. Franckfort an der Oder: Johan Eichorn, [ca. 1550]

Anon.
Ain kostlicher vnd ‖ fast gründtlicher Spruch / wie ‖ man sich zů der zeyt der ‖ Pestilentz mit allen ‖ dingen hal- ‖ ten soll [ca. 1550]

Anon.
Dat Remediū ‖ Radt vnde hülpe / vor ‖ de erscreckliken / vnde ‖ vör hen by vns Düdeschen vn ‖ erhöreden / hastigen / dötlick- ‖ en kranckheit / de Engeli- ‖ sche Sweethsüke genömet / ‖ Daruör vns Godt de al- ‖ mechtige genedichlicken ‖ behöden vnde bewa- ‖ hren wolde [ca. 1550]

Caspar Kegler
Ein nutzlichs ‖ vnd tröstlichs Regiment ‖ wider die Pestilentz / vnd giff- ‖ tige Pestilentzisch Feber / die Schweis- ‖ sucht genant / Vnd sonst mancher ‖ ley gifftig vnd tödtlich ‖ kranckheit / ‖ Durch ‖ Casparum Kegler / der ‖ Ertzney Doctorn / zusammen ‖ gebracht / vernewet / vnd mit viel ‖ tröstlichen Experimenten gebessert / ‖ die zuuor heimlich gehalten / vnd an ‖ den tag nie gegeben sein / Anno ‖ 1529. ausgegangen. ‖ Auffs newe widerumb ‖ gedruckt / im Jhar ‖ M. D. LI. (Leipzig: Wolff Günter), 1551

Georgius Pictorius
Von der pe- ‖ stilentz. ‖ Ganz kurtzer bericht ob ‖ zů der ziet so die pestilentz regiert zů ‖ fliehent sey / wie auch iedes standes ‖ personen reich vnd arm / iung vnd ‖ alt so nit fliehen könend / sich / da- ‖ mit sy gesundt bleibē / halten sollēd... Basel: (Henrich Petri, April 1551)

Christophorus Stathmion (Christoph Mass)
Ein kůrtzer doch ‖ volkümlicher bericht / Wie man sich in ‖ sterbens leufften halten sol / jedermenig ‖ lichen zu gut / Beden denen so von Ampts ‖ oder Berůffs wegen nicht gebüret vnd ‖ auch denen so Armut vñ not hal- ‖ ben nicht müglich ist zuweichen / sehr ‖ nützs vnnd gantz tröstlich. Coburg: Ciriacus Schnauß Apotecker, 1551

Anon.
Infection Ordnung / der Stat Wienn. Vienna: Hanns Syngrienner, 1551

Georg Honderlagius
EYN NVTZ ‖ lich kurtz Vnd Trostliche ‖ vnderrichtunge Wie sich ein Jder Jn zeitt ‖ der Sorgfeltigenn Vnd Graussamen ‖ kranckheitt der Pestilentz preser- ‖ ueren vnnd Bewarenn sall: ‖ Auch ob Jemant darmit ‖ beladē: Wie em durch ‖ Rechtscaffene Ar- ‖ tznei erreth vnd ‖ geholffen ‖ Werden soll:... Dortmund: Philip Maurer, 1552

Martin Luther
Ob man fur ‖ dem sterben fliehen ‖ möge. ‖ Martinus Luther. Leipzig: Georg Hantzsch, 1552

Lorenz Misch
Für die Pestilentz ‖ Zweyer köstlichen Latwergen ‖ rechter Brauch. ‖ Eine des hoch vnd weithberümpten Herrn Doctor ‖ Mangolts seligen / weilandt der Stadt ‖ Costnitz Physici. ‖ Die Ander des Hochgelarthen Herrn D. Caspar ‖ Keglers / des eltern / seligen / die so er fur seinen besten ‖ schatz stets gehalten / vnd in den büchlein sonst nicht ‖ gefunden wirt / mit welchen von beiden ‖ Doctoribus zur zeit der Pestilentz ‖ an vielen glücklichen practicirt… Leipzig: Valentin Bapst, 1552

Johann Rympffer
Ein kůrtz regiment ‖ Wider die grausame plag der Pesti- ‖ lentz / Wie sich der Mensch vor solch ‖ er plage teglichs vber bewaren sol / vnd ‖ so ein Mensch damit begrieffen wirt / wie ‖ jme vnter xix (ehe dann ers be- ‖ schlaffenn hat) mit Gottes hilff durch vormitt- ‖ lůng der Ertzney one zweiffel geholffen ‖ mag werdenn. rc.‖ Durch Johañ Rympffer der ‖ Ertzney Doctor / allenn fromen Christen ‖ zu nůtz außgegangen / 1552. Coburg: (Ciriaco Schnauß Apotecker), 1552

Cyriacus Spangenberg
Historia von der flechtender Kranckheit der Pestilentz / wie die von anfang her umb vnser Sünde willen inn der Welt gewütet hat / Das ist. Alle schwinde Pestilentzische sterben derer inn Historien vnd Chroniken gedacht wird / zu sammen gebracht. 1552

St. Cyprianus
Ein sehr nützli- ‖ ches / tröstliches vnnd ‖ geistliches regiment wieder die Pe- ‖ stilentz / vnd sonst allerely gifftig vnd ‖ tödliche kranckheitten / allen ‖ fromen Christen frucht- ‖ barlich zulesen. ‖ Zusamen gebracht vnnd ‖ gepredigt durch den heiligen Bi- ‖ schoff vnd Merterer S. Cy- ‖ prianum. ca. 1552

Magnus Hundt
Wie sich ein ie- ‖ der in der zeit der Pesti- ‖ lentz mit den seinen in sei- ‖ ner Behausung halten soll / durch ‖ den Hochgelarten Herrn Magno ‖ Hund / der Ertzney Doctor von ‖ Magdeburg in vita sua ‖ Ordinirt. Magdeburg: Christian Rödinger, 1553

Caspar Kegler
Ein nutzlichs ‖ Vnd tröstlichs Regiment ‖ wider die Pestilentz / vnd giff- ‖ tig pestilentzisch Feber / die schweis ‖ sucht genant / Vnd sonst mancher ‖ ley gifftig vnd tödlich ‖ kranckheit ‖ Durch Casparum Kegler ‖ der Ertzney

Doctorn / zusammen ‖ gebracht / vernewet / vnnd mit viel ‖ tröstlichen Experimenten gebessert / die zu- ‖ uor heimlich gehalten / vnd an den tag ‖ nie gegeben sein / Anno. 1529. ‖ ausgegangen. Leipzig, 1553

Paracelsus
Ain kurtzer begrif zůerkhennen / Ob ‖ ain Mensch in disen geschwinden leüffen den gebre- ‖ chen der pestilentz hab oder nit. D. Philip- ‖ pum Theophrastium beschriben. Salzburg: Hans Bauman, [1553] Single-leaf broadside

Hieronymus Weller
Ein Recept / ‖ oder PRAESERVATIVE ‖ Wider die Pestilentz / Ge- ‖ stellet aus der Heili- ‖ gen Schrifft. (Lepizig: Jacob Berwald, 1553)

Jodocus Willich
Wie man sich ‖ vorhalten vnnd bewaren ‖ sol in den Heuseren / in wel- ‖ chen jemandes an der Pesti- ‖ letz gestorben ist / ‖ Auff das es nicht leicht- ‖ lich einreissen vnd weiter ‖ schaden thun möge. ‖ Item ein Radtschlag / vor ‖ die schwangere weiber vnd ‖ die kleine Kinder / Leipzig: Wolff Günter, 1553

Anon.
Regiment / ‖ Gestelt allain für die / so vn- ‖ uermeydenlich in Pestilentzischen lüfften ‖ verharren vnd beleiben müssen. Salzburg: Hans Bauman, 1553

Johann Dryander
Von dem ytzi- ‖ gen Sterben oder ‖ Pestilentz. ‖ D. Jo. Eychmans genant Dryan- ‖ der / Ordinarij zů Marpurg / ‖ bedenckens. ‖ Sampt D. Luthers / vnd D. Jodoci ‖ Wilichii zweyen Büchlin von ‖ dem Sterben. Marburg: Andreas Colben, 1554

Paracelsus
AIN seer nützlich- ‖ er vnnd bewerter Tractat / ‖ der Christlichen gemayn zů nutz vnd wolfart / auß ‖ deß weitberüembten vnd hocherfarnen Doctoris Philippj ‖ Theophrastj Paracelsj Bůch gezogen. Welches Er / von ‖ diser Khranckhait beschriben. Dariñ vil vnnd manicherlay ‖ Latwergen / Püllel / Wasser / Confect vnd Pulver / Sampt ‖ anndern̄ Preseruatifen erfunnden werden. Damit sich die ‖ Gesunden in disen geschwinden leüffen der regieren- ‖ den Pestilentz bewaren mügen: Auch / wie den ‖ Khrannckhen / so mit disem Gebrechen be- ‖ hafft / soll geholffen werden rc. Diß ‖ alles / nach ordnung jnnhalt vol- ‖ gunds Registers / jñ sechs ‖ Thayl: Vormals in ‖ Truckh nye kom ‖ men: ver- ‖ fertigt. Salzburg: Hans Bawman, 1554

Martin Paeonius
Ein Tröstlicher vn- ‖ terricht / wie sich ein jeder Mensch / ‖ Wenn die grewliche kranckheit der Pestilentz ‖ regieret / halten / vnd was für ordnung ‖ vñ Ertzney er gebrauchen soll. Allen ‖ Menschen / welchs standts die ‖ sein mögen zu sondern dienst ‖ vnd Christlicher war- ‖ nung / auffs trewlichste vnd mit ‖ gantzem fleiß ‖gestellet ‖ Durch ‖ Martinum Paeonium ‖ Diner des Herrn vnd pfarhern ‖ zu Büllenhouen. ‖ ANNO ‖ 1555. Regensburg: Hans Kohl, 1555

Johannes Crato
Ordnung der preserua- ‖ tion / wie man sich wider die erschreckliche ‖ seuche der pestilentz verwahren / auch rath wie die ‖ erkant vnd curiert werden sol / Mit einerlehr ‖ von dem vorsorg der geschwir / rc. Breslau: Crispinus Scharffenberg, 1555

Anon.
Bericht auff dis neben gestelt bilde / von wegen des Aderlassens / welche ‖ Ader / vnd wo man die selben / in zeit der Pestilentz / nach jedes malns der fürgefallen note ‖ gelegenhait / zulassen pflegt / vnd lassen soll. Regensburg: Hans Khol, 1555?

Anon.
Ein Kurz Regiment wie ‖ man sich zur zeit der Pes- ‖ tilentz halten sol. Regensburg: Hans Khol, ca. 1555

Johannes Gigas
Wieder die unchristli- ‖ che / vnerhörte furcht der Pestilentz ‖ halben / sonderlich inn der ‖ Schlesien. ‖ Item ‖ Woher diese sech fürnemlich jren ‖ vrsprung habe / Vnd warumb ‖ Christen nicht so verzagt ‖ sein sollen. Frankfurt/Oder: Johann Eichorn, 1556

Johan Ulenbeck
Ein schön vnd ‖ Christlich Gespreche / eines ‖ Jüngern vnd Meisters / wie ‖ sich ein jeder Christ in ster ‖ benden nöten / auch zur ‖ zeit der Pestilentz ‖ halten ‖ sol. ‖ Durch M. Johan Ulen- ‖ beck / Pfarherr vnd Hoffpre- ‖ diger zu Seeburgk / gestel- ‖ let. Vom selbigen auch ‖ ins Latein ge- ‖ bracht. ‖ Allen Christen / in diesen ‖ letzten vnd gefehrlichen zeiten ‖ zu lesen sehr tröstlich. [1556?]

Georg Pictorius
Von der Pestilentz. ‖ Notwendiger ‖ bericht was die pestilentz ‖ sey / ob die zů fliehen / vnd wie sich ‖ yedes stands personenn / reych / arm / jung ‖ vñ alt die nit fiehen könden damit sy der ‖ sucht ledig bleyben / halten sollen / vnnd ob ‖ einer angriffen wurd / wie er sich durch mit ‖ tel der artzney

ledigen möge / sampt an ‖ gehenckter ordnung so mit den ‖ beulen vnd blateren zů ‖ gebrauchen. (Mülhusen: Peter Schmid, 1558)

Matthias Boeham
Ain nutzliche / vnnd für ‖ den gemainen Mann / genůgsam ‖ gegründte vnderricht / wie sich dieser ‖ zeyt der Pestilentz halben ‖ zuhalten sey... (Augsburg: Phillip Ulhart), 1559

Tilemann Breul
Von der Pe- ‖ stilentz / vnd anderen ‖ Kranckheiten / kurtzer bericht aus Hei ‖ liger Schrifft gestellet / vnd in 22 cap. geteylet / ‖ Durch M. Tilemannum Breul Pfarr ‖ herrn zu Spangenberg. Frankfurt: Petro Brubach, 1559

Johann Hebenstreit
Aderlaß buch / ‖ Für XXX. Jahren aus- ‖ gangen / Darinne angezeigt wird / wie ‖ man die Aderlasse / Ventosen / oder Köpffe / recht / in ‖ der noth / die Gesundheit zu erhalten / ‖ gebrauchen sol. ‖ Jetzt wider auffs new vbersehen / ge- ‖ bessert / vnd gemehrt / Sampt einem Bericht / Wie ‖ sich ein jeder Mensch / für / in / vnd nach der Ader- ‖ lasse / Auch zu Pestilentz zeiten / halten sol... M.D.LIX. (Erfurt: Georg Bawman), 1559

Sebald Nebelius
Ein kurtz ge- ‖ mein vnderricht / wie ‖ man sich zur zeit der Pestilentz hal- ‖ den sol / mit einem kleinen anhang der zufelle / ‖ so sich ynn sterbs leufften / nach vñ vor pfle- ‖ gen zu ereugen. An den Erbarn Radt vñ ‖ gantze gemein Churfürstlicher Stad ‖ Aldenburgk / durch Magistrum ‖ Sebaldum Nebelium Bür- ‖ ger daselbst / Zu samen ‖ gebracht. 1559

Anon.
Einfeltige doch hoch- ‖ nutzliche Hausartzney / wider die Erschrockh- ‖ lich Kranckheit der Pestilentz / die Ime ein yeder ‖ Hausßvatter oder haußmutter selbst machen / ‖ oder in der Apoteckhen umb gering gelt machẽ ‖ lassen Gemeiner Burgerschafft zu Amberg zu ‖ gutem / aus ettlicher gelerter Doctorn der ‖ Artzney schrifften / zusamen gezogen. (Amberg: Wolf Gulden), 1560

Matthias Boeham
Ain anzaigung ainer gegründte / Warhaffte / und Erfarne Ertzney vnd Cur / Etlich vnd dreissig Jar her / von meinem Herr ‖ Vatter D. Johann Vogt / der loblichen statt Vlm bestellter Brechen Doctor / in vilen löblichen Stetten gebraucht und erfaren ... (Ulm: 1560?)

Ulrich Wolfhart
Ain kurtzer bericht von D. Vlrich Wolfhart ‖ zů Memmingen / wie man sich vor der erschröcklichen kranckhait ‖ des gebrechens der Pestilentz

preseruiern vnd bewaren mög / Auch ‖ wann ains darmit angriffen / wie es sich halten / vnd die bewärten ‖ kostlichen stuck / dar zů dienstlich / so er auf das best in seiner Apotek / ‖ so die Alt genennt wirdt / hat lassen zůrichten / gebrauchen / Gott zů ‖ lob vnd ehr / gemainer statt Memmingen / auch mänigklich zů nutz ‖ vnd wolfart. (Augsburg: Philipp Ulhart), [ca. 1560]

Paracelsus
Von der Pestilentz. ‖ Ein seer Nutzlichs / ‖ vnnd bewertes Büchlein der ‖ Christlichen gemein zu nutz vnd wolfart / auß des ‖ weitberümbten vnd hocherfarnen Doctoris Phi- ‖ lippj Theophrastij Peracelsi Buch so er von diser ‖ kranckheit beschriben / gezogen den gesunden / ‖ sich in den geschwinden leüffen der regiren ‖ den Pestilentz / zuuerwaren / auch den ‖ krancken so mit disem brechen be- ‖ hafft / zur hilff vnd retrung / ‖ sonderlich nutz vnd ‖ dienstlich. (Straubing: Hans Burger), 1561

Anon.
Die weil der beschwerlich seuch der ‖ Pestilentz sich an vil orten ereügt / vnd nit minder alhie zu Nürn- ‖ berg zu regiren auch eingebrochen / hat ein Erber Rathe guter ‖ mainung fürgenomen… [Nuremberg?, 1561?]

Johann Lonaeus Boscium (Bosch)
Rathschlag. ‖ Wie man sich zů disen gefährlichen zei- ‖ ten / vor der Pestilentz hütten ‖ Vnd ‖ Wie dieselbig so sie eingerissen / wider zů ‖ vertreiben / vnd zů curieren sey. Ingolstadt: Alexander and Samuel Weyssenhorn, 1562

Balthasar Conradinus
Kurtze vnd nutze gegründte vnder- ‖ richt / für den gemainen Mañ / wie er ‖ sich in den geferlichē leüffen der Pesti- ‖ lentz halten sol / auff das fleissigst ‖ zůsamen getragē / Durch ‖ D. Balthasarem ‖ Conradinum ‖ Medi- ‖ cum zů Schwatz. ‖ M. D. LXII. Innsbruck: Ruprecht Höller, 1562

Veit Dietrich
Der XCI. Psalm. ‖ Wie ein Christ ‖ in Sterbßleufften sich ‖ trösten soll. Nuremberg: Valentin Newber, 1562

Johann Hebenstreidt
Regiment ‖ Pestilentzischer giff- ‖ tiger Fieber / so jetzundt in Düringen / auch vmb ‖ ligenden örthern / die Menschen plötzlich vber- ‖ fallen / Wie sich allerley Stende / jung vnd alt / Mañ vnd ‖ Weib / schwanger Weiber / Witfrawen / Jungfrawen / ‖ vnd Kinder / dafür bewa- ‖ ren sollen. (Erfurt: Georgium Bawman), 1562

Mathias Kornax
Rathschlag wie man ‖ mit der hülff Gottes sich vor der ‖ Infection hüten vnd er- ‖ wehren soll. Ingolstat: Alexander und Samuel Weissenhorn, 1562

Georg Phaedro
GE. PHAEDRONIS ‖ RHODOCHAEI MEDICI HA- ‖ lopyrgice siue Iatrochemica pe- ‖ stis epidemicae curatio. ‖ Oder ‖ Warhaffte Cur der erschröcklichen sucht ‖ der Pestilentz / an den Hochwürdigsten in Gott ‖ Fürsten vnd Herrn Johann ‖ Jacob Ertzbischoff zů ‖ Saltzburg rc. Ingolstat, 1562

Anon.
Ains Erbern Raths der ‖ Stadt Nürmberg / ver- ‖ newete Gesetz und Ord- ‖ nung / in gegenwer- ‖ tigen sterbsleufften ‖ diß M.D.LXII. ‖ Jars auffge- ‖ richt. (1562)

Anon.
Einfeltige doch hoch- ‖ nutzliche Hausartzeney / wider die Erschrockh- ‖ lich Kranckheit der Pestilentz / die Jme ein yeder ‖ Haußvatter oder haußmutter selbstmachen / ‖ oder in der Apoteckhen vmb gering gelt machē ‖ lassen mag Gemeiner Burgerschafft zu Am- ‖ berg zu gutem / aus etlicher gelerter Doctorn der ‖ Artzney schrifften / zusamen gezogen. (Amberg: Wolfgang Guldemundt, 1562)

Anon.
Ein kurtz Regiment / ‖ wie man sich in zeit Regierender ‖ Pestilentz halten soll. ‖ Durch die Hochgelerten vnd erfarnen der ‖ Ertzney Doctores / zusammen gefast ‖ vnd gebessert. / Anno 1562. Nuremberg: Valentin Geyßler, 1562

Anon.
Ein kurtz Regiment / ‖ Wie man sich zur zeit ‖ der Pestilentz hal- ‖ ten sol. Regensburg: Heinrich Geisler, 1562

Anon.
Ein kurtzes / doch ‖ sehr nutzliches Regiment / ‖ Wie sich zun zeyten der Pesti- ‖ lentz / zuhalten sey. ‖ Durch etliche Liebha- ‖ ber der Artzney / mänigklichem ‖ zů gůttem gestellt. ‖ M. D. LXii. [Landshut?]: 1562

Ambrosius Jung
Ain nutzliche trostliche / vñ ‖ kurtze vndterrichtung / wie ‖ man sich in den schwären ‖ leüffen der Pestilentz hal- ‖ ten solle / Durch Ambro- ‖ sium Jungen / der Artznej ‖ Doctor zů Augsburg / dē ‖ gemainen Mann zůhilff ‖ vñ gůtem / der nit andern ‖ beystanddt hat / ‖ verordnet. Innsbruck: Ruprecht Höller, [ca. 1562]

Michael Ostendorfer
Wie ein jeglicher Haußvater vnd Haußmutter in disen ‖ jetzigen / letzten / aller gefehrligsten / vnd geschwinden Zeitten / vnd grawsamer straffe der ‖ Pestilentz / sich selbs / jre Kinger vnd Hausgesinde / zum Gebet / vnd

Christlicher war- ‖ hafftiger Busse / vermahnen sollen. Regensburg: Heinrich Geißler, [ca. 1562] Single-leaf broadside

Johannes Lonaeus Bosch
Rathschlag ‖ Wie man sich zů disen gefährlichen zei- ‖ ten / vor der Pestilentz hütten ‖ Vnd ‖ Wie dieselbig so sie eingerissen / wider zů ‖ vertreiben / vnd zů curieren sey. Ingolstatt: Alexander and Samuel Weyssenhorn, 1563

Johann Hebenstreit
Regiment. ‖ Pestilentzischer ‖ gifftiger Fieber / so jetzund ‖ in Düringen / auch vmbligen- ‖ den örthern / die Menschē plötzlich vberfallen / Wie sich allerley Stand / Jund vnnd Alt / Mann vnd ‖ Weyb / schwanger Weyber / Witfrawen / ‖ Jungkfrawen / vnd Kinder / ‖ dafür bewaren sollen... Augsburg: Matteum Francken, 1563

Ambrosius Jung
Ain nutzliche trostliche ‖ vnd kurtze vnnderrichtung / wie man sich in di- ‖ sen schweren leüffen der Pestilentz halten solle / ‖ durch Ambrosium Junngen / der Artzney ‖ Doctor zů Augsburg / dem gemainen ‖ mann zů hilff vnd gůtem / der nit ‖ anndern beystand hat / ‖ verordnet. (Augsburg: Valentin Ottmar), 1563

Paracelsus
Von der Pestilentz. ‖ Ein seer Nutzlichs / ‖ vnnd bewertes Büchlein der ‖ Christlichen gemein zu nutz vnd wolfart / auß des ‖ weitberümbten vnd hocherfarnen Doctoris Phi- ‖ lippj Theophrastij Peracelsy Buch so er von diser ‖ kranckheit beschriben / gezogen den gesunden / ‖ sich in den gschwinden leüffen der regiren- ‖ den Pestilentz / zuuerwaren / auch den ‖ krancken so mit disem brechen be- ‖ hafft / zur hilff vnd rettung / ‖ sonderlich nutz vnd ‖ dienstlich. Straubing: Hans Burger, 1563

Valentin Trutiger
Regiment. ‖ Wider die Pe- ‖ stilentz in dieser gefehrlich- ‖ ne zeit / wie sich die gemeine bür- ‖ gerschafft der löblichen vnd Chur- ‖ fürstlichen / beider Art / vnd New- ‖ enstadt Brandbenburg / vnd an- ‖ dere etc. in solcher zeit ‖ verhalten sollen. Wittenberg: Veit Creutzer, 1563

Johann Wonecker
Regiment ‖ vnd Ordnung wider die ‖ schwere sucht der Pestilentz / nit ‖ allein wie man sich daruor ‖ hüten / sonder auch wie man dieselbi ‖ gen Curieren sol / auffs kürtzest ver- ‖ fast vnd gestelt / durch Johannem ‖ Woneckern der Artzney Doctorn / ‖ vnd Ordinarium Professo- ‖ rem zu Meyntz. Mainz: Franciscus Behem, 1563

Anon.
Von der Pestilentz. ‖ Kurtzer nütz ‖ licher vnd einfältiger be- ‖ richt / wie sich ein jeder zu zeit der re- ‖ gierenden Pestilentz verhüten ‖ vnd halten soll. ‖ Item / Wie die jhenigen ‖ sollen gehalten werden / welche mit ‖ solcher plag angriffen ‖ worden. ‖ Jetzo New verteutscht. (Frankfurt: Christian Ege. Erben), 1563

Christoff, Duke of Württemberg
Ein sehr gewisse ‖ vnnd vilbewerte Artzney ‖ für den grausamen bresten der yetz ‖ schwälbenden Pestilentz / meiglich vnd sonder- ‖ lich aber den Armen vnnd veruerstendi- ‖ gen gmeinen Volck im fürstenthumb ‖ Württemberg / zů nutz vnnd ‖ trost publiciert vnd ‖ außgangen. Tübingen: Ulrich Morharts, 1564

Joachim Cirenberger
Wider alle Pestilen- ‖ tzische geschwinde vnd gifftige Fieber / ‖ Ein gründtlicher volkömlicher Bericht / ‖ raht vnd hülffe vor Jdermenniglich / ‖ Was standts / geschlechts oder alter ‖ die sein / mit sonderm fleis ‖ trewlich an tag ‖ gegeben / (Leipzig: Rhambaw), 1564

Balthasar Conradinus
Kurtzer / doch ay- ‖ gentlicher vnd gegründter vn- ‖ terricht / Regiment vnd ordnung / wie ‖ man sich inn zeiten der Pestilentzischen leuffen ver- ‖ halten / praeseruieren oder bewaren / vnd wie man solche ai- ‖gentlich erkennen soll: Auch wie die selbige / so man ‖ damit behafft / durch hülff des Allmächtigen ‖ Gottes / vnd durch die darzů von Gott verordnete ‖ mittel der Artzney abgewendet werden ‖ mag: für den gemeynen ‖ Mann gestelt / Augsburg: Mattheus Franken, 1564

Achilles Pirmineus Gasser
Vnterricht / Wider ‖ die Pestilentz / So jtzt an allen ‖ örtern einreisset / Gestellet / ‖ Durch ‖ Den Herrn D. Achillem Pirmineum Gassarum Lindoen- ‖ sem / der Stad Augsburg ‖ Phisicum. [Augsburg?], 1564

Johann Gwynther von Andernach
Bericht / Regiment ‖ vnd Ordnung / wie bei disen sterben- ‖ den leüffen / die Pestilentz vnnd Pestilentzische Fie- ‖ ber zůerkennen / wes sich inn solliche zeitten zůhal- ‖ ten / auch wie man sich vor diser kranckheyt be- ‖ waren soll / vnd mit was Artzney die- ‖ selb zů curieren vnd zů- ‖ heylen seye. (Strassburg: Josiam Rihel, 15 January), 1564

Johann Gwynther von Andernach (Johannes Guinterius)
Bericht vnnd Ord- ‖ nung / in disen sterbenden leüf- ‖ fen der Pestilentz / auß befelch ei- ‖ nes Ersamen Rahts der ‖ Statt Straßburg. (Straßburg: Josiam Rihel), 1564

Johann Hebenstreit
Artzney Schutz: ‖ Wie der Newen jetztregierenden erschrecklichen / gifftigen ‖ gen / vnd tödtlichen Pestilentz / durch ein ordentlich Regiment / al- ‖ lerley Samen / Blumen / Kreutter / Wurtzeln / Früchte / Wasser Oel / etc. zubegeg- ‖ nen / Damit allerley Stende der Menschen / sich vermittelst Göttliches ‖ Segens / durch solcher natürlicher mittel hülffe / mö- ‖ gen errettet werden. (Erfurt: Georg Bawman, 1564)

Ludwig Lavater
Von der Pe- ‖ stilentz ‖ Zwo predginen / die ein ‖ vom vrsprung der Pestilentz / wo- ‖ har die sye / item warumb sy regier- ‖ re / vnnd wie man sich darinen hal- ‖ ten sölle: Die ander deß säligen Bischoffs vnd martyrers Cypria- ‖ ni von jm zů Carhtago / als auch ‖ ein grosser sterbend was / gethan / ‖ zů vnser zyt gantz notwändig vnd ‖ trostlich zeläsen / beschriben durch ‖ Ludwigen Lafater die- ‖ nern der kilchen zů ‖ Zürych. Zürich: Christoffel Froschower, 1564

Sebastian Mayr
Ein newer nutzli- ‖ cher / vnd grundtlicher Tra- ‖ ctat / von der Pestilentz / Item we- ‖ sen / vrsachen / fürsehung ‖ und Cur. ‖ Darinn auch ‖ vil schädlicher jrthumb / wölche in der gemeinen ‖ Cur im schwanck gehn / entdeckt vnd wi- ‖ derlegt werden / der massen ‖ bißher nie gesche- ‖ hen ist. Tübingen: (Ulrich Morharts), 1564

Burckhard Mithobius
Wie man sich für ‖ der hefftigen vnd tödlichen ‖ seuche der Pestilentz bewaren soll / Vnd so ‖ einer damit angegriffen / oder auch mit andern zůfelliger ‖ kranckheiten behafft / mit was Artzney dem zůhelffen. ‖ Beyde Reichen vnd Armen auß langer erfarung vnnd ‖ den fürtrefflichen Ertzten zůsamen getragen. ‖ jetzung von neuwem übersähen / vnd ‖ gebessert. Marpurg: Andreas Kolben, 1564

Christoph Ostwald
Nutzlicher vnd ‖ kurtzer Bericht / einem jeden ‖ in der Zeit der Pestilentz sehr von ‖ nöten zuwissen / mit anzeigung et- ‖ licher stuck / welche bey vi- ‖ len in grosser achtung ‖ gehalten seind ‖ worden. ‖ Jetzt durch Christopho- ‖ rum Ostwald / der Freyen Kün ‖ ste vnnd Artzney Doctor zů Co- ‖ nstentz / dem gemainen Mann ‖ zů trost / nutz und wol- ‖ fart beschriben. Dilingen: Sebald Mayer, 1564

Paracelsus
Zwey Bücher ‖ Theophrasti ‖ Paracelsi des erfar- ‖ nesten Artzets / von der ‖ Pestilentz vnd ihren ‖ zůfällen. ‖ Durch den Edlen vnd ‖ Hochgelerten Adamen von ‖ Bodenstein / in Druck ‖ verfertiget. (Strasburg: Paulo Messerschmidt), 1564

Jacob Theodorus Tabermontanus
Gewisse vnnd ‖ erfahren Practick / Wie ‖ man sich mit Göttlicher hülff / ‖ vor der Pestilentz hüten vnd bewaren / ‖ vnnd so einer damit behafft / wie demselben ‖ zuhelffen. Es seyen alte oder junge / arme ‖ oder reiche leuth. Gepracticiert vnd ‖ beschrieben in Anno 1551. ‖ 52. vnd nachfolgende ‖ Jar... (Heidelberg: Johann Mayer), 1564

Johannes Vogt
Ein nutzliche anzei- ‖ gung gebrauchter Artzneyen / von ge- ‖ lerten Doctoribus in der hohen Not der Pestilentz / ‖ wie die Exempla außweisen / auch yetzunder zů Straß- ‖ burg in der hohen Not in Brauch geordnet: Bey jnen ‖ Diastimios vnd precipitatis cum Auro genannt / die ‖ beide fast einer Würckung / Ich aber habs mein Au- ‖ rum vitae / auch Confectionem vitae ettlich vnd dreis- ‖ sig Jar in meinen Schrifften genannt vnd gebraucht: ‖ Die Ertzney würt gebraucht wider allerley verborgne ‖ vnbekannte / wie sie genannt mügen werden / Kranck- ‖ heitten... Ulm: (Oßwald Gruppenbacher), 1564

Leonhard Werner
Der Geistliche Bisemknopff ‖ Wider die Er- ‖ schröcklichen Plag unnd ‖ Straff der Pestilentz. Woher ‖ auch solche Plag / sampt andern ‖ Kranck- ‖ heyten und Leiblichen schmerzen jhren ur- ‖ sprung haben / und was für hulffliche mit ‖ tel / wege und Artzney (zu abwendung sol- ‖ cher straffen)... Frankfurt, 1564

Jodocus Willich
Von der Pestilentz ‖ ein nützlich Regiment. ‖ Erstlich wie man sich in einer Stat für ‖ der Pestilentz behüten sol vnd möchte. ‖ Item / wie man sich verhalten sol in heusern / ‖ in welchen jemands gestorben ist / auff das es nicht leichtlich weiter schaden thu. ‖ Item / wie man den helffen sol / welche mit der ‖ Pestilentz ischen gifft begriffen sind. ‖ Item / Ein Radtschlag vor schwangere wei- ‖ ber vnd kleine Kindlein. Frankfurt/Oder: Johann Eichorn, 1564

Anon.
Ein Kurtzer ‖ Bericht / wie sich der gemeine ‖ Man in Zeiten der Pesti- ‖ lentz halten soll. ‖ Durch des Durchleuchtigen vnd ‖ Hochgebornen Fürsten vnd Herrn / Herrn ‖ Philipsen / Landgrauen zu Hessen / Grauen ‖ zu Catzenellnbogen ‖ Dietz / Zigenhain ‖ vnd Nidda etc. Medicos be- ‖ ratschlagt vnd gestellt. 1564

Heimeran (Hemeranus) Bulderkar (and Lucas Gercke)
Kurzer Nützlicher vnd ‖ Nötiger Bericht / wie man sich jtziger zeit ‖ der Pestilentz verhalten / vnd die Ertzney / so einem ‖ Erbarn Rathe in der

Altenstadt Magde- ‖ burgk / durch jre Medicos veror- ‖ denet ist / gebrauchen ‖ sol. Magdeburg: Joachim Walden, 1565

Achilles Pirmineus Gasser
Vnterricht / Wieder die ‖ Pestilentz / So jtzt an allen ör- ‖ tern einreisset / Gestellet / ... 1565

Caspar Kegeler
Ein nützliches ‖ vnd tröstliches Regiment / ‖ wider die Pestilentz / vnd gifftig ‖ pestilentzisch Fieber / die Schweissucht ‖ genant / Vnd sonst mancherley ‖ gifftige vnd tödliche ‖ Kranckheit. (Eisleben): Andreas Petri, 1565

Lorenz Misch
Eine Tröstliche / be- ‖ werte Kunst / in sterbens nöten / wie- ‖ der die Pestilentz / die alte güldene Pillen genant / ‖ Verordtnet / durch den künstreichen / Meister Lorentz ‖ Misch / inn der Churfürstlichen Stadt Leipzig / ‖ Wundt vnd Schneidtartzt / jetzo in der Pe- ‖ terstras / Wonhafftig da- ‖ selbst zu finden. 1565

Simon Musaeus
Kurtze Ausle- ‖ gunge des ein vnd neun- ‖ tzigsten Psalms / vnd Simeons ‖ Gesangs / Zu trost vnd vnter- ‖ richt / wider die geschwin- ‖ de seuche der Pe- ‖ stilentz. 1565

Ernst Reuchlin
Zwey kurtze Büchlein / ‖ Aus welchen ieder- ‖ menniglich Arm vnd Reich lernen ‖ kan / wie er sich jtziger zeit in der Schrecklichen ‖ straffe der Pestilentz vorhalten sol. Dem durch- ‖ leuchtigsten / Hochgebornen / Fürsten vnd ‖ Herrn / Herrn Joachim des Namens dem ‖ andern / Churfürsten zu Brandenburg / ‖ etc. Zu gehorsamer vnd vnderthe- ‖ nigster dienstbarkeit... Madgeburg: Andreas Ghene, 1565

Nicolaus Selnecker
Christlicher bericht / ‖ Wie sich ein jeder Christ / inn ‖ Sterbensleufften trösten vnnd ‖ halten soll. ‖ Der XCI. Psalm ausgelegt / Wer ‖ vnter dem Schirm des höchsten sitzt. ‖ Von Sterbsleufften / Ein trost ge- ‖ schriben an einem guten Freundt. ‖ Von Viererley losem Gesinde in Sterbsleufften. ‖ Kurtze Kinder Fragstůcke von der ‖ Pestilentz / aus dem 91. Psalm Dauids / ‖ sampt schönen tröstlichen Gebetlein. (Leipzig: Jacob Berwaldt), 1565

Jodocus Willich
Von der Pestilentz ‖ ein nützlich Regiment ‖ Erstlich wie man sich in einer Stad für ‖ der Pestilentz behüten sol vnd möchte... Frankfurt/Oder: Johann Eichorn, 1565

Jobus Fincelius
Von der Pestilentz. ‖ CVRA PRAESERVATIVA. ‖ Das ist / Wie man sich vor der Pe- ‖ stilentz bewaren sol. ‖ CVRA CVRATIVA. ‖ Das ist / Wie man sich die Pesti- ‖ letnzt heilen sol. 1566

Matthaeus Flaccus
Ein Erinnerung: ‖ was die Oberkeit zur ‖ Pestilentz zeit bestellen / vnd wie ‖ sich menniglich fur solcher grausamer Seuch pre- ‖ seruirn / auch aus rechtem grund der Ertzney cu- ‖ rirn sol / der gantzen Marck zu Brandeburg / ‖ Sonderlich aber beiden Stedten / ‖ Berlin und Cöln an der Sprew ‖ zu nutz gestellt / Wittenberg: Hans Lufft, 1566

Caspar Kegeler
Ein Nützliches vnd ‖ Tröstlichs Regiment wider die Pesti- ‖ lentz / vnd gifftig Pestilentzisch Feber / ‖ die Schweissucht genant / Vnd sonst ‖ mancherley gifftige vnd todt- ‖ liche Kranckheit. Leipzig: Johan Rhambaw, 1566

Johann Neeffen
Ein kurtzer Bericht: ‖ Wie man sich in denen jtzo vorstehen- ‖ den Sterbensleufften / mit der Praeseruation ‖ oder vorwahrungen / Dornach auch der ‖ Curation der Pestilentz / vnd etzlicher ‖ jrer accidentien / oder zufellen / ‖ verhalten sol. ‖ Zu dienste den Einwohnern der ‖ Churfürstlichen Stadt Dreßden / ‖ vnd andern / so Berichtes not- ‖ türfftig / zusammen ‖ getragen / (Dresden: Matthes Stöckel), 1566

Johannes Schröter
Kurtzer einfelti- ‖ ger / doch gründtlicher Be- ‖ richt / Wie man durch Gottes ‖ gnedige hülff vnd gute ordnung / ‖ in diesen schweren Leufften der ‖ Pestilentz / sich halten vnd bewa- ‖ ren / Auch so jemand damit be- ‖ fleckt / wie er damit gebaren ‖ sol / Menniglich zu hülf- ‖ fe vnd gutem ge- ‖ stellet. Jena: Donatum Richtzenhayn, 1566

Johannes Schröter
Johannis Schröteri ‖ DOCTORIS ‖ Einfeltiger / Doch ‖ Gründtlicher Bericht vnd Ratschlag / ‖ Wie man durch Gottes gnedige hülffe und gute ‖ Ordnung / in diesen schweren Leufften der Pesti- ‖ lentz / sich halten und bewaren / Auch so jemandt ‖ damit befleckt / wie er damit gebaren sol. ‖ Menniglichen zu trost / hülffe ‖ vnd gutem gestellet. Leipzig: Johan. Rhambaw, 1566

Eusebius Wildeck
Kurtzer vnd einfelti- ‖ ger Bericht / doch aus rechtem grun- ‖ de der Artzney / Wie man sich für der schreck- ‖ lichen Seuche der Pestilentz bewaren / ‖ vnd sie Curiren sol. Leipzig: Johan Rhambaw, 1566

Johann Winter
Bericht / Re- ‖ giment 1566 v-nnd Ordnung ‖ wie bei disen sterbenden leüffen ‖ die Pestilentz vnd Pestilentzische Fieber zů- ‖ erkennen / wes sich inn sollichen zeitten zů- ‖ halten / auch wie man sich vor diser kranck- ‖ heit bewaren soll / vnd mit was Artz- ‖ ney die selb zů curieren vnd ‖ zůheylen seye. (Strasburg: Josiam Rihel), 1566

Anon.
Ein Kurtzer ‖ Bericht / wie sich der ge- ‖ meine Man in zeiten der ‖ Pestilentz halten sol. ‖ Durch des Durchleuch- ‖ tigen vnd Hochgebornen Für- ‖ sten vnd Herrn / Herrn Philipsen / Lan- ‖ grauen zu Hessen / Grauen zu Catzen- ‖ ellnbogen / Dietz / Ziegenhain vnd ‖ Nidda / etc. Medicos berath- ‖ schagt vnd gestellt. ‖ M. D. LXVI. 1566.

Anon.
Kurtzer be- ‖ richt: wes sich ‖ der Gemeine Man zu ‖ Wittemberg in zeit vorstehender ‖ gefahr der Pestilentz zuuerhal- ‖ ten / durch den Medicum Physi- ‖ cum daselbst gestelt / vnd von ‖ einem Erbarn Rath ‖ Publiciret. Wittenberg: Hans Lufft, 1566

Philip Imsser
Klein Pestilentzbüchlin / ‖ Für die armen ‖ Handwercks vñ Baurs ‖ Leut / wölche den Artzten vnnd ‖ Apotecken zů weit gesessen / oder ‖ sich Armůt halben schlech- ‖ ter ding behelffen ‖ müssen. ‖ In gegenwertiger Gefahrli- ‖ cheit auffs kürtzest beschriben. Tübingen, 1567

Paracelsus
MEDICI LIBELLI, ‖ Des hocherfarnesten ‖ Herrn THEOPHRASTI PARACEL- ‖ SI, beyder Artzeney Doctoris / vorhin ‖ niemals in Truck aus- ‖ gangen. Cöln: Gerhart Vierendunck (in verlegung Arnoldt Birckmans Erben), 1567

Wilhelmus Triphyllodaenus
GIFFTIAGER, ‖ Das ist: ‖ Von vrsach / ‖ reynigung / bewahrung ‖ vnd Cur Pestilentzischer lufft / fürne- ‖ mer Artzten rath vnd bedencken / mit ange- ‖ hencktem vnterschied der Schüler Para- ‖ celsi vnd Galeni / in der Cur gemel- ‖ ter Kranckheyt. Franckfurt: (Martin Lechler in verlegung Sigmund Feyrabends and Simon Hüters), 1567

Christoph Vischer and Ortolphum Maroldt
Kurtzer vnter- ‖ richt / Wie man sich mit ‖ Gottes hülffe vor der Pestilentzi- ‖ schen vergifftung bewaren / Vnd auch ‖ den behafften Personen wider ‖ helffen solle. (Schmalkalden: Michel Schmuck), 1567

Johann Kentmann
Ein kurtz / nütz / vnd sehr tröstlich Regiment / wie man sich ‖ mit der hülffe Gottes / vor der schwinden vnd giff- ‖ tigen Seuch der Pestilentz behüten / vnd so jemand damit ‖ angegriffen würde / was mittel man daruor brauchen ‖ sol... Wittenberg: Peter Seitz, 1568

Johann Spremberg
Kurtzer Bericht / ‖ Von Zweyerley Ge- ‖ schlecht der Pestilentischen ‖ Febern. Emes / ‖ Das sich mit Beulen / ‖ Mackeln oder Geschwieren erzeigte ‖ Das Ander / so man die Schweiß- ‖ sucht nennet... Breslau: (Crispinus Scharffenberg), 1568

Anon.
Der Kayserlichen ‖ Stadt Breßlaw / ‖ new auffgerichte ‖ Infection Or- ‖ dnung. (Breslau: Crispinus Scharffenberg), 1568

Zacharias Kempe
Oration vnd Predig / ‖ Welche in die- ‖ sem geschwinden sterben / ‖ auff dem newen Gottesacker / ‖ zu Ellinhausen gehalten. ‖ Darinnen gemelt wird / was die ‖ Pestilentz sey / vnnd warumb sie komme / ‖ Woher / oder von wem sie vber die Menschen ‖ gerathe / Vnd endtliche vrsachen / wie ‖ man diser plag auß dem land ‖ loß werde. Frankfurt am Mayn: (Thomam Rebart in verlegung Simon Hutters), 1569

Anon.
Wie man sich zu zeit- ‖ ten der Pestilentz fürsehen vnd ‖ erhalten mög. Vienna: Caspar Stainhofer, 1569

Leonhart Werner
BVLLA CHRISTIANA, ‖ Das ist / ‖ Der Geistliche ‖ Bysemknopff / wider die Ge- ‖ schwinde / Schreckliche Plage vnd ‖ Straff der Pestilentz / Woher auch solche ‖ Plage / sampt anderen Kranckheiten vnnd Leiblichen ‖ Schmertzen jren Vrsprung haben / Vnd was für hülffli- ‖ che mittel / Wege vnd Artzney / Zu abwendung solcher ‖ Straffen / sich die guthertzigen Christen haben zugebrau- ‖ chen / vnd zu getrösten / für den armen Wehestandt / vnder ‖ welchen die Armen / hochbetrübten Eheleut / in diesen ‖ Sterbens leufften müssen schwerlich seufftzen / ‖ und offtermals Heulen und Weinen / ‖ Mit sampt gar schönen Tröst- ‖ lichen vnd nützlichen ‖ Gebättlin. Frankfurt: [?], 1571

Georgius Phaedro
GEORGII PHAE- ‖ DRONIS RHODOCHAEI ‖ MEDICI HALOPYRGICE ‖ SIVE IATROCHEMICA ‖ pestis epidemicae cu- ‖ ratio. ‖ Oder ‖ Warhaffte Cur der erschrockenlichen ‖ sücht der pestilentz an den Hochwirdigen in ‖ Gott Fürsten vnnd Herren / Herrn ‖ Johan Jacob Ertzbishof- ‖ fen zû Saltzburg. (Basel, 1571)

Theobald Fettich
Ordnung ‖ Vnd Regiment / wie ‖ man sich vor der scharpffen vnd giff- ‖ tigen kranckheit der Pestilentz bewaren ‖ sol: Auch wie denen / so dar- ‖ mit begriffen / zuhelf‖ fen sey. ‖ Sampt den natürlichen vrsachen ‖ des Englischen Schwaiß. München: (Adam Berg), 1572

Adam Lonitzer
Ordnung ‖ Für die Pe- ‖ stilentz. ‖ I. PRAESERVATIVA. ‖ Wie sich ein jeder in zeit Regierender Pe- ‖ stilentz halten / vnd sich darfür bewaren soll. ‖ II. CVRATIVA. ‖ Von Cur der Pestilentz / vnnd von man- ‖ cherley zufallen / so sich darbei zutragen. ‖ III. ANTIDOTARIVM. ‖ Beschreibung der Artzneien vnd für- ‖ nemen Compositionen etc. (Frankfurt: Christian Egenolff), 1572

Adolph Occo
Was die Pestilentz an jr selbs ‖ sey / mit jren vrsachen vnd Ertzneyen / Den Er- ‖ samen vnd Weysen Burgermaister vnd Rathe / auch gantzer ‖ gemain der statt Augspurg / durch die bestelten Doctores da- ‖ selbst / zů nutz vnd gůt gemacht vnd beschriben. [Augsburg?]: (Philipp Ulhart), [1572?]

Anon.
Anzaig vnd bericht der Statt Nürmberg verodenten vnnd ge- ‖ schwornen Doctorn der Artzney / die jetztregierende ‖ geuerliche Haubtkranckheit belangend / woher die ‖ selbig vermutlich entspringt / vnd wie sich darinnen / ‖ auch sonst zuuerkomung derselben zuhalten sey / ‖ auß beufelch eines Erbern Raths daselbst / ‖ jrer Burgerschafft vnd Vnterthanen ‖ zu gutem gestelt / im Jar ‖ M.D. LXXII. Nuremberg: Dieterich Gerlatz, 1572

Caspar Macer
Drey kurtze bittpredig. ‖ I. ‖ Von der grossen Theu- ‖ rung und hungers noth. ‖ II. ‖ Von der grausamen Kranckheit vnd ‖ plag der Pestilentz / zur zeit des sterbens läufft. ‖ III. ‖ Vom Krieg vnd Blutvergiessen / mit ‖ angehengter starcker gegenwehr. Munich: Adam Berg, 1572

Christoff Vischer
Christliche ‖ Erklerung des Ein ‖ vnd neutzigsten Psal- ‖ men / in 21. Predigten ver- ‖ fasset / Deren man sich in Ster- ‖ bens leufften oder auch sonst bey ‖ Christlichen Begrebnissen ‖ nutzlichen gebrau- ‖ chen mag. (Schmalkalden: Michel Schmuck), 1572

Anon.
DIeweil [sic] der almechtig Got / kurtz verschiner zeit / dise Stat… [1572]

Jacob Theodorus (Tabernomontanus)
Kurtzer vnder- ‖ richt vnd Rahtschlag / wie ‖ man dem jetzigen Pestilentzischē ‖ gifftigen vnd hitzigen Feber / in welchem ‖ groß Hauptwehthumb / Breün vnd andere ‖ gefärliche zufäll mit vnderlauffen / begeg ‖ nen vnd vorkommen

/ auch wie man ‖ das so jetzt vorhanden abwen- ‖ den vnd Curieren soll. Heidelberg: Johann Maier (in Verlegung Matthei Harnisch), (1573)

Georg Fraunberger
Ain Gaistliches ‖ Regiment / fürzukommen vñ ‖ zü vertreiben den vnhailsamen vnd ‖ gifftigen Gebresten der Pestilentz / ‖ Leibs vnd der Seelen / vnd ‖ den ewigen Tod. ‖ Volgt hernach ain leiblich Regi- ‖ ment / das ain yeder Christen ‖ mensch in solcher not vnd ‖ zeyt / zů gebrauchen ‖ waiß. 1573

Georg Fraunberger
Ein Geistlich ‖ Regiment / für zu kom- ‖ men vñ zuuertreiben den vn- ‖ heilsamen vñ Gifftigen gebre- ‖ sten der Pestilentz / leibs vñ ‖ der Seelen / vnnd den ‖ Ewigen Todt. ‖ Volgt hernach auch ein ‖ Gemein Leiblich Regiment / ‖ das ein jeder Christen mensch ‖ in solcher Not und zeit der ‖ Pestilentz / zu brauchen ‖ waißt. (Landshut), [1573?]

Theobald Fettich
Ordnung ‖ Vnd Regiment / wie ‖ man sich vor der scharpffen vnd gifftigen kranckheit der Pestilentz bewaren ‖ sol: Auch wie denen / so darmit begriffen / zuhelf‖ fen sey. ‖ Sampt den natürlichen vrsachen ‖ des Englischen Schwaiß. München: (Adam Berg), [1573?]

Anon.
Ein kurtz Regi- ‖ ment / wie man sich in zeit ‖ Regierender Pestilentz ‖ halten soll. ‖ Durch die Hochgelerten vnd er- ‖ farnen der Ertzney Doctores / zu- ‖ samen gefast vnd gebessert. Nuremberg: Dieterich Gerlach, 1574

Paul Heusler
Der Ein vnd ‖ neunzigste Psalm / tröstlich ‖ zu dieser zeit / wider die Seuche ‖ der Pestilentz vnd anders anlie- ‖ gen / in gesangsweise ‖ verfasset. ‖ Im Thom / Es spricht der vnwei- ‖ sen Mund wol / etc. (Leipzig: Jacob Berwaldte Erben, 1575)

Andreas Langner
Promptuarium. ‖ Wie zur Zeit der Pesti- ‖ lentz / ein jeder Gesunder und Krancker / ‖ Jungk oder Alt / Man vnd Weibsperson / sich mit ‖ allem Praeseruiren vnd Curirn sol / Vor des- ‖ gleichen nie auffkommen noch gesehen worden / ‖ Sampt ‖ Beyligenden seer nützlichem Process / ‖ von der Aderläß ... Item / ‖ Verzeichnus vnd warhafftiger bericht / ‖ was ein jedes Himlisch Zeichen in Zodiaco für ‖ Glieder im menschlichen Cörper regierte... (Leipzig: Johan Rhambaw), 1575

Bartholomeus Scultetus, ed. (Paracelsus and Bodenstein)
Vom urspurng ‖ der Pestilentz udn jhren zu- ‖ fallenden Kranckheiten / Auch ‖ derselbigen fürkom-ung / unnd ‖ heilung / Doctoris Para- ‖ celsi schreiben. Basel: Peter Perna, 1575

Nicolaus Selnecker
Kurtze / Ein- ‖ feltige / Ware / Christliche ‖ vnd gantz notwendige Warnung / ‖ fromen Christen zu gut vnd nutz geschrie- ‖ ben das sie sich vorsehen vnd hüten für ‖ dem ergernis / gifft / vnd gemechlich ein- ‖ schleichenden pestilentz der Sacraments- ‖ schwermer / vnd zugleich ein richtige vn- ‖ terweisung / wie sie sich für jhren gelerten ‖ klugen / vnd doch faulen vnd nichtigen ‖ gründen / argumenten / folgern / vnd ‖ einreden / aus Gottes Wort ver- ‖ waren / vnnd gefasset ‖ machen können. (Leipzig), 1575

Johann Wittich
Hausartzney / ‖ vnd Notwendiger kurtzer ‖ Vnterricht / wie man sich jtzt / in ‖ anhebender Pestilentzseuche / ‖ mit Göttlichem beystan- ‖ de schützen / Vnd da ‖ man darein gera- ‖ then / auch Cu- ‖ rieren ‖ sol. ‖ Alle Hausuetern vnd ‖ armen Leuten nützlichen. (Eisleben: Urban Gaubisch), 1575

Anon.
Eins Erbern Raths ‖ der Statt Nürmberg / ‖ vernewte Gesetz vnd Ordnung / von we- ‖ gen besorgender einreissender ‖ Sterbsleufft, 1575

Anon.
Ein kurz Regi- ‖ ment / wie man sich in diesen ‖ gegenwertigen Sterbsleuff- ‖ ten halten sol. Nuremberg: Katharinam Gerlachin und Johans vom Berg Erben, 1575

Anon.
Kurzer und Einfelti- ‖ ger Bericht: ‖ Wie sich in die- ‖ sen jetzigen Sterbensleuff- ‖ ten der gemeine Man zu- ‖ uerhalten habe. ‖ Auff beger ei- ‖ nes Erbarn Wolweisen ‖ Raths zu Halle / von den ‖ Medicis daselbst / gemei- ‖ ner Stadt zunutz ‖ gestellet. (Eisleben: Andream Petri), 1575

Anon.
Kurtzer vñd ‖ notwendiger Be- ‖ richt / ‖ Wie sich Junge vnd Alte / ‖ Arme vnd Reiche Leut / in Ster- ‖ bensleufften verhalten / Auch womit sie sich ‖ vor der grausamen Plag der Pestilentz ver- ‖ waren / Oder do sie nach Gottes wil- ‖ len damit angegriffen / sich ‖ widerumb curirn ‖ vnd haylen ‖ sollen. Zum Hoff: Mattheum Pfeilschmidt, 1575.

Adam Lonitzer
Ordnung ‖ Für die Pe- ‖ stilentz. (Frankfurt: Christian Egenolff's Erben), 1576

Paracelsus and Michael Toxites
De Peste ‖ PHILIPPI THEO- ‖ phrasti Paracelsi, des hoch- ‖ erfarnen Teutschen Philosophi / vñ ‖ beyder Artzney Doctoris / an die ‖ Statt Stertzingen ‖ geschriben. ‖ Item, ‖ Etliche Consilia Theophrasti ‖ Paracelsi. ‖ Apologia Doctoris Toxite des Bassauischen ‖ Cantzlers tödtlichen abgang

belangen. ‖ Vorhin nie getruckt / jetztunder aber alles durch ‖ Doctorem Toxiten gefertigt. Strassburg: Niclauss Wyriot, 1576

Gervasius Marstaller
Kurtzer vnd einfeltiger ‖ Bericht / ‖ Wie man / so viel Gott ‖ gefellig / sich für der grawsamen vnd ‖ schrecklichen Pestilentz bewaren / Oder so man ‖ damit behafft / sie vertreiben müge... (Ulssen: Michel Kröner), 1576

Heinrich Wolffius (Arnaldus de Villa Nova)
Herliche Medi- ‖ cische Tractat / vor nie ‖ in truck kommen ‖ Von Cur des Podagrams / ‖ des Hocherfarnen alten Medici / Arnaldi ‖ de Villa Nova. ‖ Item... ‖ Vor der Pestilentz: vnd andern nützlichen ‖ materien / welche die vorred andeitet... Strasburg: Bernhart Jobin, 1576

Christoph Fischer
Ein Geistliche ‖ bewerte Artzney aus der ‖ Himlischen Apotecken des Götlichen ‖ Worts genommen / Wie sich ein Christ in ‖ den ganzt beschwerlichen leufften der Pesti- ‖ lentz verhalten / was er dafür für ein heil- ‖ sam Praeservatiu / für ein heilwertig Cu- ‖ ratiu / vnd wenn er genesen / für ein ‖ Regiment brauchen solle / ‖ damit er nicht vbel ‖ erger mache. 1577

Christoph Fischer
Ein Geistliche ‖ bewerte Artzney / aus der ‖ Himlischen Apotecken des Gött- ‖ lichen Worts genommen / Wie sich ein ‖ Christ in den gantz beschwerlichen leuff- ‖ ten der Pestilentz verhalten / was er dafür ‖ für ein heilsam Praeseruatiu / für ein heil- ‖ wertig Curatiu / vnd wenn er genesen / ‖ für ein Regiment brauchen solle / ‖ damit er nicht vbel erger ‖ mache. Ulssen: Michel Kröner, 1577

Georg Friderau
Ein kurtzer Bericht / ‖ Wie ein jeder in die- ‖ sen fürstehenden Sterbens leufften ‖ der Mittel vnnd Artzneyen / so in der Apoteck zu ‖ Halberstadt aus Beuehlich eines Hochwirdigen ‖ Thumcapittels / vnd eines Erbarn / Weisen ‖ Raths daselbst zu gebrauchen gestel- ‖ let vnd geordnet. Magdeburg: Wilhelm Ross, 1577

Gervasius Marstaller
Kurtzer vnd einfeltiger ‖ Bericht / ‖ Wie man / so viel Gott ‖ gefellig / sich für der grawsamen vnd ‖ schrecklichen Pestilentz bewaren / Oder so man ‖ damit behafft / sie vertreiben müge... (Ulssen: Michel Kröner), 1577

Gervasius Marstaller
Kurtze Summa / Wie man sich in Pestilentz zeitten zur ‖ vorsorg vnd in der not verhalten sol / in Reimen gefast / durch ‖ Gervasium Marstaller / der Artzney Doctorem, vnd Fürstlichen ‖ Lünebergischen Medicum. Ulssen: Michel Kröner, 1577 Single-leaf broadside

Johann Neeffen (Naeve)
Ein kurtzer Bericht: ‖ Wie man sich in denen jtzo vorstehen- ‖ den Sterbensleufften / mit der Praeseruation ‖ oder vorwahrungen / Dornach auch der ‖ Curation der Pestilentz / vnd etzlicher ‖ jrer accidentien, oder zufellen / verhalten sol. (Dresden: Söckel), 1577

Andreas Pangratius
Funffzehen Predigten ‖ Voñ der Schrecklichen ‖ Plage der Pestilentz / Was sie sey / Woher ‖ sie komme / Vnd wie wir vns ‖ drein schicken sollen. Hoff: Mattheus Pfeilschmidt, 1577

Ernst Reuchlin
Zwo Haußtafeln und underricht vor die Reichen unnd Armen / zur Sommer und Winter zeit / wider die fürstehende / schreckliche und wegkfressende Pestilentz / die nicht allein (wie der Königkliche Prophet / Psal: 91 saget) im finstern schleichet / sondern auch im Mittage / als ein wütender Mörder eilends unzeliche Menschen tödet. Lübeck: Asswerus Kröger, 1577

Anon.
Ein kurtzer bericht ‖ wie man sich mit der hilff Gottes ‖ vor der Pestilentz hütten / vnnd so der Mensch ‖ darmit angrieffen / was mittel er darfür brauchen ‖ sölle: mennigklichem zum gutten / Durch die ‖ Stadtartzte zu Zůrich Anno M. D. ‖ LXiiij. Gestelt / vnnd druch den Druck ‖ daselbs außgangen / jetzt aber auß dringender not mit Rath Einer ‖ E. L. Artzte in der Steyr- ‖ marck / wider auffs ‖ new gedruckt. Graz: Zacharias Bartsch Formschneider, 1577

Joachim Aue (Awe)
Einfeltiger Bericht aus Gottes Wort / wie sich ein fromer Christ / in der zeit der Pestilentz / mit heilsamer Ertzney / beide an Leib und Seel verwaren sol / auff das er mit gutem frölichem gewissen leben / und / so es Gott verhenget / seliglich sterben / und zum weigen leben erhalten werden möge. Magdeburg, 1578

Johannes Bökel
Gründtlicher bericht / ‖ von der Pestilentz / welche für Zwölff ‖ Jaren in der löblichen Stadt Hamburg ‖ grewlichen hat regieret. Heinrichsstadt: Conradus Horn, 1578

Johannes Neander
Ein kurtz doch noth- ‖ dürfftig Regiment / De prae- ‖ seruatione & curatione Pe- ‖ stis, aus eigener obseruation vnd ‖ erfarung / an vielen Menschen frucht- ‖ barlichen befunden. ‖ Sampt fleissiger verzeichnus der ‖ vielfeltigen Tugendt vnd Operation ‖ des Börnstein Oeles am endt ‖ hinzugedruckt. (Magdeburgk: Joachim Walden), 1579

Jakob Schade
Kurtzer bericht wie ‖ sich ein jeder in Sterbens leufften ‖ nechst Gott / recht praeseruiren vnd Cu- ‖ riren möge. ‖ Der Erbarn vnd Christlichen gemei- ‖ ne diser Königlichen Stadt Dantzigk zum ‖ besten gestellet vnd in Druck verfertiget ‖ Durch Iacobum Schaden der Artzney ‖ D. vnd verordenten Phisicum ‖ daselbst. (Danzig: Jacob Rhodus), 1579

Anon.
Ein neu Klag ‖ vnd Trostlied / inn gegen- ‖ wertiger Theuerzeit vñ sterbs- ‖ leufften / damit vnns GOtt [sic] an man- ‖ chem ort Strafft vnnd heimsucht / u. ‖ Im Thon: Warumb betrübstu ‖ dich mein Herz. ‖ Hierbey auch ein schönes Ge- ‖ sprech / deß sterbenden armen Sünders ‖ mit Christo. Auch ge- ‖ sangweiß. ‖ Im Thon. Auß tieffer noth. / rc. (Nürnberg: Valentin Fuhrmann), [1580?]

Balthasar Brunner
Kurtzer vnd einfeltiger Bericht / ‖ Wie man sich / in jetzo ‖ verfallender Sterbenßzeit / prae- ‖ seruiren vnd verhalten sol. ‖ Gestellet vor die Gemeine zu Halle / Leipzig: Jacob Berwaldts Erben, 1581

Georg am Wald
Bericht vnd Erklerung ‖ Georgij am Wald / der ‖ Rechten Licentiaten / Philosophie vnd beyder Ar- ‖ tzeneyē Doctoris an jetzo bestalten Physici deß H. Reichs ‖ Statt Thonawerdt / Wie vnd was gestalt das new von jm erfunden ‖ Terra Sigillata vnd vniuersal Artzeney / wider die Pestilentz vnnd dero zu- ‖ fellen / auch allerley eingenommen Gifft / biß vnnd stich der Gifftigen Thie- ‖ ren / für das Viertäglich vnd allerely Fieber / Seitten stechen / oder geschweh- ‖ ren / auch andern innwendigen geschweren mehr / neuw Haupt oder Vnge- ‖ risch Kranckheit / Wassersucht / Gelbsucht / Wührm / Grimmen / Sandt / ‖ Harnwindt / Contractur oder Lem-e… (St. Gallen: Leonhard Straub), 1581

Job Fincel
Von der ‖ Pestilentz ‖ Notwendiger Unterricht ‖ der Praeseruation unnd Cur ‖ sampt etzlichen der Artzney ‖ heimligkeiten. (Leipzig: Johann Beyer in verlegung Simon Hütters and Sigmund Feyrabends, 1582)

Johann Gryneus
Ein Trost ‖ Büchlein / dariñen ‖ anzeigt wirt / auß was ‖ vrsachen Gott der Herr als ‖ ein gerechter Vatter / mit Pestilentz ‖ vnd ander noht / vnß seine Kinder ‖ heimsůche / wessen wir vns in allem ‖ anligen zů trösten haben: vnd wirt ‖ auch der xcj. Pslame Davids / kürtz ‖ lich erklert. Gestellt zů ehren / trost / ‖ vnd dienst einer loblichen Burger ‖ schafft der Christenlichen vnnd ‖ weitberümten Statt ‖ Basel, (1582)

Philip Imsser
Pestilentzbüchlin / ‖ Für die armen ‖ Handwercks vnd Baurs ‖ Leut / welche den Artzten vnd Apo‖ tecken zu weit gesessen / oder sich ‖ Armut halben schlechter ding ‖ behelffen müssen. ‖ In gegenwertiger Gefahrlichkeit ‖ auffs kürtzest beschriben / Strassburg: Christian Müllers Erben, 1582

Johann Pomarius (Johann Baumgartner)
Pestilentz Büchlein. ‖ VOn [sic] der Pe- ‖ stilentz vnd jhren vrsa- ‖ chen / Auch von gewisser Ertzney / wie ‖ man dawieder praeseruirt vnd Cu- ‖ riret werden sölle. ‖ Von dem höchsten Doctore ‖ Gott dem H. Geist / in der Geistli- ‖ chen Officina vnd Himlischen A- ‖ poteken heiliger Schrifft / allen ‖ Christen zu gut verordnet vnd praepariret. Magdeburg: Johan Francken, 1582

Jacob Theodorus
Regiment ‖ Vnd kurtzer Be- ‖ richt / wie man sich in Ster- ‖ bensläuffen / da die Pestilentz ein- ‖ reisset halten / auch wie man sich durch ‖ Gottes hülff vor dieser Sucht bewaren / vnd mit ‖ welchen Artzeneyen dieselbe zu curi- ‖ ren vnd zu heylen sey. Frankfurt: (Nicolaus Bassaeum), 1582

Jakob Theodorus (Tabernomontanus)
Gewisse Practick / ‖ Wie man sich ‖ mit Göttlicher hülff / ‖ vor der Pestilentz hüten vnd be- ‖ waren / vnnd so einer damit be- ‖ hafft / wie dem selben zuhelffen / Es sey- ‖ en alte oder junge / arme oder reiche leut. ‖ Gepracticiert vnnd beschrieben in ‖ Anno 1551/ 52. vnd nachfol- ‖ genden Jaren / Newstatt an der Hardt: Matteum Harnisch, 1582

Georg am Wald
Bericht vnd Erklerung ‖ Georgij am Wald / der ‖ Rechten Licentiaten / Philosophie vñ beyder Ar- ‖ tzeneyē Doctoris an jetzo bestaltē Physici des H. Reichs ‖ Statt Thonawerdt / Wie vnd was gestalt das new von jm erfundē ‖ Terra Sigillata vnd vniuersal Artzeney / wider die Pestilentz vnd dero zu- ‖ fellen… (St. Gallen: Leonhart Straub), 1582

Anon.
Die Pestilentz ‖ Ob sie eyn anfällige Seüchte ‖ sey: Vnd wie ferr sie eyn Chri- ‖ sten mensch weichen möge: ‖ Zwo Fragen. ‖ Deßgleichen / ‖ Zwen gründtlicher Rhatschläg ‖ vnnd vnderricht für den gemeinen ‖ Mann / wie er sich inn zeit der Pestilentz ‖ halten / vnd mit geringem vnkosten eyn köst- ‖ liche Artzney zů bereiten soll / auff das ‖ er mit der hilff Gottes diser ‖ Seüchte möge entrin- ‖ nen / rc… Basel: (Samuel Apiario), 1582

Anon.
Ein kurtz Re- ‖ giment / wie man sich in di- ‖ sen gegenwertigen Sterbsleuff- ‖ ten halten soll. Nuremberg: Katharinam Gerlachin and Johans vom Berg Erben, 1582

Anon.
Kurtzer Nützlicher ‖ vnd nötiger bericht / Wie man sich zur zeit ‖ der Pestilenz vorhalten / vnd die Ertzeney / so Anno ‖ 76. auff des Rahts der Altenstadt Magdeburgk Apoteck vor- ‖ ordnet / vnd jtzo dieses 82. Jahres daselbst auch ‖ zubekommen / gebrauchen sol. [Magdeburg]: Wolffgang Kirchner, 1582

Gallus Emmen
Einfeltiger / kurtzer ‖ nothwendiger vnd gründt- ‖ licher Bericht / wie man sich jetziger Zeit / ‖ weil das Sterben in der Chron Behmen / ‖ vnd anderßwo mit gewalt vberhandt ‖ nimpt / vormittels Göttlicher ‖ hülff vorwahren vnd ‖ halten soll. (Görlitz: Ambrosius Fritzsch), 1583

Ludwig Grave
Regiment / ‖ Vnd ‖ Kurtzer Bericht ‖ was man sich in sterbens läuff- ‖ ten zur Praeseruation vnd Curation ‖ der Pestilentz kranckheyten / habe zuverhalten: ‖ Was auch für Artzneyen darzu dienlich / in die Apotecken ‖ zu Heydelberg geordnet / vnd wie dieselbigen zu fordern / ‖ Auch nützlich vnd ordentlich zu ge- ‖ brauchen seyen. Heidelberg: Jacob Müller, 1583

Melchior Klesel
WIR Melchior Klesl / der heiligen Schrifft Licentiat. Thumbprobst vnd der Hochlöblichen Vniuersitet zu Wienn Cancellarius vnd Canonicus zu Preßlaw / Auch des Hochwirdigen Fürsten vnd Hewrrn / Herrn Urban Bischouen zu Passaw / etc. Rath / vnd Official in Österreich vndter der Ennß... 1583
Single-leaf broadside

Valentin Leucht
Zwo Christliche Ca- ‖ tholische vnd in Gott reinem wort ‖ wollgegründte Predigten vber das Acht vnd ‖ zwantzigste Capitel des trewen Propheten Ezechielis / ‖ Darinnen die scheinbarliche Hoffart / so jetzundt ge- ‖ waltig im schwange gehet / vnd mit macht von jedermann gepfle- ‖ get wirt / mit jhrer schönen Hoffarbe / eigener art / rechter weiß vnd ‖ Staffeln / als die fürnembste ursach in stehender Petsilentzischer ge- ‖ fährlicher zeit angezogen vnd erwiesen. Vnd was hiergegen für ‖ mittel / geistliche Praeservatiff vnd Antidota wider den schädlichen ‖ gifft der Pestilentz... Mainz: Caspar Behem, 1583

Wolfgang Peristerus
Das Geistliche ‖ ANTIDOTVM, ‖ Das ist / ‖ Ein Uberaus ‖ krefftiges vnd heilwertiges ‖ Recept / Praeservativ oder Ertzney / ‖ Wider ‖ Die Pestilentzische Seuche / vnd an- ‖ dere tödliche Kranckheiten.‖ Durch ‖ Vuolfgangum Peristerum, der H. S. ‖ Docotrn / zum theil gestellet / zum teil auch ‖ aus andern Bet vnd Psalm Büchern / vnd zuvorab ‖ aus der ganzen

Biblischen Schrifft beider ‖ Testamenten zuhauff getragen. Berlin: Nicolaus Voltzen, 1583

Johann Reusch
Regiment / ‖ Wie man sich zur ‖ zeit der Pestilentz halten sol / ‖ Der Stadt Leipzig vnd deren Ein- ‖ wohnern vornemlich / Vnd denn auch son- ‖ sten jedermenniglichen zum besten mit son- ‖ derm fleis geschrieben / Im Jhar ‖ nach der Geburt CHristi [sic] / ‖ 1539. durch weiland ‖ Den Achtbarn / Hochgelarten ‖ vnd wolerfahrnen Herrn Johan Reuschen / ‖ Der freyen Künste vnd Ertzney Doctorem / ‖ Auch Professorem vnd bestalten im ‖ Hospital zu S. Georgen / ‖ Medicum / rc... (Leipzig: Johan Beyer), 1583

Johann Rodius
Von Pestilentz / vnd ‖ Sterbensläufften. ‖ Ein Christliche ‖ Erinnerung / mit waserley ‖ Sünden / die schreckliche Straffe der ‖ Pestilentz verursachet / in Lender / Stedte vnd ‖ Dörffer bracht / Was fur naturliche Zeichen gemei- ‖ niglich als verboten Göttliches Zorns vorher lauf- ‖ fen... (Erfurt: Johann Beck), 1583

Philipp Schopf
DE PESTE ‖ Ein kurtz metho- ‖ disch Tractätlein vnnd Vnter- ‖ richt / wie man sich von solcher beschwer- ‖ lichen erblichen Sucht durch natürliche Mittel ‖ vnd Artzney / neben Göttlicher Hülff / preseruieren vnd ‖ bewahren / Auch die jenige / so von solcher an- ‖ gegriffen / curieren vnd jhnen wi- ‖ der helffen solle. Heidelberg: Johan Spies, 1583

Johannes Schröter.
Johannis Schröteri ‖ DOCTORIS ‖ Einfeltiger / Doch ‖ Gründtlicher Bericht vnnd Rath- ‖ schlag / Wie man durch Gottes gnedige hülffe ‖ vnd gute Ordnung / in diesen schweren leufften der ‖ Pestilentz / sich halten und bewaren / Auch so jemandt ‖ damit befleckt / wie er damit gebaren sol. ‖ Menniglichen zu trost / hülffe vnd ‖ gutem gestellet. ‖ Auffs newe wider vbersehen / vnd ‖ mit vielen bewerten Ertzneyen... (Leipzig: Jacob Berwaldts Erben), 1583

Johann Ewich
Pestilentzordenunge: ‖ Nützer vnd not- ‖ wendiger vnderricht / von ‖ dem Ampt der Obrigkeit / in Pestilentzzeit- ‖ ten / wie durch jhren fleis die Pestilentz ‖ verhütet / vnd da dieseble ein- ‖ gerissen / gedempfft wer- ‖ den könne. (Leipzig: Grosse, Mülhausen), 1584

Michael von Glaubitz
Zwo Haußtaf- ‖ feln vnd vnderricht fur die ‖ Reichen vnd Armen / zur sommer ‖ vnd winterzeit wider die für?ehende schreck ‖ liche vnd

wegfressende Pestilentz die nicht allein ‖:wie der Königlich Prophet Psalm 91. sagt: im ‖ finstern schleicht / sondern auch vmb Mit- ‖ tag alß ein wütendter Mörder ei- ‖ lendts vnzehliche Men- ‖ schen tödtet. Mainz: Casparum Behem, (1584)

Johann Hildebrand
Regiment. ‖ Wie sich allerley ‖ Stände / Jung vnnd Alt / Manns ‖ vnd Frawens Personen / in diesen gefehrli- ‖ chen Zeiten / vor der Pestilentz / so jetzund im Land zu ‖ Österreich / Behäm / auch andern vmbligenden ‖ örtern / die Menschen plötzlich vber- ‖ fellet / bewaren sol. (Nuremberg: Niclas Knorr), 1584

Caspar Kegler
Ein Regiment / ‖ Durch Doctorem Caspa- ‖ rum Kegeler gemacht / Darinnen ‖ angezeiget / wie man sich für der erschrecklichen seuche der Pestilentz / praeseruiren vnd ‖ bewaren / Vnd do eins dardurch inficiret oder ver- ‖ gifftet wurden / wie man dem / mit ausserlesenen ‖ Medelen vnd Ertzneyen / zu hůlffe / zu seiner vori- ‖ gen gesundheit wider bringen / vnd ‖ jhn retten sol. Dresden: (Gimel Bergen), 1584

Victorinus Schönfeldt
CONSILIVM oder ‖ Rathschlag ‖ VOr {sic} die be- ‖ schwerliche jetz re- ‖ gierende Plage der Roten Ruhr / vnd ‖ andere schädliche Bauchflüsse. ‖ Daneben ein kurtzer Bericht wie ein ‖ jeder sich vor der Pestilentz bewahren / ‖ vnd von derselbigen sich er- ‖ ledigen soll. Frankfurt: Christian Egenolffs seligen Erben, 1584

Clement Chelner
Kurtzer bericht / von jtzo regieren. ‖ der Kranckheit der Pestis. ‖ Was sie sey / woher sie ‖ komme / vnd wie man sich dafür ver- ‖ waren / vnd do einer damit beladen / ‖ Curirt werden soll. Eisleben: Andream Petri, 1585

Johannes Crato (von Crafftheim)
Ordnung der Praeservation: ‖ Wie man sich zur zeit ‖ der Infection verwahren / Auch be- ‖ richt / wie die rechte Pestilentia erkandt / vnd ‖ curirt werden sol: Mit einer lere / von dem ‖ vorsorg der Geschwieren. Nuremberg: Katharina Gerlachin, 1585

Theobald Fettich
Ordnung ‖ Vnd Regiment / ‖ wie man sich vor der scharpf- ‖ fen vnd gifftigen Kranckheit der Pe- ‖ stilentz bewahren soll: Auch wie de- ‖ nen / so darmit begriffen / zu- ‖ helffen sey. ‖ Sambt den natürlichen vrsachen ‖ des Englischen Schwaiß. Munich: Adam Berg, 1585

Andreas Langner
PROMPTVA- ‖ RIVM ‖ Wie zur zeit der ‖ Pestilentz / ein jeder Gesunder ‖ vnd Krancker / Jungk oder Alt / Mann ‖ vnd Weibspersonen / sich mit allem prae- ‖ seruiren vnd Curirn sol / vor des gleichen nie ‖ auffkommen noch gesehen worden. ‖ Sampt ‖ Beyligendem sehr nützlichem ‖ Process von der Aderläß… 1585

Johann Pontani (Johann Wittich, ed.)
Iohannis Pontani ‖ DOCTORIS ‖ Einfeltiger vnd gar ‖ kurtzer bericht / was man in den ‖ schweren Pestilentz leufften gebrauchen sol / ‖ beydes zur Praeservation vnd curation. Leipzig cum privilegio: (Hans Steinmann), 1585

Bartholomaeus Schualb
Gründtlicher vnterricht / ‖ Wie sich gesunde vnd kran- ‖ cke / diesen Herbst vnd Winter / so Sterbensleufft ‖ (da Gott für sey) gefehrlichen einrissen / ‖ verhalten sollen. ‖ Zu nutz und wolfahrt / ‖ Der Einwoner vnnd grantzen Bürgerschafft / ‖ Obrigkeit vnnd Underthanen / Geistliches vnnd ‖ Weltliches standes / Edel vnd Unedel / Reich vnd ‖ Arm / Mann uvd Weib / Alt vnd Jung / rc. ‖ Der Kayserlichen Stadt Großglogaw / vnd derselben ‖ zugehörungen / rc. In eyl auffs trewlichste ‖ verordnet den ersten Octobris / Im ‖ 1585 Jahr. Neiße: [Joh. Creutziger], 1585

Anon.
Ein kurtz Regiment / wie man sich in di- ‖ sen gegwertigen Sterbs- ‖leufften halten soll. Nuremberg: Katharinam Gerlachin, 1585

Anon.
Einfeltiger vnd kurtzer ‖ Bericht / von Praeseruation, Erkentnuß ‖ vnd heylung / der erschröcklichen Kranckheit ‖ der Pestilentz / Sampt derselbigen gifftigen ‖ Peulen vnd Plattern / dem gemeinen Mann ‖ vnd fürnemlich den Palbiren vnd ‖ Badern / Nothwendig ‖ zu wissen. Regensburg: Johann Burger, 1585

Anon.
Eins Erbarn Raths ‖ der Stadt Nüremberg / verneute Ge- ‖ setz vnnd Ordnung / inn gegen- ‖ wertigen sterbsleufften diß ‖ M D LXXXV ‖ Jars auffge- ‖ richt. 1585

Anon.
Wie sich mit ‖ Artzney / vnd all ander ‖ dingen / zu diser gefahrlichen zeit ‖ der Pestilentz / zuhalten: vnd wie diesel- ‖ big / da sie eines angreifft / zuuertreiben sey / ‖ guter vnd kurtzer Bericht / meniglich / so ‖ nicht weichen wöllen / sollen oder ‖ könden / zu gutem beschri- ‖ ben / vnnd durch den ‖ Truck mitge- ‖ theilt. Tübingen, 1585.

Johann Haym von Themar
S. Sebastiani ‖ fürbitt / wider die erschröck- ‖ lichen Kranckheit / auch andere Ca- ‖ tholische Gebet / auff den Cantzlen / in den ‖ Häussern / jetzigen Sterbens vnd gefärlichen ‖ zeiten / Gott vmb dessen abwendung täglich ‖ zu bitten / Auch dañ 7. Pater noster, in die 7. Blutsuergiessung ‖ Jesu Christi zu spre- ‖ chen / rc. Munich: Adam Berg, 1586

Mattheus Sebisch
Ein kurtzer ‖ vnd gegründter be- ‖ richt / raht vnd hilff wider ‖ die Pestilentzische ‖ Kranckheit. Augsburg: Valentin Schönigk, 1586

Jakob Theodorus (Tabernaemontanus)
Regiment ‖ Vnd kurtzer Be- ‖ richt / wie man sich in Ster- ‖ bensläufften / da die Pestilentz einreis- ‖ set / halten / auch wie man sich durch Gottes ‖ deß Allmächtigen hülff vor dieser vergifften Sucht ‖ mit guten erfahrnen Mitteln bewahren / vnnd wie die Infi- ‖ cirten durch bewerte Artzeneyen curirt vnd geheylet werden ‖ sollen. Auß langwiriger erfahrung auffs kürtzest ‖ vnd fleissigst gestellt / (Frankfurt: Nicolaum Basseum), 1586

Petrus Victorius Welsenacensus (Pietro Vettori)
Amphialtos. Das ist Beyde Leibes unnd Seelen Artzney für die schedliche Gifft der Pestilentz / allen frommen Christgleubigen Menschen zu gute gestellet und geprediget. Magdeburg: Johan Francken, 1586

Wolfgang Peristerus
SUPPLEMEN- ‖ TVM. ‖ Zusatz oder Verfüllung deß ‖ Geistlichen Antidoti wider ‖ die Pestilentz ‖ Das ist / ‖ Noch zwee vbrige gar gehei- ‖ me vnnd Geistreiche auch zu wissen ‖ Hochnötige Artikel vnser Christlich- ‖ en Lehre / vom ewigen Leben / aus Gottes ‖ wort zusamen getragen vnd erkleret / so noch ‖ zu dem Geistlichen Antidoto D. Wolf- ‖ gangi Peristeri, gehörig… 1587

Johannes Pontanus (Johann Wittich, ed.)
Iohannis Pontani ‖ DOCTORIS ‖ Einfeltiger vnd gar ‖ kurtzer bericht / was man in den ‖ schweren Pestilentz leufften gebrauchen sol / byedes zur praeseruation vnd curation. ‖ Das erste Tractetlein / ‖ Der mal eins zu Weymar in gefehr- ‖ lichen anfallenden sterbens leufften gestelt / ‖ vnd vielen guten feunden mitgeteilet… Leipzig: (Hans Steinman), 1587

Henrich Rantzau (Johann Wittich, trans.)
De conseruanda valetudine. ‖ Das ist: ‖ Von erhaltung menschli- ‖ cher gesundheit: Ein sehr nützliches Hand- ‖ buch / allen menschen hohes vnd niedriges standes / ‖ auch dem wanders vnd kriegsleuten gantz ‖ dienstlichen. ‖ Vor dieser zeit von dem Edlen / gestrengen / hochge- ‖ larten Herrn Henrich Rantzau / Holsteinischen Stadt- ‖ halter / in Latein gebracht. ‖ Jetzt aber gantz trewlich verdeutscht… Leipzig, 1587

Jakob Theodorus
Rathschlag / ‖ Wie der jetzigen ‖ Pestilentzischen Seucht / vnd ‖ vergifften schnellen tödtlichen Feber / ‖ in welchem groß Hauptwehthumb / Bräun / ‖ faslche schmertzliche Seitenstechen pleuritides men- ‖ dosae, vnnd andere sorgliche Zufäll mit vnterlauffen / ‖ begegnen vnd vorkommen soll. Vnd wie denen ‖ zu helffen / so damit inficiert vnnd be- ‖ hafft seindt. Frankfurt: Nicolaum Bassaeum, 1587

Ludwig Echer
Ein bewert Artzneybüch- ‖ lein von dem vberauß köstlichen vnd bewer- ‖ ten aquavitae vnd Wacholder Oel / wider die jetzige pla- ‖ ge der Pestilentz zu gebrauchen / auch andern zu- ‖ felligen kranckheiten / wie hierinn zu sehen ist. ‖ M. D. LXXXVIII. 1588

Caspar Kegler
Ein Nützliches vnd ‖ tröstlichs Regiment wider die Pesti- ‖ lentz / vnd gifftig Pestilentzische Fieber / ‖ die Schweissucht genant / Vnd sonst ‖ mancherley gifftige vnd todt- ‖ liche Kranckheit. ‖ Durch Casparum Kegeler / der Artz- ‖ ney Doctorn zusamen gebracht / vernewet / vñ mit ‖ viel tröstlichen Experimenten gebessert / die zuuorn heim- ‖ lich gehalten vnd an den tag nie gegeben sind / Anno ‖ 1529. ausgegangen / vnd denn folgens ‖ Anno 53. zu Leipzig wider ‖ nachgedruckt. ‖ Jtzt aber in diesen gefehrlichen ster- ‖ bensleufften dem gemeinen Man zum be- ‖ sten wider auffgelegt / vnd gedruckt. Königsberg in Preussen: Georg Osterberger, 1588

Wolfgang Peristerus
Noch Etliche ‖ mehr besondere / auserwehl- ‖ te / Ausbůndige / schöne andechtige ‖ vnnd jnnigliche Gebete / wieder die ‖ Pestilentz / vnd in andern ‖ fellen zubeten. 1588

Anon.
Kurtzer vnterricht in ‖ Sterbensläuffen. ‖ So wol für kran- ‖ cke Inficierte, als andere Per- ‖ sonen so den Krancken zu warten be- ‖ stellt / mit angehengkter Praeseruatif vnd ‖ nutzlicher vorsehung für die Pestilentz. ‖ Menigklichen zu gutem. Munich: Adam Berg, 1589

Anon.
Regiment vnd ‖ Ordnung in zeit der Pesti- ‖ lentz vnd wie man sich dar- ‖ inn verhalten soll. ‖ Von ‖ Einem andern wolerfahr- ‖ nen Doctor der Artzney zu- ‖ sammen getragen. [1580s?]

Georg am Wald
Kurtzer Bericht / ‖ Wie / was gestlat vnd ‖ warvmb das Panacea am Waldina / ‖ als ein einige Medicin / wider den Aussatz / Fran- ‖ tzosen / Zauberische Zuständt / Pestilentz / Gifft / Gewalt ‖ Gottes / kleinen Schlag

/ Freyß / hinfallendt Sucht / Beraubung der Vernunfft ... Frankfurt: Nicolaus Basseum, 1591

Anon.
Von Gottes genaden wir Wilhelm Pfaltzgraue ‖ bey Rhein / Hertzog in Ober vnnd Nidern Bayrn / etc. 1592? Single-leaf broadside

Jacob Hornstein
Sterbens flucht: ‖ Das ist / ‖ Christlicher vñ ‖ Catholischer Bericht / von ‖ Sterbensläuff der Pest: ‖ Sampt angehengter frag ‖ vnd antwort / ob man dersel- ‖ bigen Zeit fliechen soll ‖ oder nit: ‖ Auffs kurzest vnd einfaltigest ‖ zusammen getragen vnd ‖ gepredigt. Ingolstatt: Wolffgang Eder, 1593

Martin Ruland
Kurtze ‖ Instruction vnd ‖ Ordnung / wie sich Reiche ‖ vnd Arme hüten vnd hailen sollen / ‖ an der schrecklichen Pestilentz / mit ‖ gewisen vnd bewerten ‖ Artzneyen. Nuremberg: Christof Lochner, 1593

Joachim Landolt
Christliche ‖ Antwort von ‖ der Flucht zur Zeit regie- ‖ render Pestilentz. ‖ Genom-en auß dem Wort ‖ Gottes / vnnd Lehr etlicher be- ‖ wehrten Theologen: ‖ Vnd in offentlichen Truck ver- ‖ fertiget / Durch Herrn Joachim ‖ Landolt / H. Schrifft Doctor / etc. Freyburg im Breisgau: Martin Böckler, 1594

Georgius Bartholdus Pontanus
Christengebett / ‖ So wider den Tür- ‖ cken vnd andere Feind / ‖ wider Pestilentz / Thewrung / ‖ vnd allerley mitlauffende Noth in ‖ gemein von jeden insonderheit ‖ mögen gebraucht wer ‖ den. Ingolstadt: Wolffgang Eder, (1594)

Henrik Rantzau and Johann Pontanus (Johann Wittich, trans.)
De conseruanda valetudine. ‖ Das ist: ‖ Von erhaltung menschli- ‖ cher gesundheit: Ein sehr nutzlichs Hand- ‖ buch / allen menschen hohes vnd niedrigs standes / ‖ auch den wanders vns kriegleuten gantz ‖ dienstlichen. ‖ Vor dieser zeit von dem Edlen / gestrengen / hochge- ‖ larten Herrn Henrich Rantzau / Holsteinischen Stadt- ‖ halter / in Latein gebracht / ‖ Jetzt aber gantz trewlich verdeutscht / zum andernmal ‖ vbersehen / vnd mit vielen herrlichen Experimentlein (als Aqua vitae, weiß vnd gelb / gülden Carfunckelwasser / Hewpt / Apostemen vnd Cappaunwasser / Zimmet vnd Augenwassern / Gifftlatwergen vnd Puluer / Waffen vnd sonsten an- ‖ dern heilsamen Salben / Pfalstern / vnd vielen stücken mehr / so biß daher in geheim ‖ von grossen Herren gehalten) vermehret... Leipzig: Valentin Vögelin, 1594

Georg am Wald
Kurtzer vnd zum andernmal ge- ‖ mehrter Bericht. ‖ Wie / was Gestalt vnd ‖ warumb das Panacea am Waldina / ‖ als ein eynige Medicin / wider den Aussatz / Frantzo- ‖ sen / Zauberischer Zuständt / Pestilentz... Ursel: (Nicolaus Henricus), 1594

Johann Graman
Warhafftige Ursachen / ‖ Warumb auff Theriac / ‖ Mithridat / Gülden Ey vnd andere Opiatas ‖ Confectiones sich in nöthen empfangener Gifften / Pesti- ‖ letzen / Sterbens Leufften / vnnd jetzigen grassirende / newen Kranckheiten / nicht zu verlassen: Sondern wie an derselbigen ‖ stadt mit hundertfältigern Kräfften / das Spagirische / ‖ extrahirte / essentialische Alexipharmacum, ‖ oder Widergifft zu gebrauchen... Erfurt: Johann Beck, 1596

Moysen Staffelsteiner and Cornelius van der Hamsport
Twe korte einfoldige Recept ‖ jegen die Pestilentz / ‖ Dat Erste / ‖ eines Olden ‖ hochgelerden vnd wolerfar- ‖ nen / der Kön. May. tho Dennemar- ‖ cken / wilandt Lyff Medici vnd Doctoris ‖ Corneli van der Hamsport / vor ‖ den simpelen vnd gemeinen ‖ Man gestellet. ‖ Dat Ander / ‖ Uthgegan dörch Moysen ‖ Staffelsteiner Jödē Medicus / wan- ‖ hafftich tho Weymar / vth den olden Jö- ‖ deschen Böken ynt Düdesch geta- ‖ gen / allen Minschen tho ‖ nütte. Hamburg: Hinrich Binder, 1596

Johannes Böckel
Pestordnung / ‖ in der Stadt Ham- ‖ burg. Hamburg: Jacobus Lucius, 1597

Joachim Camerarius
SYNOPSIS ‖ COMMENTARIORVM DE PESTE ‖ Das ist / ‖ Kurtzer / Doch beständiger Begriff / ‖ dreyer Außbündiger Tractätlein / von der Pesti- ‖ lentz / deren Natur / Praeservation, Curation, vnd sonsten in ge- ‖ mein von allerhand diß fals bedencklichen Sachen. ‖ Von Dreyen Vorneh- ‖ men Hochgelahrten Medicis, Als D. ‖ Hieronymo Donzellion Veronensi, D. Ioanne Philippo Ingrassia ‖ Italis: Vnd dann von dem vortrefflichen weitberhümbten Herrn / ‖ D. Ioachimo Camerario Noribergensi Medico zum ‖ fleissigsten beschrieben... Lich (in der Grafschaft Solmß): Nicolaus Erbenius, 1597

Johann Graman
Extract vnd kurtzer außzug ei- ‖ nes in heiliger Schrifft / vnnd dem Liecht ‖ der Natur gegründten Regiments / wie man sich durch ‖ Gottes segen für der Pestilentz praeserviren vnd bewaren / auch ‖ die inficierten krancken curiren vnd wieder zur gesundheit ‖ bringen soll / nach altem Spagirischen vnd newen ‖ Paracelsischen Styol gesetzet vnd ‖ zusammen getragen... Erfurt: Johann Beck, 1597

Heinrich Julius (duke of Braunschweig and Lüneburgk)
Des Hochwir- ‖ digen / Durchleuchtigen / ‖ Hochgebornen Fürsten ‖ vnd Herren / Herrn Hein- ‖ richs Julij / Postulirten ‖ Bischoffen zu Halberstadt / vnd Hertzo- ‖ gen zu Braunschweig und Lüne- ‖ burgk / etc. ‖ Constitution vnd ‖ Ordnunge / ‖ Wie es bey diesen gefehrlichen Sterbens- ‖ leufften in jrer Fürstl. G. Stifft Halber- ‖ stadt gehalten werden ‖ solle. Halberstadt: Georg Koten, 1597

Jakob Horst
Rath in Pestilentz zei- ‖ ten / Wie man die verhüten / vnd in noth- ‖ fall Curiren sol / zu nothurfft aller bußfertigen ‖ Christen. Heinrichstadt: Conrad Horn, 1597

Caspar Kegler
Nützlicher vnd ‖ wahrer Bericht wider die ‖ Pestilentz / vnnd wie man sich in zeit ‖ dero erschrecklichen regierung preseruiern / ‖ bewahren vnnd erhalten. Neben etlichen ‖ tröstlichen vnd vnder andern außerlesenen ‖ mittelen / hůlff vnnd Artzneyen / so man ‖ alsdann zugebrauchen / vnd mit Gött- ‖ licher gnaden zur voriger ge- ‖ sundtheit gerathen möge. ‖ Imgleichen wie man die wahre Ter-‖ ra Sigillata zugebrauchen habe. Cölln: Wilhelm Lützenkirchen, 1597

Paul Simler
Kurtzer / einfeltiger und wol- ‖ gegründter Bericht / ‖ Wie man sich in die- ‖ sen beschwerlichen Leufften der Pe- ‖ stilentzischer seuchen praeserviren... (Coburg: Valentinus Krönern), 1597

Johann Schwartz
Christlicher Unterricht / von dem graw- ‖ samen unnd tödtlichen Pesti ‖ lentzgifft. ‖ Darinnen auß Gottes ‖ Wort gründtlich angezeigt wirdt... Frankfurt: Johann Spieß, 1597

Andreas Starck
Von der Pestilentz ‖ Kurtzer vnd einfeltiger ‖ Bericht / wie man sich mit Gottes hülffe ‖ durch Mittel von jm gnedig geschaffen / dafur ‖ bewaren / vnd die auch heilen möge. ‖ Darneben auch ein Harmspiegel / darinnen ‖ gewiesen wird / das dem Harm vnd Vrinschawen in ‖ Pestilentz Zeit nicht zu trawen sey / vnd solches nicht allein betrieg- ‖ lichen / sondern auch in andern Kranckheiten sehr vngewis ‖ vnd gefehrlichen / furnemlich wenn man dorauff ‖ allein sol Artzney ordenen. Erfurt, 1597

Caspar Strubius
Kurtzer Bericht vnd ‖ Ordnung / wie men- ‖ niglich / besonders aber auch der ge- ‖ meine Man / in jtzo gefehrlichen sterbensleufften / sich solle ver- ‖ halten / vnd mit was Mitteln vnd artzneyen / vorm anfal solcher ‖

geschwinder Seuche vnd Kranckheit / ein jeder sich durch ‖ Gottes hülffe / müge verwaren. Wittenberg: Zacharias Lehman, 1597 Gewise vnd bewehrte ‖ Artzney vnd Ordnung ‖ wider die Vngerische newe ‖ Kranckheit. ‖ Item / für die Pestilentz. ‖ Alles auß bewehrten vnd erfahrnen Autoribus ‖ zusamen gezogen / vnd männiglich zu diser jetzigen ‖ gefährlichen / grassierenden Pestilentz zeit zu ‖ gutem in Druck verfertigt. Regensburg: Bartholome Gräf, 1597

Anon.
Kurtzer vnd einfeltiger bericht / ‖ Wie man in zeit der ‖ jetzo regierenden Pestilentz / ‖ beydes in der Praeservation / vnd ‖ auch Curation sich verhalten soll. Auff eines Hoch- ‖ würdigen Thumb Capittels / vnd auch eines Erbaren ‖ Rahts zu Halberstadt befehlich / von den Me- ‖ dicis daselbst / der Gemeine zu gut ‖ angeordnet. Halberstadt: Georg Koten, 1597

Anon.
Von der Pestilentz / vnd deren ‖ Curation / wie sich hiebey gesunde ‖ vnd krancke zu verhalten: ‖ Dem gemeynen Mañ im Fürstenthumb Hessen ‖ gegen die jetzo hin vnd wider einstehende Pestilen- ‖ tzische Feber vnnd Schwachheiten zu gu- ‖ tem gestellet / Marburg: Paulus Egenolff, 1597

Johann Bauhin
Kurtzer bericht / ‖ Wie man sich ‖ mit Göttlicher hülff vor ‖ der Pestilentz verhüten vnd bewah- ‖ ren sol / vnd so einer damit behafftet ‖ jhme geholffen werden ‖ möge: ‖ Gestelt vnnd erfahren zu ‖ Leon / Genff / vnnd Mümpelgart ‖ durch den Hochgelehrten D. Ioan. Bau- ‖ hinum, des Hochgebornen vnd Durchleuchti- ‖ gen Fürsten vnd Herrn / Herrn Fridrichen Her- ‖ tzogen zu Würtemberg vnd Teck / Graf- ‖ fen zu Mümpelgart / rc. Leibs ‖ Medicum. Mümpelgart: Jacob Foillet, 1597?

Kaspar Bucha
Kurtzer bericht ‖ Wie man in jetzo vnd ‖ künfftigen sterbensleufften / welches Gott gnedig ab- ‖ wenden wolle / sich vorhalten / vnd durch Gottes gnade für der gifftigen ‖ Seuche der Pestilentz vorwahren / vnnd was man teglich gebrau- ‖ chen / vnd womit man reuchern sol. Magdeburg: Johann Francke, 1598

Guillaume Bude
Guill. Budaei Saxonis ‖ Gründtlicher Bericht / vnd ‖ rahtsames bedencken / ‖ Von der sehr gefehrlichen seuche ‖ der Pestilentz / wie diesel- ‖ be gewiß zuerkennen sey / woher sie entstehe / ‖ auch wie man sich dawieder (vermittelst Göttli- ‖ cher hülff vnd segen) mit der Artzney / vnd sonsten ‖ eusserlichem Wesen / der gebür nach verhalten / ‖ sichern vñ verwaren / In fall aber jemandt ‖ damit begriffen / er deroselben wie- ‖ der vmb entlediget werden ‖ möge. Halberstadt: Georg Koten, 1598

Caspar Kegler
Ein Nützliches vnd ‖ Tröstliches Regiment wider die Pe- ‖ stilentz / vnd gifftig Pestilentzisch Feber / die ‖ Schweißsucht genandt / Vnd sonst mancherley ‖ gifftige vnd tödliche Kranckheit / ‖ Durch ‖ Casparum Kegeler der Artzney Do- ‖ ctorn / weilandt zusammen gebracht / vnd mit ‖ viel tröstlichen Experimenten / Anno 1529. zum ‖ andermal von jhm selber vernewert ‖ vnd gebessert. ‖ Nun aber auffs new / nach dem alten ‖ Exemplar vbersehen vnd corrigiret, vnd in disen ge- ‖ fehrlichen Sterbensleufften mennigklichen ‖ zu Nutz in Druck verfertiget. Leipzig: Abraham Lamberg, 1598

Matthaeus Martini
Außführlicher und Grundlicher Bericht / ‖ DArauß menniglich ‖ vernemen kan / welcher gestaldt ‖ er in gegenwertigen geschwinden ‖ Sterbensleufften… Eisleben: Vartholomaeus Hörnigk, 1598

M. Paulus Nicandrus
Geistliche Praeseruativa, ‖ Das ist / ‖ CHristlicher [sic] ‖ vnterricht auß dem Fünfften ‖ Bußpsalm König Davids / welcher ‖ in der ordnung ist der hundert vnd ander / wie sich ‖ ein Christ in der jetzt schwebenden Pestilentzseuch / vnd ‖ in andern flectenden Kranckheiten verhalten sol / ‖ darmit die Seel vnverletzt bleibe. ‖ Gottseligen Predigern vnd Christen in ‖ diesen gefehrlichen Sterbensleufften / sehr nützlich ‖ zu lesen und zu gebrauchen / In vnterschiedliche ‖ Predigten verfast. Leipzig: Abraham Lamberg, 1598

Johann Rubinger
Ordnung ‖ Zur Praeservation und ‖ Vorsorg jtztiger hin und wider ‖ schwebenden Sterbens- ‖ leufften. ‖ Vor gemeine Stadt und Land ‖ des Kraiß Egers… Hof: Mattheus Pfeilschmidt, 1598

Johann Werner
Bericht / Regiment / vnd ‖ anordnung: ‖ Wie man sich in jtzo ‖ schwebenden sterbens leufften / wider ‖ die Pest praeseruirn oder bewahren: ‖ Vnd da man / durch Gottes willen / von ‖ deroselbigen inficirt oder angesteckt würde / wie man jr ‖ durch vernünfftige Cur / vnd heilsame Mittel bege- ‖ gnen vnd widerstreben sol. Leipzig: (Frantz Schnelboltz), 1598

Anon.
Für die Pestilentz / ‖ Die besten be- ‖ wehrtesten Praservativen ‖ vnnd Curierung / wie sich hiebey ‖ Gesunde vnnd Krancke zuverhalten / ‖ mit Enderung vnd Wählung deß Luffts / mit ‖ Speiß vnnd Tranck / Gebrauch der Artz- ‖ neyen zu den Bewlen / Pestilentzmah- ‖ len / Blutschweren / vnnd dann ‖ zu dero zufällen. ‖ Dem gemeinen Mann bey inn- ‖ stehenden gefährlichen Zeiten der ‖ Pestilentz / von Gelehrten Leuthen zu ‖ gutem gestellet / vnd nun auch ‖ in Truck verfer- ‖ tiget. Steinfurdt in Westphalen: Theophilum Keiser, 1598

Johann Steinmetz
Kurtze / nothwendige vnd Nützliche ‖ Instruction oder Anleitung ‖ Wie sich Reich vnd ‖ Arm / zu diesen gefehrlichen Zeiten / vor ‖ der abschewlichen Seuchen vnd gefehrlichen ‖ Kranckheit der Pestilentz / mit bewehrten ‖ Schutzmitteln bewahren… Leipzig: Frantz Schnelboltz, 1599

Anon.
Kurtzer vnderricht in ‖ Sterbensläuffen. ‖ So wol für kran- ‖ cke Inficierte, als andere Perso- ‖ nen so den Krancken warten sollen / ‖ mit angehenckter Praeseruatif vnnd nüz- ‖ licher vorsehung vor der ‖ Pestilentz. ‖ Menigklichen zu gutem… Munich: Nicolaus Heinricus, 1599

Anon.
Kurtzer vnd gründlicher ‖ Bericht ‖ Wie sich jedermen- ‖ niglich für der erschröckenlichen seu- ‖ che der Pestilentz praeserviren; Auch wie ‖ solche schädliche Kranckheit sampt jhren gifftigen ‖ Beulen vnd Blattern ordenlich vnd recht ‖ curirt werden soll. (Regensburg: Bartholomeus Gräf), 1599

Hermann Muenster
Alexipharmacum ‖ Das ist ‖ Heylsame Artze- ‖ ney auß den bewerten Sepcie- ‖ bus der Himlischen vnde Irrdischen ‖ Apoteck / wieder das schedtlichen Gifft der Pe- ‖ stilentz zugerichtet / vnd in Fünff ‖ Predigten verfasset / Lemgo, (1600)

Anon.
Eins Erbarn Raths ‖ der Statt Nüremberg / verneute Ge- ‖ setz vnd Ordnung / in gegenwerti- ‖ gen Sterbsläufften diß ‖ M D C. ‖ Jars / auffgericht. Nuremberg: Paul Kauffmann, 1600

Anon.
Kurtzer Bericht / ‖ Was man sich zur ‖ zeit der Sterbensläufft zuverhalten / ‖ die schwere Seuch der Pestilentz durch ‖ Gottes Gnade zuver- ‖ hüten. ‖ Gestellt durch die verordneten ‖ Doctores der Artzney / diser ‖ Statt Nüremberg. Nuremberg: Paul Kauffmann, 1600

Anon.
Kurtzer Bericht / ‖ WAs [sic] man sich zur zeit ‖ der Sterbensläufft zuverhalten / die ‖ schwere Seuch der Pestilentz durch Got- ‖ tes Gnade zuverhüten. ‖ Gestellt durch die verordneten ‖ Doctores der Artzney / diser ‖ Statt Nürnberg. Nuremberg: Balthasar Scherffen, 1600

Georg am Wald
Gemehrter Bericht / ‖ WIe [sic] vnd was gestalt ‖ die new erfundne / vnnd nicht allein in ‖ Teutscher Nation / Sonder auch andern weit auß- ‖ ligenden Ländern / von Sieben vnd Zweintzig Jahren hero / viel ‖ probierte Terra Sigillata am – Waldina / wider die Pestilentz ‖ Zauberisch vnnd andere

empfangne Gifften / Fieber / Schlag / ‖ Fallendtsucht / Freyß... ‖ ...ohne alle gefahr zu ge- ‖ brauchen sey. Stuttgart: Marx Fürstern, 1601

Johann Pontanus (Johann Wittich, ed.)
Iohannis Pontani ‖ DOCTORIS ‖ Einfeltiger vnd gar kur- ‖ tzer bericht / was man in den schweren ‖ Pestilentzischen gebrauchen soll / beydes ‖ zur praeservation vnd curation. 1601

Tobias Dornkrell
Kurtzer / ‖ Doch gründtlicher ‖ vnd vollnkömlicher ‖ Bericht ‖ Von ‖ Der angehen- ‖ der bereit grassirenden Pestilentz ‖ dieses 1603. Jahrs / ‖ Wie sich ein jeder insonderheit / mit Got- ‖ tes hülff dafür bewahren: Oder da jemandt da- ‖ mit behafft ... Hamburg: (Paul Langen) in verlegung M. Frobenij, 1604

Heinrich Decimator
LeichPre- ‖ digten ‖ ZUr [sic] zeit der gras- ‖ sirenden Pestilentz / vnd sonst in aller- ‖ ley anliegen / aus dermassen nützlich zu gebrau- ‖ chen / aus Gottes Wort zusammen gezogen. Magdeburg: Johan Francken, 1606

Maximilian, duke of Bavaria
Von Gottes genaden wir Wilhelm Pfaltzgraue ‖ bey Rhein / Hertzog in Ober vnnd Nidern Bayrn / etc. 1606 Single-leaf broadside

Andreas Pangratius
Geistliche Seelenartzney ‖ Wie man zur Zeit ‖ der schrecklichen Plage der ‖ Pestilentz die Seelen bewaren ‖ vnd Curiren sol. ‖ In welcher die Pest sampt jhren ‖ Vrsachen vnd Zeichen beschrieben / Vnd ‖ wie man bewerte Hülffmittel / aus der heiligen ‖ Schrifft / die Seelen zu beschützen / vnnd ‖ sie zu heilen / finden sol. Leipzig: Johan Rosen Buchhänd. in Vorlegung, 1606

Heinrich Schiller
Von der Pestilentz. ‖ Erster Tractat: ‖ Von den Pesti- ‖ letzischen Funcken / jhrer ‖ Art / Vnderschiedt / Zunder ‖ vnd Schweffel. ‖ I. Vom Regiment oder Lebens-Ord- ‖ nung bey der Pest. ‖ II. Von den Bezoartischen Gifftreibern / ‖ beyde zur Versicherung vnnd zur Hey- ‖ lung. ‖ Ins gemein vnd auch in sonderheit / gegen jetzo an- ‖ schwebende gifftige Seuche / Hanauwischen Ange- ‖ hörigen / zu Vnterricht vnd nutzli- ‖ chem Gebrauch. Hanaw: Johann Halbeyen, 1606

Anon.
Eines E. Rahts der Statt Speyer ‖ Gebott vnd Ordnung ‖ wegen sterbender Lufft. Speyer: Melchior Hartmans seligen hinterlassenen Wittib., 1606

Anon.
Einfeltiger / Kurtzer ‖ BEricht [sic] von der Ab- ‖ scheulichen Seuch der Pestilentz / ‖ wie solche mit der Hilff Gottes nicht allein zu ‖ verhüten / sondern auch zu curirn seye:... Lauingen: Jacob Winter (the princely Pflaz-Graf's Truckerey), 1606

Anon.
Kurtzer vnd sehr nützlicher ‖ Vnterricht / ‖ Von Praeserva- ‖ tion vnnd Curation Mit- ‖ teln / in jetzo eynschleichender Pestilen- ‖ tzischer Seuch / Nothwendig zugebrau- ‖ chen / rc. Von einem berühmbten vnd ‖ erfahrnen Medico zusammen ‖ getragen. Speyer: (gedruckt und verlegt von) Johann Taschner, 1606

Anon.
Kurtzer vnderricht in ‖ Sterbensläuffen. ‖ So wol für kran- ‖ cke inficierte, als andere Perso- ‖ nen / so den Krancken warten sollen / ‖ mit angehenckter Praeservatif vnd nütz- ‖ licher vorsehung vor der ‖ Pestilentz. Munich: Nicolaus Heinricus, 1606

Anon.
Tractätlein ‖ Vnd kurtzer Bericht / ‖ wie man sich in Sterbens Läuf- ‖ fen verhalten / auch durch GOttes [sic] Hülff / vor ‖ dieser bösen Seucht / bewahren / vnd mit ‖ welchen Artzneyen dieselbige zu curiren sey. ‖ Auffs kürtzest vnd fleissigst gestellt / ‖ dessen sich das arme gemeine Volck / im ‖ gantzen Churfürstenthumb Maintz / vnd ‖ andere nechst Benachbarte zu ge- ‖ trösten haben. ‖ Ex mandato Reuerendissimi. Mainz: Johann Albin, 1606

Anon.
Tröstliche vnd andächtige ‖ Geseng vnnd ‖ Gebett / ‖ Zu diesen vorfallenden gefährli- ‖ chen sterbens Läufften bey Gott dem All- ‖ mechtigen vmb linderung der wolver- ‖ dienten straff demütiglich ‖ zu bitten. ‖ Vor die liebe Jugend in den Schulen zu- ‖ sammen gelesen / vnd besonder in ‖ Druck gegeben... Speyer: verlegt durch Johann Taschnern, 1606

Andreas Brentius
Kurtze anordnung / ‖ Wie sich mäñig- ‖ l iche zur zeit der Abschewlichen ‖ Seuch der Pestilentz verhalten: ‖ mit Gottes hülff verwahren: vnd ‖ heylen möge. Amberg: Michael Forstern, 1606?

Christoff Heinrich Ayrer
Regiment vnd ‖ Ordnung / ‖ WIe [sic] sich in den je- ‖ tzigen gefährlichen Zeiten / vor ‖ den zweyen Erschröcklichen Seuchen der Pesti- ‖ lentz / vnd ansteckenten rote Ruhr / zu ver- ‖ wahren / vnd den Krancken mit Artzneyen widerumb zu ‖ helffen. Onolzbach: Paulus Böhem, 1607

W. Budeaus.
D. Guill. Budaei Saxonis anjetzo be- ‖ stallten Stiffts vnd StadtMedici zu ‖ Halberstadt ‖ Gründtlicher Be- ‖ richt vnd Rathsames Be- ‖ dencken / ‖ Von der hochschädlichen vnd ‖ gantz gefährlichen Seuche der Pesti- ‖ lentz / wie dieselbe gewiß zu erkennen sey… Leipzig: Thomae Schürer, 1607

Achilles Gasser
Kurtzer vnd General vnderricht wider die Pestilentz. Augsburg: David Francken, 1607 Single-leaf broadside

Rudolph Goclenius
Weiß vnd Weg / ‖ SIch [sic] for der ‖ schweren Seuche der ‖ Pestilentz / so nun mehr hin vnd wieder ‖ einschleichet / zubewahren / Auch wie denen / so da- ‖ mit beladen / durch darzu dienende Artz- ‖ neyen zu helffen seye / … Marburg: Rudolff Hutwelcker, 1607

Johann Hiltprandus
Ein sehr nutzliche Ordnung ‖ vnd Regiment / ‖ Wie man sich zu ‖ disen jetzigen gefährlichen Zeiten ‖ vor der Pestilentz / welche in Oesterreich ‖ diß Jar / auch vmb vns herumb vnd anderer Or- ‖ then eingerissen / hüten soll / vnnd wie dieselbige zuuer- ‖ treiben vnd zucuriern sey: Jetzt zum andernmal gemeh- ‖ ret vnd gebessert in Truck geben: … [Ingolstat?]: Ederischen Truckerey / druch Andreas Angermayer, 1607

Caspar Kegler (the grandson)
Ein heilsam / nutzbar vndhülffreichs ‖ Regiment ‖ Wieder die Pestilentz vnd das ‖ gifftige Pestilentz Fieber (die Schweissucht ‖ genant) vnd sonsten mancherley gifftige vnd ‖ todtliche Krankheiten / Anfengklich ‖ Durch ‖ Herrn Caspar Keglern / der artzeney Doctorn / weiland ‖ Professoren vnd Physicen zu Leipzig / mit vielen gewissen Exper- ‖ menten zusammen gebracht… Dresden: Christian Bergen, 1607

Johann Malsius
Ein Christliches demütiges Gebet / aus Gottes Wort ‖ zusammen getragen / vnd sonderlich auff das Hertzrühende Gebet des Propheten Danielis ‖ Cap. 9. gerichtet / wider die Seuch der Pestilentz / Allen andechtigen vnd einfeltigen ‖ Christen / sonderlich aber den betrübten Jacobiten / als seinen lieben Pfarkindern ‖ vnnd Zuhörern vorgeschrieben / ‖ Durch ‖ Iohannem Malsium Diac. zu S. Jacob. Magdeburg: Salomon Richtzenhan, 1607

Johann Malsius
Ein kurtzer vnterricht ‖ aus Gottes Wort / Wie man in ‖ Sterbensluefften sich Christlich ‖ verhalten soll. Magdeburg: Salomon Richtzenhan, 1607 Single-leaf broadside

Christoph Meurer
Kurtz vnd nützlich ‖ Haußregiment / ‖ Darinnen gründtlichen vermeldet vnd an- ‖ gezeiget wird / Wie ein Haußvater sich vnd sein Gesind vor der schrecklichen Seuche der Pestilentz hüten sol / Oder / So je- ‖ mandes von derselben angriffen / Wie jhm zu rettung seines Lebens vermit- ‖ tels Göttlicher Gnaden zu helffen / Vnd da auch letzlichen eines oder mehr aus ‖ einem Hause gestorben / das es nicht weiter einreisse / vnd fer- ‖ ner mehr schaden thun möge. Leipzig: in verlegung Abraham Lamberg, 1607

Martin Ruland
LOIMAGOGVS ‖ Kurtzer vnd doch ge- ‖ grundter Vnterricht Regiments vnd Ord- ‖ nunge / wie man sich in jetzt grassierenden Pestilentz leufften ‖ ten verhalten / praeserviren / vnd wie man ‖ solche eigentlich erkennen ‖ soll: ‖ Auch wie dieselbige / so man damit behafft / ‖ durch hülff des Allmechtigen / vnnd durch die dar zu von ‖ GOtt [sic] verordneten Mittel abgewendet ‖ werden mag. Leipzig: Valentin am Ende (in vorlegung Jacob Apels, Buchhändler), 1607

Bonifacius Sauter
Regiment / ver- ‖ hütung vnd Curation, der ‖ erschröcklichen Kranckheit ‖ der Pestis. ‖ Zu Nutz vnd Nachrichtung / ‖ Den Edlen / Ehrnvesten / ... Munich: Nicolaus Henricus, 1607

Matthais Untzer

Kurtzer und einfältiger doch nützlicher und nothwendiger Bericht Von der Pestilentz / Darin nicht allein gründlichen un außführlichen vermeldt un angezeiget wird / was die Pest sey / woher sie eigentlich entspringe / und wo bey sie soll erkandt werden / sonder auch wie vor derselbe beydes Reiche und Arm / Manns un Frawenspersonen / junge Kinder / und schwangere Frawen mit Artzneyen sich praeserviren und verwahren... Hall in Sachsen: Erasmum Hynitzsch, 1607

Anon.
Bericht: ‖ WIe [sic] man sich inn ‖ vorstehendē Pestilentz ‖ zeiten mit Artzeneyen / so in Holtzwir- ‖ tischer Apotecken zu finden / verwah- ‖ ren soll. Hall in Saxony: Erasmus Harnitzsch, 1607

Anon.
Kurtzer Bericht / ‖ Wie die Artzneyen / ‖ welchen in vorstehender sterbens ge- ‖ fahr / alheir zu Wittenberg / in der ‖ Apotheken angeordnet / ‖ Nützlich mit Gottes hülff zu ge- ‖ brauchen sind. Wittenberg: (Martin Henckel) / In verlegung Paul Helwigs Buchführers, 1607

Anon.
Kurtzer Bericht / ‖ Wie man sich in ‖ Sterbensleufften verhal- ‖ ten / vnd was man im fall der noth gebrauchen soll: ‖ Gestellet ‖ Durch die Medicos zu Heydelberg. Heidelberg, 1607

Anon.
Kurtzer Nützlicher ‖ vnd Nötiger Bericht / Wie man die Me- ‖ dicamenta praeservativa curativa Pestis, so Anno ‖ 97. auff des Raths Apoteken der Alten Stadt Mag- ‖ deburgk verordnet / vnnd jtzo dieses 1607. Jahrs ‖ aus Befehl eines Erbarn Raths von jhren ver- ‖ ordneten Medicins revidirt vnd verbessert / ‖ gebrauchen sol. (Magdeburg): Ambrosius Kirchner (Salomon Kichtzenhan), 1607

Anon.
Kurtze PestOrdnung / vnd ‖ Verzeichnuß der Artzneyen / welche von den ‖ Medicis alhie angeordnet auff der Apoteken in der Heinrichstadt zu finden / vnd ‖ in bevorstehender Sterbens gefahr / mit Gottes Hülffe können nützlich gebraucht werden. Wolffenbüttel, 1607 Single-leaf broadside

Anon.
Kurtzer vnd Notdürfftiger ‖ Vnterricht / ‖ Wie man bey vor ‖ stehen der erschrecklichen Pestilens ‖ Zeit / mit göttlicher Hülffe / sich durch ordentliche ‖ Mittel verwahren / vnd in der Curation ‖ verhalten möge. ‖ Allen begierigen Leuten zu Hülff vnd Trost:... Jena: Johann Weidner, 1607

Anon.
Kurtzer vnderricht in ‖ Sterbensläuffen. ‖ So wol für kran- ‖ cke inficierte, als andere Perso- ‖ nen / so den Krancken warten sollen / ‖ mit angehenckter Praeservatif vnd nutz- ‖ licher Vorsehung vor der ‖ Pestilentz. Munich: Nicolaus Heinricus, 1607

Anon.
Ordnung ‖ Eines Erbarn Hochweisen ‖ Raths der Stadt Leipzig... Leipzig: Michael Lantzenberger, 1607

Bibliography

Manuscript sources

Stadtarchiv Leipzig

Richterstube Inventarien und Hilfsbuch
Ratsbuch Bd. 7
Ratsbuch Bd. 8
Ratsbuch Bd. 9
Tit. XLIV B Nr. 3 (F)
Tit. XLIV B Nr. 4 (F)

Universitätsarchiv Leipzig

Film 538, Nr. 80

Sächsische Landes- und Universitätsbibliothek Dresden

B201

Kantonsbibliothek St. Gallen

VadSlg. Ms. 455

Printed primary sources (works not included in Appendix 2)

Alexander Seitz Sämtliche Schriften, 3 Vols., Ed. Peter Ukena. Berlin: Walter de Gruyter, 1975.

Apoteck für den gmeynē man. der die Ertzte zuersuchen. am gůt nict vermügens / oder sonst in der not allwege nicht erraychen kan. Augsburg?: Heinrich Stainer?, 1530?

Apoteck für den gmeynen Mann / der die Artzte zuersůchen am gůt nicht vermag / oder sunst in der not allwegen nit erreychen kan. Fleissig Corrugieret / vnd mit vil gůten stücken gemehret. Marburg: Kleeblat, 1560.

Apoteck für den gemeinen Mann… Erfurt: Singe, 1619.

Baierland, Ortolf von. *Arzneibuch*. Nuremberg: Anton Koberger, 1477.

Brunschwig, Hieronymus. *Hauß apoteck. Zu yeden leibs gebresten für den gemainen man[n] und dz arm Landvolck*. Augsburg: Stainer, 1545.

— *Haußarmen Schatz. Gute gebreuchliche vn- bewerte Artzneien / zu Allerhandt gebrechen des gantzen Leibs / Für den gemeinen Mann insonderheit / so die Apotecken nit erreychen / oder die Artzte zuersuchen am gut nicht vermag / gestellt vnd mit fleiß zusamen getragen / jetzt von newem in truck verfertigt.* Frankfurt, 1568.

Compendium de epidemia, Ed. H. Emile Rebouis. Paris: Alphonse Picard, 1888.

D. Martin Luthers Werke: Kritische Gesammtausgabe, 72 vols. Weimar: Hermann Böhlau, 1883.

D'Agramont, Jacme. Regiment de Preservacio a Epidemia o Pestilencia e Mortaldats, Trans. C.-E. A. Winslow and M. L. Duran-Reynals, *Bulletin of the History of Medicine* 23 (1949): 57–89.

Die Messkataloge des sechzehnten Jahrhunderts, Vol. V. Hildesheim: Georg Olms Verlag, 1972.

Dr. Martin Luthers Sämmtliche Schriften, Ed. Johann Georg Walch, Vol. XXI, Pt. 2, *Dr. Luthers Briefe*. St. Louis: Concordia Publishing, 1904.

Dryander, Johannes, Ed., *Opusculum praeclarum de omni Pestilentia, sive sit ab aere corrupto, sive ab aquis putridis, aut a cadaveribus: & de diuturna peste morbi Gallici...* Cologne, 1537.

E. E. Hochweisen Raths der Stadt Leipzig Verneuerte und verbesserte Ordnung / Wie es bey besorgenden ansteckenden Seuchen / da GOtt [sic] *dergleichen über diese Stadt verhängen sollte / ...* Leipzig: Christoph Günther, 1680.

Ellenbog, Ulrich. *Von den gifftigen besen Tempffen und Reuchen*, Eds. Franz Koelsch and Friedrich Zoepfl. Munich: Verlag der Münchner Drucke, 1927.

Erasmus, Desiderius. *Collected Works of Erasmus*, Vol. XXIX, Eds. Elaine Fanthan and Erika Rummel. Toronto: University of Toronto Press, 1989.

Folz, Hans. *Die Reimpaarsprüche*, Ed. Hanns Fischer. Munich: C. H. Beck, 1961.

Guaineri, Antonio. [*De peste; de venenis*]. Venice: Reynaldus de Novimagio, 1487?

Girtanner, Christoph. *Abhandlung über die venerischen Krankheit*, Vol. II. Göttingen: Johann Christian Dieterich, 1793.

Herbarius Moguntinus (or) *[R]ogatu plurimo[rum] inopu[m] num[m]o[rum] egentiu[m] appotecas refuta[n]tiu[m] occasione illa, q[uia] necessaria ibide[m] ad corp[us] egru[m] specta[n]tia su[n]t cara simplicia et composita...* Mainz: Peter Schöffer, 1484.

Jacobi, Joannes. *Ad honore[m] sancte & i[n]diuidue trinitatis, gloriosq[ue] virginis marie & ad utlititatem rei publice, pro [con]seruatione sano[rum] ac reformatione lapsorum...* Nuremberg: Conrad Zeninger, ca. 1482.

Jung, Ambrosius. *Tractatulus perutilis de pestilentia ex diuersis auctoribus aggregatus...* Augsburg: Hans Schönsperger, 1494.

Luther's Works, Vol. LIV, *Table Talk*, Trans. Theodore G. Tappert. Philadelphia: Fortress Press, 1967.

Manlius, Johannes. *LOCORVM communium collectanea: A IOHANNE MANLIO per multos annos, tum ex Lectionibus D. PHILIPPI MELANCHTONIS, tum ex aliorum doctissimorum virorum relationibus excerpta, & nuper in odinem ab eodem redacta, iamque postremum recognita.* 1572.

Moran, Bruce T. "The Herbarius of Paracelsus," *Pharmacy in History* 39 (1993): 99–128.

Müller, Ernst. *Leipziger Neubürgerliste 1502–1556*, Vol. I, Ed. Annelore Franke. Leipzig: Stadtarchiv Leipzig, 1982.

[Pestblatt], Augsburg: s.n., ca. 1473.

Pieper, Wilhelm. *Ulrich Rülein von Calw und sein Bergbüchlein: Mit Urtext-Faksimile und Übertragnung des Bergbüchleins von etwa 1500 und Faksimile der Pestschrift von 1521*. Berlin: Akademie Verlag, 1955.

PRAESIDE IOHANNE HERMANNO ARTIS MEDICAE DOCTORE, AD SEQVENtes [sic] *propositiones pro Licentia in arte Medica consequenda, respondebunt honesti ac docti Viri. Ad Priores XLI. (DE FLVXIONIBVS ALVI) MAGISTER CLEMENS CHELNERVS ISLEBIENSIS. Ad Posteriores et Practicas. (CVRATIO FLVXIONVM ALVI.) MAGISTER ERNESTVS REVCHLINVS GEVSINGIVS Die primo Octobris. Anno 1563*. Wittenberg: Jakob Lucius, 1563.

Rebouis, H. Emile. *Etude historique et critique sur la peste*. Paris: Alphonse Picard, 1888.

Rhegius, Urbanus. *Underricht Wie ain Christenmensch got seinem herren teglich beichten soll Doctoris Urbani Regij Thůmpredigers zů Augspurg rc. M.D.XXI.* Augsburg: Silvanum Ottmar, 1521.

— *Geystlich ärtzney für gesund vnd krancken zů disen gefärlichen zeyten gemert vnd gebessert*. Augsburg: Alexander Weyssenhorn, 1530.

Ryff, Walther Hermann. *Warhafftige / künstliche / gerechte vnderweisung vnnd anzeygung Alle Latwergen / Confect / Conseruen / einbeytzungen vnd einmachungen / von mancherley früchten / blůmen / kreütern vnnd wurtzeln / sampt andern künstlichen vnd anmütigen stucken / wie solche in den Apotecken gemacht*. 1542.

Sender, Clemens, Ed. *Die Chroniken der deutschen Städte vom 14. bis ins 16. Jahrhundert*, Vol. XXIII. Leipzig: Verlag von S. Hirzel, 1894.

Sonnemann, Andreas. *Elegia ad clarissimum & integerrimum virum, D. Ernestum Reuchlinum Geusingensem ordinarium medicus veteris Marchiae...* Wittenberg: Laurentus Schwenk, 1564.

Spengler, Lazarus. *Lazarus Spengler Schriften*, Vol. I., Eds. Berndt Hamm and Wolfgang Huber. Gütersloh: Gütersloher Verlagshaus, 1995.

Stahleder, Helmuth. *Chronik der Stadt München*, Vol. II, *Belastungen und Bedrückungen: Die Jahre 1506–1705*. Ebenhausen: Dölling und Galitz Verlag, 2005.

Stepner, Salomon. *Leipzigische Lorbeer-Blätter / das ist Alte und neue denckwürdige Uberschrifften / Grab- und Gedächtniß-Mahle...* Leipzig: Lanckischen Buchladen, 1690.

Sudhoff, Karl. "Pestschriften aus den ersten 150 Jahren nach der Epidemie des 'schwarzen Todes' 1348," I–XX, *Archiv für Geschichte der Medizin* 4, 5, 6, 7, 8, 9, 11, 14, 16, 17 (1911–1925).

Theophrast von Hohenheim gen. Paracelsus Sämtliche Werke, 14 Vols., Ed. Karl Sudhoff. Munich: Otto Wilhelm Barth, 1922–33.

Verzeichnis der im deutschen Sprachbereich erschienenen Drucke des XVI. Jahrhunderts, 25 Vols. Stuttgart: Anton Hiersemann, 1983–2000.

Vochs, Johann. *De pestilentia Anni p[raese]ntis et ei[us] cura*. Magdeburg, 1507.

Winslow, C.-E. A., and M. L. Duran-Reynals, Trans., "Texts and Documents. Regiment de Preservacio a Epidemia o Pestilencia e Mortaldats," *Bulletin of the History of Medicine* 23 (1949): 57–89.

Woodcut, Nuremberg: Dürer School, ca. 1505.

Wustmann, Gustav, Ed., *Quellen zur Geschichte Leipzigs*, Vol. I. Leipzig: Duncker & Humblot, 1889.

Zedler, Johann Heinrich. *Grosses völlständiges Universal-Lexicon*, Vol. E (VIII). Halle: J. H. Zedler, 1734.

Secondary sources

Allgemeine Deutsche Biographie, 56 Vols. Leipzig, 1875–1912.

Arber, Agnes. *Herbals, Their Origin and Evolution: A Chapter in the History of Botany 1470–1670*, 2nd Edn. Cambridge: Cambridge University Press, 1938.

Arrizabalaga, Jon. "Facing the Black Death: Perceptions and Reactions of University Medical Practitioners," in *Practical Medicine from Salerno to the Black Death*, Eds. Luis Garcia-Ballester, Roger French, Jon Arrizabalaga, and Andrew Cunningham: 237–288. Cambridge: Cambridge University Press, 1994.

Arrizabalaga, Jon, John Henderson, and Roger French. *The Great Pox: The French Disease in Renaissance Europe*. New Haven, CT: Yale University Press, 1997.

Assion, Peter. "Geistliche und weltliche Heilkunst in Konkurrenz," in *Bayerisches Jahrbuch für Volkskunde 1976/77*: 7–23. Würzburg: Kommissionsverlag Karl Hart, 1978.

— "Ambrosius Jung," in *Die deutsche Literatur des Mittelalters, Verfasserlexikon*, Vol. IV, Ed. Kurt Ruh: 905–907. Berlin: Walter de Gruyter, 1983.

Baker, Patrick. *Italian Renaissance Humanism in the Mirror*. Cambridge: Cambridge University Press, 2015.

Baldwin, Martha. "Danish Medicines for the Danes and the Defense of Indigenous Medicines," in *Reading the Book of Nature: The Other Side of the Scientific Revolution*, Eds. Allen G. Debus and Michael T. Walton: 163–180. Kirksville, MO: Sixteenth Century Journal Publishers, 1998.

Barkai, Ron. "Jewish Treatises on the Black Death (1350–1500): A Preliminary Study," in *Medicine from the Black Death to the French Disease*, Eds. Roger French, Jon Arrizabalaga, Andrew Cunningham, and Luis García-Ballester: 6–25. Aldershot, UK: Ashgate, 1998.

Barnes, Robin Bruce. *Prophecy and Gnosis: Apocalypticism in the Wake of the Lutheran Reformation*. Stanford, CA: Stanford University Press, 1988.

—"Astrology and the Confessions in the Empire, c. 1550–1620," in *Confessionalization in Europe, 1555–1700*, Eds. John M. Headley, Hans J. Hillerbrand, and Anthony J. Papalas: 131–153. Aldershot, UK: Ashgate, 2004.

Barrera, Antonio. "Local Herbs, Global Medicines: Commerce, Knowledge, and Commodities in Spanish America," in *Merchants and Marvels: Commerce, Science, and Art in Early Modern Europe*, Eds. Pamela H. Smith and Paula Findlen: 163–181. New York: Routledge, 2002.

Baumann, Brigitte, and Helmut Baumann. *Die Mainzer Kräuterbuch-Inkunabeln: Herbarius Moguntinus, Gart der Gesundheit, Hortus Sanitatis*. Stuttgart: Anton Hiersemann, 2010.

Behrend, Fr. J., Ed. *Archiv für Syphilis und Hautkrankheiten*, Vol. I. Berlin: August Hirschwald, 1846.

Behringer, Wolfgang. "Weather, Hunger and Fear: Origins of the European Witch-Hunts in Climate, Society and Mentality," *German History* 13 (1995): 1–27.

— *Witchcraft Persecutions in Bavaria*, Trans. J. C. Grayson and David Lederer. Cambridge: Cambridge University Press, 1997.

—"Die Krise von 1570: Ein Beitrag zur Krisengeschichte der Neuzeit," in *Um Himmels Willen: Religion in Katastrophenzeiten*, Eds. Manfred Jakubowski- Tiessen and Hartmut Lehmann: 51–156. Göttingen: Vandenhoeck & Ruprecht, 2003.

Benedictow, Ole J. *The Black Death, 1346–1353: The Complete History*. Woodbridge, UK: Boydell Press, 2004.

Berger, Beate, Bodo Gronemann, and Jakuf Pacer. *Vom Aderlass zum Gesundheitspass: Zeittafel zur Geschichte d. öfftentl. Gesundheitswesens in Leipzig*. Leipzig: Leipziger Universitätsverlag, 2000.

Biereye, Johannes. *Erfurt in seinen berühmten Persönlichkeiten*. Erfurt: Stenger, 1937.

Biraben, Jean-Noël. *Les hommes et la peste en France et dans les pays européenes et méditerranéens*, 2 Vols. Paris: Moulton, 1975–76.

Boeckl, Christine M. *Images of Plague and Pestilence: Iconography and Iconology*. Kirksville, MO: Truman State University Press, 2000.

Boettcher, Susan R. "The Social Impact of the Lutheran Reformation in Germany," in *Lutheran Ecclesiastical Culture, 1550–1675*, Ed. Robert Kolb: 305–359. Leiden: Brill, 2008.

Bonorand, Conradin. *Vadians Humanistenkorrespondenz mit Schülern und Freunden aus seiner Wiener Zeit: Personenkommentar 1–4 zum Vadianischen Briefwerk*. St. Gallen: Verlagsgemeinschaft St. Gallen, 1988.

Breher, Anton. *Der Memminger Stadtarzt Ulrich Ellenbog und seine Pestschriften*. Kempten: Oechelhäuser, 1942.

Breuer, Dieter. *Oberdeutsche Literatur 1565–1650: Deutsche Literaturgeschichte und Territorialgeschichte in frühabsolutischer Zeit*. Munich: Beck, 1979.

Brevart, Francis B. "Between Medicine, Magic and Religion: Wonder Drugs in German Medico-Pharmaceutical Treatises of the Thirteenth to the Sixteenth Centuries," *Speculum* 83 (2008): 1–57.

Bröer, Rald, and Ralf Hofheinz. "Gesundheitspädagogik statt Tröstung: Die theologische Bewältigung von Krankheit bei Philipp Melanchthon und Caspar Peucer," *Sudhoffs Archiv* 85 (2001): 18–44.

Brown, Christopher Boyd. *Singing the Gospel: Lutheran Hymns and the Success of the Reformation*. Cambridge, MA: Harvard University Press, 2005.

Brunner, Otto. "Das 'ganze Haus' und die alteuropäische 'Ökonomik,'" in *Neue Wege der Sozialgeschichte: Vorträge und Aufsätze*: 33–61. Göttingen: Vandenhoeck & Ruprecht, 1956.

Bulst, Neithard. "Die Pest verstehen: Wahrnehmungen, Deutungen und Reaktionen im Mittelalter und in der Frühen Neuzeit," in *Naturkatastrophen: Zu ihrer Wahrnehmung, Deutung und Darstellung von der Antike bis ins 20. Jahrhundert*, Ed. Dieter Groh: 145–164. Tübingen: Gunter Narr Verlag, 2003.

Burke, Peter. *Popular Culture in Early Modern Europe*. New York: New York University Press, 1978.

Burke, Peter, and R. Po-chia Hsia, Eds. *Cultural Translation in Early Modern Europe*. Cambridge: Cambridge University Press, 2007.

Burmeister, Karl Heinz. *Achilles Pirmin Gasser 1505–1577*, Vol III. Wiesbaden: Guido Pressler, 1975.

Cameron, Euan. *The European Reformation*, 2nd Edn. Oxford: Oxford University Press, 2012.

Carmichael, Ann G. "Universal and Particular: The Language of Plague, 1350–1500," in *Pestilential Complexities: Understanding Medieval Plague*, Ed. Vivian Nutton: 17–52. London: Wellcome Trust Center, 2008.

Chase, Melissa P. "Fevers, Poisons, and Apostemes: Authority and Experience in Montpellier Plague Treatises," in *Science and Technology in Medieval Society*, Ed. Pamela O. Long: 153–171. New York: New York Academy of Sciences, 1985.

Chrisman, Miriam. *Lay Culture, Learned Culture: Books and Social Change in Strasbourg, 1480–1599*. New Haven, CT: Yale University Press, 1982.

— *Conflicting Visions of Reform: German Lay Propaganda Pamphlets, 1519–1530*. Atlantic Highlands, NJ: Humanities Press, 1996.

Claus, Helmut. *Das Leipziger Druckschaffen der Jahre 1518–1539: Kurztitelverzeichnis*. Gotha: Forschungsbibliothek Gotha, 1987.

Clemen, Otto. "Johannes Reusch von Eschenbach: Humanist, Theolog, Mediziner," *Neues Archiv für Sächsische Geschichte* 21 (1900): 111–145.

— "Zur Lebensgeschichte Heinrich Stromers von Auerbach," *Neues Archiv für sächsische Geschichte* 24 (1903): 100–110.

— "Zur Literatur über den englischen Schweiß von 1529," *Archiv für Geschichte der Medizin* 15 (1923): 85–97.

Cohn, Samuel K., Jr. *Cultures of Plague: Medical Thinking at the End of the Renaissance*. Oxford: Oxford University Press, 2010.

Collins, David J. *Reforming Saints: Saints' Lives and Their Authors in Germany, 1470–1530*. Oxford: Oxford University Press, 2008.

Cook, Harold J. *Matters of Exchange: Commerce, Medicine, and Science in the Dutch Golden Age*. New Haven, CT: Yale University Press, 2007.

Cooper, Alix. *Inventing the Indigenous: Local Knowledge and Natural History in Early Modern Europe*. Cambridge: Cambridge University Press, 2007.

Coste, Joël. *Représentations et comportements en temps d'épidémie dans la littérature imprimée de peste (1490–1725)*. Paris: Editions Champion, 2007.

Crawshaw, Jane L. Stevens. *Plague Hospitals: Public Health for the City in Early Modern Venice*. Farnham, UK: Ashgate, 2012.

Crisciani, Chiara, and Michela Pereira. "Black Death and Golden Remedies: Some Remarks on Alchemy and the Plague," in *The Regulation of Evil: Social and Cultural Attitudes to Epidemics in the Late Middle Ages*, Eds. Agostino Paravicini Bagliani and Francesco Santi: 7–39. Sismel, Belgium: Edizioni del Galluzzo, 1998.

Cunningham, Andrew, and Ole Peter Grell. *The Four Horsemen of the Apocalypse: Religion, War, Famine and Death in Reformation Europe*. Cambridge: Cambridge University Press, 2000.

Curth, Louise Hill. *English Almanacs, Astrology and Popular Medicine: 1550–1700*. Manchester: Manchester University Press, 2007.

Dannenfeldt, Karl H. "The Introduction of a New Sixteenth-Century Drug: 'Terra Silesiaca,'" *Medical History* 28 (1984): 174–188.

— "Wittenberg Botanists during the Sixteenth Century," in *The Social History of the Reformation*, Eds. Lawrence P. Buck and Jonathan W. Zophy: 223–248. Columbus, OH: Ohio State University Press, 1972.

Deason, Gary B. "Reformation Theology and the Mechanistic Conception of Nature," in *God and Nature: Historical Essays on the Encounter between Christianity and Science*, Eds. David C. Lindberg and Ronald L. Numbers: 167–191. Berkeley, CA: University of California Press, 1986.

De Waardt, Hans. "Chasing Demons and Curing Mortals: The Medical Practice of Clerics in the Netherlands," in *The Task of Healing: Medicine, Religion and Gender in England and the Netherlands, 1450–1800*, Eds. Hilary Marland and Margaret Pelling: 171–203. Rotterdam: Erasmus Publishing, 1996.

Dicke, Gerd. "Heinrich Steinhöwel," in *Die deutsche Literatur des Mittelalters: Verfasserlexikon*, Vol. IX: 258–278. Berlin: Walter de Gruyter, 1995.

Dienel, Sigrid. *Die Pestschrift des schlesischen Arztes Heinrich Cunitz (1580–1625) aus dem Jahr 1625: Ein zeitgenössisches medizin-pharmazeutisches Dokument? Eine vergleichende Untersuchung mit Pestschriften aus dem 16. und 17. Jahrhundert*. Munich: Technischen Universität München, 2000.

Dinges, Martin. "Süd-Nord-Gefälle in der Pestbekämpfung: Italien, Deutschland und England im Vergleich," in *Das europäische Gesundheitssystem: Gemeinsamkeiten und Unterschiede in historischer Perspektive*, Eds. Wolfgang U. Eckart and Robert Jütte: 19–51. Stuttgart: Steiner, 1994.

Dinzelbacher, Peter. "Die tötende Gottheit: Pestbild und Todesikonographie als Ausdruck der Mentalität des Spätmittelalters und der Renaissance," in *Zeit, Tod und Ewigkeit in der Renaissance Literatur*, Vol. II: 5–138. Salzburg: Universität Salzburg, 1986.

Dormeier, Heinrich. "Laienfrömmigkeit in den Pestzeiten des 15./16. Jahrhunderts," in *Maladies et Société (XIIe–XVIIIe siècles)*, Eds. Neithard Bulst and Robert Delort: 269–306. Paris: Centre National de la Recherche Scientifique, 1989.

— "Die Flucht vor der Pest als religiöses Problem," in *Laienfrommigkeit im späten Mittelalter*, Ed. Klaus Schreiner: 331–397. Munich: R. Oldenburg Verlag, 1992.

— "'Ein geystliche ertzeney fur die grausam erschrecklich pestilentz': Schutzpatrone und frommer Abwehrzauber gegen die Pest," in *Das große Sterben: Seuchen machen Geschichte*, Eds. Hans Wilderotter and Michael Dorrmann: 54–93. Berlin: Jovis, 1995.

— "Pestepidemien und Frömmigkeitsformen in Italien und Deutschland (14.–16. Jahrhundert)," in *Um Himmels Willen: Religion in Katastrophenzeiten*, Eds. Manfred Jakubowski-Tiessen and Hartmut Lehmann: 14–50. Göttingen: Vandenhoeck & Ruprecht, 2003.

Döring, Thomas. "Der Buchdruck in Leipzig zu Lebzeiten Luthers," in *Luther und Leipzig: Beiträge und Katalog zur Ausstellung*, Eds. Ekkehard Henschke and Klaus Sohl: 25–50. Leipzig: Universitätsbibliothek Leipzig, 1996.

Duden, Barbara. *Geschichte unter der Haut: Ein Eisenacher Arzt und seine Patientinnen um 1730*. Stuttgart: Klett-Cotta, 1987.

Eamon, William. "Alchemy in Popular Culture: Leonardo Fioravanti and the Search for the Philosopher's Stone," *Early Science and Medicine* 5 (2000): 196–213.

— *Science and the Secrets of Nature: Books of Secrets in Medieval and Early Modern Culture*. Princeton, NJ: Princeton University Press, 1994.

Eckert, Edward A. *The Structure of Plagues and Pestilences in Early Modern Europe: Central Europe, 1560–1640*. Basel: Karger, 1996.

— "The Retreat of Plague from Central Europe, 1640–1720: A Geomedical Approach," *Bulletin of the History of Medicine* 74 (2000): 1–28.

Effra, Hans Martin von. "Christus als Arzt," in *Reallexikon zur deutschen Kunstgeschichte*, Vol. III, Eds. Ernst Gall and L. H. Heydenreich: 639–643. Stuttgart: Alfred Druckenmueller, 1953.

Eire, Carlos. *War against the Idols: The Reformation of Worship from Erasmus to Calvin*. Cambridge: Cambridge University Press, 1986.

— "Early Modern Catholic Piety in Translation," in *Cultural Translation in Early Modern Europe*, Eds. Peter Burke and R. Po-chia Hsia: 83–100. Cambridge: Cambridge University Press, 2007.

Eisenstein, Elizabeth. *The Printing Press as an Agent of Change: Communications and Cultural Transformations in Early-Modern Europe*, Vol. II. Cambridge: Cambridge University Press, 1979.

Eisermann, Falk. "Leipziger Einblattdrucke des 15. Jahrhunderts," in *Bücher, Drucker, Bibliotheken in Mitteldeutschland*, Ed. Enno Bünz: 373–400. Leipzig: Leipziger Universitätsverlag, 2006.

Esser, Thilo. *Pest, Heilangst und Frömmigkeit: Studien zur religiösen Bewältigung der Pest am Ausgang des Mittelalters*. Altenberge: Oros, 1999.

— "Die Pest: Strafe Gottes oder Naturphänomen? Eine frömmigkeits-geschichtliche Untersuchung zu Pesttraktaten des 15. Jahrhunderts," *Zeitschrift für Kirchengeschichte* 108 (1997): 32–57.

Fabbri, Christiane Nockels. "Continuity and Change in Late Medieval Plague Medicine." Ph.D. thesis, Yale University, 2006.

— "Treating Medieval Plague: The Wonderful Virtues of Theriac," *Early Science and Medicine* 12 (2007): 247–283.

Feldhay, Rivka. "Religion," in *The Cambridge History of Science*, Vol. III, *Early Modern Science*, Eds. Katharine Park and Lorraine Daston: 727–755. Cambridge: Cambridge University Press, 2006.

Feuerstein-Herz, Petra. "Im Druck der Seuchen: Seuchen und Buchdruck in der Frühen Neuzeit am Beispiel der Bestände der Herzog August Bibliothek," in *Gotts verhengnis und seine strafe: Zur Geschichte der Seuchen in der Frühen Neuzeit*: 27–36. Wolfenbüttel: Herzog August Bibliothek, 2005.

Findlen, Paula, and Pamela H. Smith. "Commerce and the Representation of Nature in Art and Science," in *Merchants and Marvels: Commerce, Science, and Art in Early Modern Europe*, Eds. Pamela H. Smith and Paula Findlen: 1–25. New York: Routledge, 2002.

Fischer, Gerhard. *Aus zwei Jahrhunderten Leipziger Handelsgeschichte 1470–1650*. Leipzig: Felix Meiner, 1929.

Flamm, Heinz. *Die ersten Infektions- oder Pest-Ordnungen in den österreichischen Erblanden, im Fürstlichen Erzstift Salzburg und im Innviertel im 16. Jahrhundert*. Vienna: Verlag der Österreichischen Akademie der Wissenschaften, 2008.

Fleischmann, Josef. "Die Ärztefamilie Jung," *Lebensbilder aus dem Bayerischen Schwaben* 4 (1955): 14–43.

Flood, John L. "'Safer on the Battlefield than in the City': England, the 'Sweating Sickness', and the Continent," *Renaissance Studies* 17 (2003): 147–176.

Flood, John L., and David J. Shaw. *Johannes Sinapius (1505–1560): Hellenist and Physician in Germany and Italy*. Geneva: Droz, 1997.

Forbes, Robert James. *Short History of the Art of Distillation*. Leiden: Brill, 1970.

Forster, Marc R. "With and without Confessionalization: Varieties of Early Modern German Catholicism," *Journal of Early Modern History* 1 (1998): 315–343.

Franz, Gunther. *Huberinus-Rhegius-Holbein: Bibliographische und druckgeschichtliche Untersuchung der verbreitesten Trost- und Erbauungsschriften des 16. Jahrhunderts*. Nieuwkoop, Netherlands: B. De Graff, 1973.

Friedrich, Christoph, and Wolf-Dieter Müller-Jahncke. *Rudolf Schmitz: Geschichte der Pharmazie*, Vol. II, *Von der Frühen Neuzeit bis zur Gegenwart*. Eschborn: Govi, 2005.

Gemert, Guillaume van. "Tridentische Geistigkeit und Moraldidaxis in Guarinonius' 'Greweln': Der Artzt als geistlicher Autor," in *Hippolytus Guarinonius im interkulturellen Kontext seiner Zeit: Acta der Tagung Neustift 1993*, Ed. Elmar Locher: 45–63. Bolzano: Edition Sturzflüge, 1995.

Gentilcore, David. *Healers and Healing in Early Modern Italy*. Manchester: Manchester University Press, 1998.

Gnann, Martin. "Populäres Heilen im kulturellen Umfeld der Vormoderne." Ph.D. thesis, Eberhard-Karls-Universität Tübingen, 1994.

Grell, Ole Peter, and Andrew Cunningham, Eds. *Medicine and the Reformation*. London: Routledge, 1993.

Gruner, Christian Gottfried. *Scriptores de sudore anglico superstites*. Jena: Sumtibus Friderici Maukii, 1847.

Habermas, Rebekka. "Wunder, Wunderliches, Wunderbares: Zur Profanisierung eines Deutungsmusters in der Frühen Neuzeit," in *Armut, Liebe, Ehre: Studien zur historischen Kulturforschung*, Ed. Richard van Dülmen: 38–66. Frankfurt: Fischer Taschenbuch Verlag, 1988.

Hackenberg, Michael R. "Private Book Ownership in Sixteenth-Century German-Language Areas." Ph.D. thesis, University of California, Berkeley, 1983.

Hamm, Berndt. *The Reformation of Faith in the Context of Late Medieval Theology and Piety*, Ed. Robert J. Bast. Leiden: Brill, 2004.

Hammond, Mitchell Lewis. "Medicine and Pastoral Care for the Dying in Protestant Germany," in *Ways of Knowing: Ten Interdisciplinary Essays*, Ed. Mary Lindemann: 113–136. Boston: Brill, 2004.

— "Contagion, Honor, and Urban Life in Early Modern Germany," in *Imagining Contagion in Early Modern Europe*, Ed. Claire Carlin: 94–106. New York: Palgrave Macmillan, 2005.

Harkness, Deborah E. *The Jewel House: Elizabethan London and the Scientific Revolution*. New Haven, CT: Yale University Press, 2007.

Harrington, Joel F. *Reordering Marriage and Society in Reformation Germany*. Cambridge: Cambridge University Press, 1995.

Hartinger, Walter, and Winfried Helm. *"Die laidige Sucht der Pestilentz": Kleine Kulturgeschichte der Pest in Europa*. Passau: Universität Passau, 1986.

Hatje, Frank. *Leben und Sterben im Zeitalter der Pest: Basel im 15. bis 17. Jahrhundert*. Basel: Helbing & Lichtenhahn, 1992.

Hayum, Andree. *The Isenheim Altarpiece: God's Medicine and the Painter's Vision*. Princeton, NJ: Princeton University Press, 1989.

Heal, Bridget. "Images of the Virgin Mary and Marian Devotion in Protestant Nuremberg," in *Religion and Superstition in Reformation Europe*, Eds. Helen Parish and William G. Naphy: 25–46. Manchester: Manchester University Press, 2002.

Hecker, J. F. C. *Der englische Schweiß: Ein ärztlicher Beitrag zur Geschichte des funfzehnten und sechzehnten Jahrhunderts*. Berlin: Theod. Christ. Friedr. Enslin, 1834.

Heimers, Manfred Peter. *Krieg, Hunger, Pest und Glaubenszwist: München im Dreißigjährigen Krieg*. Munich: Buchendorfer Verlag, 1998.

Heinrichs, Erik A. "The Live Chicken Treatment for Buboes: Trying a Plague Cure in Medieval and Early Modern Europe," *Bulletin of the History of Medicine* 91 (2017): 210–232.

— "The Plague Cure: Physicians, Clerics and the Reform of Healing in Germany, 1473–1650." Ph.D. dissertation, Harvard University, 2009.

Heitz, Paul, Ed. *Pestblätter des XV. Jahrhunderts*. Strassburg: Heitz & Mündel, 1901.

Helm, Jürgen. "Religion and Medicine: Anatomical Education at Wittenberg and Ingolstadt," in *Religious Confessions and the Sciences in the Sixteenth Century*, Eds. Jürgen Helm and Annette Winkelmann: 51–68. Leiden: Brill, 2001.

Helm, Jürgen, and Annette Winkelmann, Eds. *Religious Confessions and the Sciences in the Sixteenth Century*. Leiden: Brill, 2001.

Heming, Carol Piper. *Protestants and the Cult of the Saints in German-Speaking Europe, 1517–1531*. Kirksville, MO: Truman State University Press, 2003.

Hendrix, Scott. "Urbanus Rhegius," in *Theologische Realenzyklopädie*, Vol. XXIX: 155–156. Berlin: Walter de Gruyter, 1998.

Herbrand-Hochmuth, Grete. "Systematisches Verzeichnis der Arbeiten Karl Sudhoffs," *Sudhoffs Archiv für Geschichte der Medizin und der Naturwissenschaften* 27 (1934): 131–188.

Hickel, Erika. *Die Arzneimittel in der Geschichte*. Nordhausen: Verlag Traugott Bautz, 2008.

Hirsch, Rudolf. "The Invention of Printing and the Diffusion of Alchemical and Chemical Knowledge," *Chymia* 3 (1950): 115–141.

Hoffmann, Julius. *Die "Hausväterliteratur" und die "Predigten über den christlichen Hausstand."* Weinheim: Verlag Julius Beltz, 1959.

Hoffmeister, Alexander von. *Das Medizinalwesen im Kurfürstentum Bayern*. Munich: Werner Fritsch, 1975.

Hofheinz, Ralf-Dieter. *Philipp Melanchthon und die Medizin im Spiegel seiner akademischen Reden*. Herbolzheim: Centaurus Verlag, 2001.

Holste, Thomas. *Der Theriakkrämer: Ein Beitrag zur Frühgeschichte der Arzneimittelwerbung*. Pattensen: Horst Wellm Verlag, 1977.

Horanin, Mariusz. "Die Pest im frühneuzeitlichen Augsburg: Soziale Konstruktion einer Krankheit." Ph.D. thesis, Georg-August-Universität Göttingen, 2011.

Hsia, R. Po-chia, Ed. *A Companion to the Reformation World*. Malden, MA: Blackwell, 2004.

Jacquart, Danielle. "Theory, Everyday Practice, and Three Fifteenth-Century Physicians," *Osiris* 2nd series 6 (1990): 140–160.

Jardine, Lisa. *Worldly Goods*. New York: Norton, 1998.

Jepson, Michael H. "From Secret Medicines to Prescription Medicines: A Brief History of Medicine Quality," in *Making Medicines*, Ed. Stuart Anderson: 223–241. London: Pharmaceutical Press, 2005.

Jöcher, Christian Gottlieb. *Christian Gottlieb Jöchers Allgemeines Gelehrten-Lexicon*. Hildesheim: Georg Olms, 1961.

Johnson, Christine. *The German Discovery of the World: Renaissance Encounters with the Strange and Marvelous*. Charlottesville, VA: University of Virginia Press, 2008.

Jones, Colin. "Languages of Plague in Early Modern France," in *Body and City: Histories of Urban Public Health*, Eds. Sally Sheard and Helen Power: 41–49. Aldershot, UK: Ashgate, 2000.

— "Plague and Its Metaphors in Early Modern France," *Representations* 53 (1996): 97–127.

Jütte, Robert. *Ärzte, Heiler und Patienten: Medizinischer Alltag in der frühen Neuzeit*. Munich: Artemis & Winkler Verlag, 1991.

— "Die Leiden der Elisabeth von Rochlitz, der Schwester Philipps des Großmütigen," in *Quantität und Struktur: Festschrift für Kersten Krüger zum 60. Geburtstag*, Eds. Werner Buchholz and Stefan Kroll: 337–356. Rostock: Universität Rostock, 1999.

Keil, Gundolf. "Das 'Costelic Laxatijf' Meister Peters von Dorth," *Sudhoffs Archiv* 50 (1966): 113–135.

— "Der Hausvater als Arzt," in *Haushalt und Familie in Mittelalter und frühe Neuzeit*, Ed. Trude Ehlert: 219–243. Sigmaringen: Jan Thorbecke Verlag, 1991.

— "Seuchenzüge des Mittelalters," in *Mensch und Umwelt im Mittelalter*, Ed. Bernd Herrmann: 109–128. Stuttgart: Deutsche Verlags Anstalt, 1986.

Keil, Gundolf, Ed. *Das Lorscher Arzneibuch*, Vol. II, Trans. Ulrich Stoll and Gundolf Keil. Stuttgart: Wissenschaftliche Verlagsgesellschaft, 1989.

Keiser, Georg R. "Two Medieval Plague Treatises and Their Afterlife in Early Modern England," *Journal of the History of Medicine and Allied Sciences* 58 (2003): 292–324.

Kinzelbach, Annemarie. *Gesundbleiben, Krankwerden, Armsein in der frühneuzeitlichen Gesellschaft: Gesunde und Kranke in den Reichsstädten Überlingen und Ulm, 1500–1700*. Stuttgart: Steiner, 1995.

— "Infection, Contagion and Public Health in Late Medieval and Early Modern German Imperial Towns," *Journal of the History of Medicine* 61 (2006): 369–389.

Klebs, Arnold C., and Karl Sudhoff, *Die Ersten Gedruckten Pestschriften*. Munich: Verlag der Münchener Drucke, 1926.

Klimpel, Volker. *Dresdner Ärzte: Historisch-Biographisches Lexikon*. Dresden: Hellerau Verlag, 1998.

Kobolt, Anton Maria. *Ergänzungen und Berichtingungen zum Baierischen Gelehrten-Lexikon*. Landshut: Franz Seraph Storno, 1824.

Koerner, Joseph. *The Moment of Self-Portraiture in German Renaissance Art*. Chicago: University of Chicago Press, 1996.

Köhler, Hans-Joachim, Ed. *Flugschriften als Massenmedium der Reformationszeit*. Stuttgart: Klett-Cotta, 1981.

— "The Flugschriften and Their Importance in Religious Debate: A Quantitative Approach," in *Stars and the End of the World in Luther's Time*, Ed. Paola Zambelli: 153–175. Berlin: Walter de Gruyter, 1986.

Koslofsky, Craig. *The Reformation of the Dead: Death and Ritual in Early Modern Germany, 1450–1700*. New York: St. Martin's Press, 2000.

Krafft, Fritz. *"Die Artznei kommt vom Hernn, und der Apoteker bereitet sie" biblische Rechtfertigung der Apotekerkunst im Protestantismus: Apotheken-Auslucht in Lemgo und Pharmako-Theologie*. Stuttgart: Wissenschaftliche Verlagsgesellschaft, 1999.

Krammer, Markus. *Die Wallfahrt zum heiligen Sebastian nach Ebersberg*. Ebersberg: Katholische Pfarrkirchenstiftung Ebersberg, 1981.

— *G'schichten aus Ebersberg*. Ebersberg: Stadt Ebersberg, 2000.

Kusukawa, Sachiko. "*Aspectio Divinorum Operum*: Melanchthon and Astrology for Lutheran Medics," in *Medicine and the Reformation*, Eds. Ole Peter Grell and Andrew Cunningham: 33–56. London: Routledge, 1993.

Lang, Matthias. "'Der Vrsprung aber der Pestilentz ist nicht natürlich, sondern übernatürlich…': Medizinische und theologische Erklärung der Seuche im Spiegel protestantischer Pestschriften 1527–1650," in *Die leidige Seuche: Pest-Fälle in der Frühen Neuzeit*, Ed. Otto Ulbricht: 133–180. Cologne: Böhlau Verlag, 2004.

Lederer, David. *Madness, Religion and the State in Early Modern Europe*. Cambridge: Cambridge University Press, 2006.

Lehmann, Hartmut. "Die Kometenflugschriften des 17. Jahrhunderts als historische Quelle," in *Literatur und Volk*, Vol. II, Eds. Wolfgang Brückner, Peter Blickle, and Dieter Breuer: 683–700. Wiesbaden: Harrassowitz Verlag, 1985.

Letter, Paul. *Paracelsus: Leben und Werk*. Krummwisch: Königsfurt Verlag, 2000.

Liess, Leonore. *Geschichte der medizinischen Fakultät in Ingolstadt von 1472 bis 1600*. Munich: Münchner Vereinigung für Geschichte der Medizin, 1984.

Lindberg, Carter. "The Lutheran Tradition," in *Caring and Curing: Health and Medicine in the Western Religious Traditions*, Eds. Ronald L. Numbers and Darrel W. Amundsen: 173–203. Baltimore: Johns Hopkins University Press, 1998.

Lindemann, Mary. *Medicine and Society in Early Modern Europe*. Cambridge: Cambridge University Press, 2010.

Linder, Gottlieb. "Doktor Alexander Sytz: Ein Lebensbild aus der Reformationszeit," *Zeitschrift für Allgemeine Geschichte, Kultur-, Literatur-, und Kunstgeschichte* 3 (1886): 224–232.

Lotz-Heumann, Ute, and Matthias Pohlig. "Confessionalization and Literature in the Empire," *Central European History* 40 (2007): 35–61.

Ludolphy, Ingetraut. *Friedrich der Weise: Kurfürst von Sachsen 1463–1525*. Göttingen: Vandenhoeck & Ruprecht, 1984.

Lutterbach, Hubertus. "Der Christus medicus und die Sancti medici: Das wechselvolle Verhältnis zweier Grundmotive christlicher Frömmigkeit zwischen Spätantike und Früher Neuzeit," *Saeculum* 47 (1996): 239–281.

McCormick, Michael. "Toward a Molecular History of the Justinianic Pandemic," in *Plague and the End of Antiquity*, Ed. Lester K. Little: 290–312. Cambridge: Cambridge University Press, 2007.

McKendrick, Neil, John Brewer, and J. H. Plumb, *The Birth of a Consumer Society: The Commercialization of Eighteenth-Century England*. London: Europe Publications, 1982.

Maeser, H. *Historisch-pathologische Untersuchungen: Als Beiträge zur Geschichte der Volkskrankheiten*, Vol. II. Dresden: Verlag von Gerhard Fleischer, 1841.

Martin, A. Lynn. *Plague? Jesuit Accounts of Epidemic Disease in the 16th Century*. Kirksville, MO: Sixteenth Century Journal Publishers, 1996.

Marxer, Norbert. *Praxis statt Theorie! Leben und Werk des Nürnberger Arztes, Alchemikers und Fachschriftstellers Johann Hiskia Cardilucius (1630–1697)*. Heidelberg: Palatina, 2000.

Mering, Friedrich Everhard von, and Ludwig Reischert. *Zur Geschichte der Stadt Köln am Rhein: Von ihrer Gründung bis zur Gegenwart*, Vol. I. Cologne: Johann Wilhelm Dietz, 1838.

Merton, Robert K. *Science, Technology and Society in Seventeenth-Century England*. Bruges: Saint Catherine Press, 1938.

Methuen, Charlotte. "Science and Medicine," in *The Reformation World*, Ed. Andrew Pettegree: 521–534. London: Routledge, 2000.

Moeller, Bernd. "Religious Life in Germany on the Eve of the Reformation," in *Pre-Reformation Germany*, Ed. Gerald Strauss: 13–31. New York: Harper & Row, 1972.

Moran, Bruce T. *The Alchemical World of the German Court: Occult Philosophy and Chemical Medicine in the Circle of Moritz of Hessen (1572–1632)*. Stuttgart: Franz Steiner Verlag, 1991.

— *Distilling Knowledge: Alchemy, Chemistry, and the Scientific Revolution*. Cambridge, MA: Harvard University Press, 2005.

Müller-Jahncke, Wolf-Dieter. *Georg am Wald (1554–1616): Arzt und Unternehmer*. Stuttgart: Franz Steiner, 1994.

Naumann, Friedrich, Ed. *Georgius Agricola 500 Jahre*. Basel: Birkhäuser Verlag, 1994.

Newman, William R., and Anthony Grafton. "Introduction: The Problematic Status of Astrology and Alchemy in Premodern Europe," in *Secrets of Nature: Astrology and Alchemy in Early Modern Europe*: 1–38. Cambridge, MA: MIT Press, 2001.

Niccoli, Ottavia. *Prophecy and People in Renaissance Italy*, Trans. Lydia G. Cochrane. Princeton, NJ: Princeton University Press, 1990.

Ninck, Johannes. *Artz und Reformator Vadian: Ein Charakterbild aus großer Zeit*. St. Gallen: Buchhandlung der Evangelischen Gesellschaft St. Gallens, 1936.

Nummedal, Tara. "Practical Alchemy and Commercial Exchange in the Holy Roman Empire," in *Merchants and Marvels: Commerce, Science, and Art in Early Modern Europe*, Eds. Pamela H. Smith and Paula Findlen: 201–222. New York: Routledge, 2002.

— *Alchemy and Authority in the Holy Roman Empire*. Chicago: University of Chicago Press, 2007.

Nutton, Vivian. "The Seeds of Disease: An Explanation of Infection from the Greeks to the Renaissance," *Medical History* 27 (1983): 1–34.

— "Murders and Miracles: Lay Attitudes towards Medicine in Classical Antiquity," in *Patients and Practitioners: Lay Perceptions of Medicine in Pre-Industrial Society*, Ed. Roy Porter: 23–54. Cambridge: Cambridge University Press, 1985.

— "The Reception of Fracastoro's Theory of Contagion: The Seed that Fell among Thorns?," *Osiris* 2nd Series 6 (1990): 196–234.

— "Wittenberg Anatomy," in *Medicine and the Reformation*, Eds. Ole Peter Grell and Andrew Cunningham: 11–32. London: Routledge, 1993.

— "Medicine at the German Universities, 1348–1500: A Preliminary Sketch," in *Medicine from the Black Death to the French Disease*, Eds. Roger French, Jon Arrizabalaga, Andrew Cunningham, and Luis García-Ballester; 85–109. Aldershot, UK: Ashgate, 1998.

O'Boyle, Cornelius. *The Art of Medicine: Medical Teaching at the University of Paris*. Leiden: Brill, 1998.

O'Connell, Marvin R. "The Roman Catholic Tradition since 1545," in *Caring and Curing: Health and Medicine in the Western Religious Traditions*, Eds. Ronald L. Numbers and Darrel W. Amundsen: 108–145. Baltimore: Johns Hopkins University Press, 1998.

Ogilvie, Brian. *The Science of Describing: Natural History in Renaissance Europe*. Chicago: University of Chicago Press, 2006.

Overfield, James. "Germany," in *The Renaissance in National Context*, Eds. Roy Porter and Mikulas Teich: 92–122. Cambridge: Cambridge University Press, 1992.

Ozment, Steven. *Magdalena and Balthasar*. New Haven, CT: Yale University Press, 1989.

— "The Social History of the Reformation: What Can We Learn from Pamphlets?," in *Flugschriften als Massenmedium der Reformationszeit*, Ed. Hans-Joachim Köhler: 171–203. Stuttgart: Klett-Cotta, 1981.

Pagel, Walter. *Paracelsus: An Introduction to Philosophical Medicine in the Era of the Renaissance*. Basel: Karger, 1982.

Palazzotto, Dominick. "The Black Death and Medicine: A Report and Analysis of the Tractates Written between 1348 and 1350." Ph.D. thesis, University of Kansas, 1973.

Palmer, Richard. "Pharmacy in the Republic of Venice in the Sixteenth Century," in *The Medical Renaissance of the Sixteenth Century*, Eds. A. Wear, R. K. French, and I. M. Lonie: 100–117. Cambridge: Cambridge University Press, 1985.

— "The Church, Leprosy and Plague in Medieval and Early Modern Europe," in *The Church and Healing*, Ed. W. J. Shields: 79–99. Oxford: Basil Blackwell, 1982.

Pantin, Isabelle. "The Role of Translations in European Scientific Exchanges in the Sixteenth and Seventeenth Centuries," in *Cultural Translation in Early Modern Europe*, Eds. Peter Burke and R. Po-chia Hsia: 163–179. Cambridge: Cambridge University Press, 2007.

Park, Katharine, and Lorraine Daston. "Unnatural Conceptions: The Study of Monsters in Sixteenth- and Seventeenth-Century France and England," *Past and Present* 92 (1981): 20–54.

—, Eds. *The Cambridge History of Science*, Vol. III, *Early Modern Science*. Cambridge: Cambridge University Press, 2006.

Peickert, Heinz. *Geheimmittel im deutschen Arzneiverkehr*. Leipzig: Alexander Edelmann, 1932.

Pomata, Gianna. *Contracting a Cure: Patients, Healers and the Law in Early Modern Bologna*. Baltimore: Johns Hopkins University Press, 1998.

— "Observation Rising: Birth of an Epistemic Genre, 1500–1650," in *Histories of Scientific Observation*, Eds. Lorraine Daston and Elizabeth Lunbeck: 45–80. Chicago: University of Chicago Press, 2011.

Porter, Roy. *English Society in the Eighteenth Century*. London: Penguin Books, 1982.

— *Health for Sale: Quackery in England 1660–1850*. Manchester: Manchester University Press, 1989.

Porterfield, Amanda. *Healing in the History of Christianity*. Oxford: Oxford University Press, 2005.

Porzelt, Carolin. *Die Pest in Nürnberg: Leben und Herrschen in Pestzeiten in der Reichsstadt Nürnberg (1562–1713)*. St. Ottilien: EOS Verlag, 2000.

Prescher, Hans, and Otfried Wagenbreth. *Georgius Agricola: Seine Zeit und ihre Spuren*. Leipzig: Deutscher Verlag für Grundstoffindustrie, 1994.

Rankin, Alisha. "Medicine for the Uncommon Woman: Experience, Experiment, and Exchange in Early Modern Germany." Ph.D. thesis, Harvard University, 2005.

— "Duchess Heal Thyself: Elisabeth of Rochlitz and the Patient's Perspective in Early Modern Germany," *Bulletin of the History of Medicine* 82 (2008): 109–144.

— *Panaceia's Daughters: Noblewomen as Healers in Early Modern Germany*. Chicago: University of Chicago Press, 2013.

Richardson, Linda Deer. "The Generation of Disease: Occult Causes and Diseases of the Total Substance," in *The Medical Renaissance of the Sixteenth Century*, Eds. A. Wear, R. K. French, and I. M. Lonie: 175–194. Cambridge: Cambridge University Press, 1985.

Riha, Ortrun. "Vom mittelalterlichen 'Hausbuch' zur frühneuzeitlichen 'Hausväterlit eratur': Medizinische Texte in Handschrift und Buchdruck," in *Die Gleichzeitigkeit von Handschrift und Buchdruck*, Eds. Gerd Dicke and Klaus Grubmüller: 203–227. Wiesbaden: Harrassowitz Verlag, 2003.

Rublack, Ulinka. *Reformation Europe*. Cambridge: Cambridge University Press, 2005.

Schanze, Frieder. "'Pestregiment Herrn Kamits' eine unbekannte deutsche Inkunabel," in *Gutenberg-Jahrbuch 1993*: 88–90. Mainz: Gutenberg Gesellschaft, 1993.

Schenda, Rudolf. "Der 'gemeine Mann' und sein medikales Verhalten im 16. und 17. Jahrhundert," in *Pharmazie und der gemeine Mann: Hausarznei und Apotheke in deutschen Schriften der frühen Neuzeit*, Ed. Joachim Telle: 9–20. Wolfenbüttel: Waisenhaus-Buchdruckerei und Verlag, 1982.

Schirmer, Uwe. "Die Leipziger Messen in der ersten Hälfte des 16. Jahrhunderts: Ihre Funktion als Silberhandels- und Finanzplatz der Kurfürsten von Sachsen," in *Leipzigs Messen 1497–1997*, Vol. I, Eds. Hartmut Zwahr, Thomas Topfstedt, and Günter Bentele: 87–107. Cologne: Böhlau Verlag, 1999.

Schlenkrich, Elke. *Von Leuten auf dem Sterbestroh: Sozialgeschichte obersächsischer Lazarette in der frühen Neuzeit*. Leipzig: Sax-Verlag Beuche, 2002.

Scribner, Robert W. "Civic Unity and Reformation in Erfurt," *Past and Present* 66 (1975): 29–60.

— "Cosmic Order and Daily Life: Sacred and Secular in Pre-Industrial German Society," in *Religion and Society in Early Modern Europe 1500–1800*, Ed. Kaspar von Greyerz: 17–32. London: George Allen & Unwin, 1984.

— *For the Sake of Simple Folk: Popular Propaganda for the German Reformation*. Cambridge: Cambridge University Press, 1981.

— *Religion and Culture in Germany 1400–1800*, Ed. Lyndal Roper. Leiden: Brill, 2001.

Scribner, Robert W., and C. Scott Dixon. *The German Reformation*, 2nd Edn. Basingstoke, UK: Palgrave Macmillan, 2003.

Seyfarth, Carly. *Das Hospital zu St. Georg in Leipzig durch acht Jahrhunderte 1212–1940*, Vol. I. Leipzig: Georg Thieme Verlag, 1939.

— *725 Jahre Hospital zu St. Georg in Leipzig*. Leipzig: Hermann-Eichblatt-Verlag, 1939.

Siebenthal, Wolf von. *Krankheit als Folge der Sünde: Eine medizinhistorische Untersuchung*. Hanover: Schmorl & von Seefeld, 1950.

Siraisi, Nancy. "'Remarkable' Diseases, 'Remarkable' Cures, and Personal Experience in Renaissance Medical Texts," in *Medicine and the Italian Universities 1250–1600*: 226–252. Leiden: Brill, 2001.

Slack, Paul. *The Impact of Plague in Tudor and Stuart England*. Oxford: Clarendon Press, 1985.

Smith, Pamela H. *The Body of the Artisan: Art and Experience in the Scientific Revolution*. Chicago: University of Chicago Press, 2004.

Soergel, Philip. *Wondrous in His Saints: Counter-Reformation Propaganda in Bavaria*. Berkeley, CA: University of California Press, 1993.

— "Die Wahrnehmung der Endzeit in monströsen Anfängen," in *Im Zeichen der Krise: Religiosität im Europa des 17. Jahrhunderts*, Eds. Hartmut Lehmann and Anne-Charlott Trepp: 33–51. Göttingen: Vandenhoeck & Ruprecht, 1999.

Spitz, Lewis W. *The Religious Renaissance of the German Humanists*. Cambridge, MA: Harvard University Press, 1963.

Steiger, Johann Anselm. *Medizinische Theologie: Christus Medicus und Theologia Medicinalis bei Martin Luther und im Luthertum der Barockzeit*. Leiden: Brill, 2005.

Stein, Claudia. *Die Behandlung der Franzosenkrankheit in der Frühen Neuzeit am Beispiel Augsburgs*. Stuttgart: Steiner, 2003.

Stolberg, Michael. "Empiricism in Sixteenth-Century Medical Practice: The Notebooks of Georg Handsch," *Early Science and Medicine* 18 (2013): 487–516.

Stolleis, Michael. "Public Law and Patriotism in the Holy Roman Empire," in *Infinite Boundaries: Order, Disorder and Reorder in Early Modern German Culture*, Ed. Max Reinhart: 11–33. Kirksville, MO: Sixteenth Century Journal Publishers, 1998.

Strasser, Gerald F. "Science and Pseudoscience: Athanasius Kircher's *Mundus Subterraneus* and His *Scrutinium...Pestis*," in *Knowledge, Science and Literature in Early Modern Germany*: 219–240. Chapel Hill, NC: University of North Carolina Press, 1996.

Strasser, Ulrike. *State of Virginity: Gender, Religion and Politics in an Early Modern Catholic State*. Ann Arbor, MI: University of Michigan Press, 2004.

Stürzbecher, Manfred. "The Physici in German-Speaking Countries from the Middle-Age to the Enlightenment," in *The Town and State Physician in Europe from the Middle Ages to the Present*, Ed. Andrew W. Russell: 123–129. Wolfenbüttel: Herzog August Bibliothek, 1979.

Sudhoff, Karl. *Deutsche Medizinische Inkunabeln*. Leipzig: Johann Ambrosius Barth, 1908.

— *Die medizinische Fakultät zu Leipzig im ersten Jahrhundert der Universität*. Leipzig: Johann Ambrosius Barth, 1909.

— *Bibliographia Paracelsica*, Reprint Edn. Graz: Akademische Druck- und Verlagsanstalt, 1958.

Talkenberger, Heike. *Sintflut: Prophetie und Zeitgeschehen in Texten und Holzschnitten astrologischer Flugschriften 1488–1528*. Tübingen: Niemeyer, 1990.

Telle, Joachim. "Das Rezept als literarische Form: Bausteine zu seiner Kulturgeschichte," *Medizinische Monatsschrift* 28 (1974): 389–395.

—, Ed. *Pharmazie und der gemeine Mann: Hausarznei und Apotheke in deutschen Schriften der frühen Neuzeit*. Wolfenbüttel: Waisenhaus-Buchdruckerei und Verlag, 1982.

Tetzner, Franz. "Zur Lebensgeschichte Schnellenbergs," *Westfälisches Magazin* (1910): 2–5.

Thayer, Anne T. *Penitence, Preaching and the Coming of the Reformation*. Aldershot, UK: Ashgate, 2002.

Thibodeau, Kenneth. "Science and the Reformation: The Case of Strasbourg," *Sixteenth Century Journal* 7 (1976): 35–50.

Thorndike, Lynn. *A History of Magic and Experimental Science*, Vol. IV, *Fourteenth and Fifteenth Centuries*. New York: Columbia University Press, 1934.

Tlusty, B. Ann. *Bacchus and Civic Order: The Culture of Drink in Early Modern Germany*. Charlottesville, VA: University Press of Virginia, 2001.

Toellner, Richard. "Die medizinischen Facultäten unter dem Einfluß der Reformation," in *Renaissance Reformation: Gegensätze und Gemeinsamkeiten*, Ed. August Buck: 287–297. Wiesbaden: Harrassowitz Verlag, 1984.

Trepp, Anne-Charlott. "Zur Pluralisierung im Luthertum des 17. Jahrhunderts und ihrer Bedeutung für die Deutungen von 'Natur,'" *Berichte zur Wissenschaftsgeschichte* 26 (2003): 183–198.

Utz, Hans. *Wallfahrten im Bistum Regensburg*. Munich: Verlag Schnell & Steiner, 1981.

Viets, Henry R., and James F. Ballard. "Notes on the Plague Tracts in the Boston Medical Library," *Bulletin of the History of Medicine* 8 (1940): 370–380.

Wandel, Lee Palmer. *The Eucharist in the Reformation*. Cambridge: Cambridge University Press, 2006.

— *The Reformation: Towards a New History*. Cambridge: Cambridge University Press, 2011.

Wear, Andrew. "Religious Beliefs and Medicine in Early Modern England," in *The Task of Healing: Medicine, Religion and Gender in England and the Netherlands, 1450–1800*, Eds. Hilary Marland and Margaret Pelling: 145–169. Rotterdam: Erasmus Publishing, 1996.

— *Knowledge and Practice in English Medicine, 1550–1680*. Cambridge: Cambridge University Press, 2000.

— "Medical Practice in Late Seventeenth- and Early Eighteenth-Century England: Continuity and Union," in *The Medical Revolution of the Seventeenth Century*, Eds. Roger French and Andrew Wear: 294–320. Cambridge: Cambridge University Press, 1989.

— "The Early Modern Debate about Foreign Drugs: Localism versus Universalism in Medicine," *The Lancet* 354 (1999): 149–151.

Webster, Charles. "Paracelsus: Medicine as Popular Protest," in *Medicine and the Reformation*, Eds. Ole Peter Grell and Andrew Cunningham: 55–77. London: Routledge, 1993.

— "Paracelsus Confronts the Saints: Miracles, Healing and the Secularization of Magic," *Social History of Medicine* 8 (1995): 403–421.

— *Paracelsus: Medicine, Magic and Mission at the End of Time*. New Haven, CT: Yale University Press, 2008.

Weeks, Andrew. *Paracelsus: Speculative Theory and the Crisis of the Early Reformation*. Albany, NY: State University of New York Press, 1997.

Werfing, Johann. *Der Ursprung der Pestilenz: Zur Ätiologie der Pest im loimographischen Diskurs der frühen Neuzeit*. Vienna: Edition Praesens, 1998.

Werner, Karl. "Ananizapta: Eine geheimnisvolle Inschrift des Mittelalters," *Sammelblatt des Historischen Vereins Ingolstadt* 105 (1996): 59–90.

Wilderotter, Hans, and Michael Dorrmann, Eds. *Das große Sterben: Seuchen machen Geschichte*. Berlin: Jovis, 1995.

Winslow, C.-E. A., and M. L. Duran-Reynals. "Jacme d'Agramont and the First of the Plague Tractates," *Bulletin of the History of Medicine* 22 (1948): 747–765.

Wulf, Rüdiger. "Tarquinius Schnellenberg alias Ocyorus: Doktor der Freien Künste und Arznei, Stadtphysikus zu Dortmund," *Heimat Dortmund* 3 (2005): 11–17.

Wunderli, Richard M. *Peasant Fires: The Drummer of Niklashausen*. Bloomington, IN: Indiana University Press, 1992.

Wüst, Wolfgang. *Die "gute" Policey im Bayerischen Reichskreis und in der Oberpfalz*. Berlin: Akademie Verlag, 2004.

Wustmann, Gustav. *Der Wirt von Auerbachs Keller: Dr. Heinrich Stromer von Auerbach 1482–1542*. Leipzig: Hermann Seemann Nachfolger, 1902.

— *Geschichte der Stadt Leipzig*, Vol. I. Leipzig: C. L. Hirschfeld, 1905.

Ziegler, Joseph. "Practitioners and Saints: Medical Men in Canonization Processes in the Thirteenth to Fifteenth Centuries," *Social History of Medicine* 12 (1999): 191–225.

Zimmermann, Birgit. "Das Hausarzneibuch: Ein Beitrag zur Untersuchung laienmedizinischer Fachliteratur des 16. Jahrhunderts unter besonderer

Berücksichtigung ihres humanmedizinischen-pharmazeutischen Inhalt." Math-Naturwiss. dissertation, Philipps-Universität Marburg, 1975.

Zimmermann, Heinz. *Arzneimittelwerbung in Deutschland vom Beginn des 16. bis Ende des 18. Jahrhunderts: Dargestellt vorzugsweise an Hand von Archivalien der Freien Reichs-, Handels- und Messestadt Frankfurt am Main*. Würzburg: Jal-Verlag, 1974.

Zupko, Ronald E. *Revolution in Measurement: Western European Weights and Measures since the Age of Science*. Philadelphia: American Philosophical Society, 1990.

Index